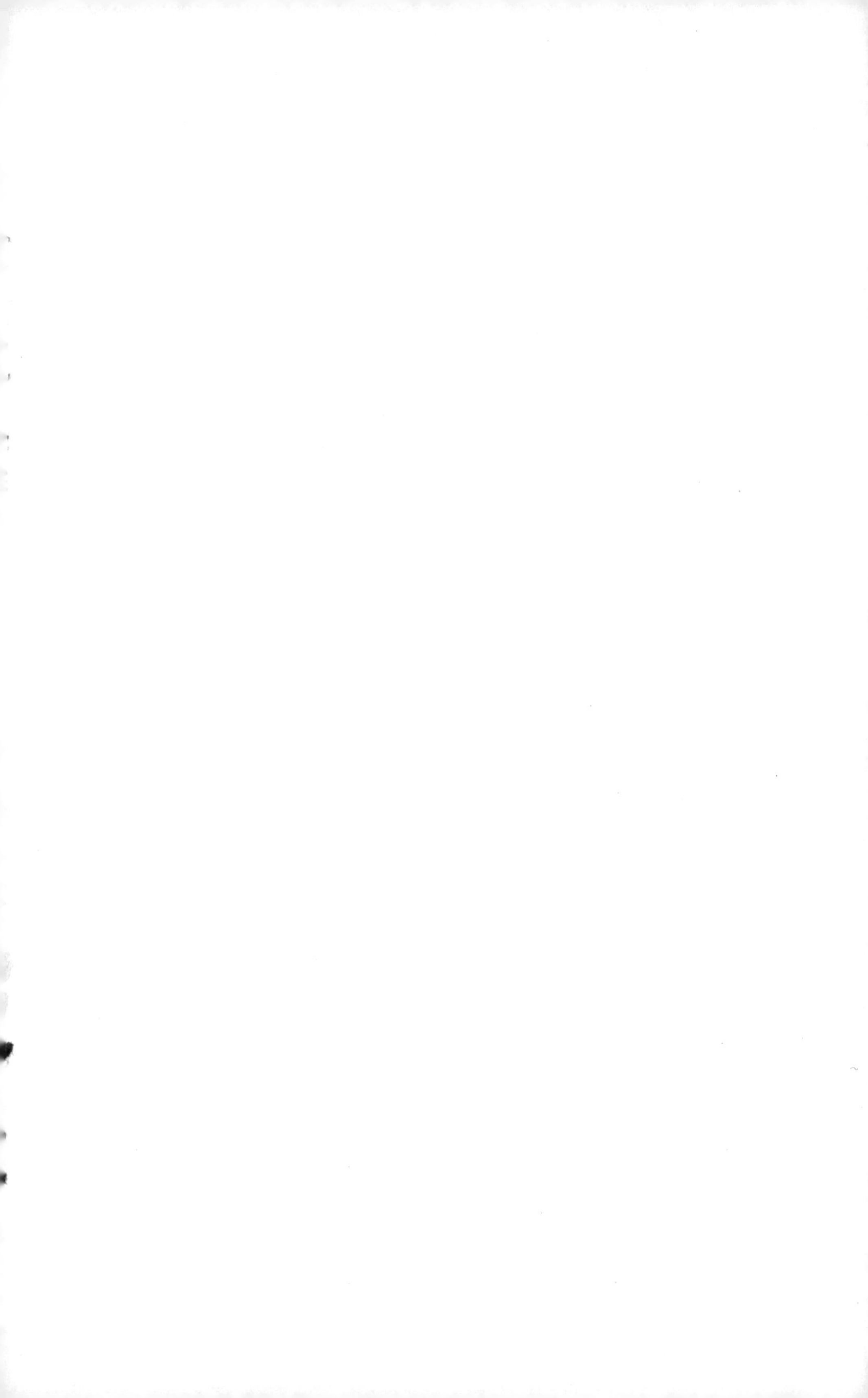

Treatment of Infective Endocarditis

Grune & Stratton Rapid Manuscript Reproduction

Treatment of Infective Endocarditis

Edited by

Alan L. Bisno, M.D.
Professor of Medicine and
Chief, Division of Infectious Diseases
Department of Medicine
The University of Tennessee Center for the Health Sciences
Memphis, Tennessee

Grune & Stratton
A Subsidiary of Harcourt Brace Jovanovich, Publishers
New York London Toronto Sydney San Francisco

Grune & Stratton, Inc.
111 Fifth Avenue
New York, New York 10003

Distributed in the United Kingdom by
Academic Press Inc. (London) Ltd.
24/28 Oval Road, London NW 1

Library of Congress Catalog Number 81-7080
International Standard Book Number 0-8089-1450-8

Printed in the United States of America

To Barbara, Susan, and Neal, with love

CONTENTS

ACKNOWLEDGEMENTS

I would like to acknowledge the invaluable assistance of a number of individuals in preparing this book. These include: Dr. Edward L. Kaplan, Chairman, Council on Cardiovascular Disease in the Young, American Heart Association; Mark Oliveira, Dale Stringfellow, Leonard Cook, Franck Cushner, and Gina Jacobs of the American Heart Association; members of the Committee on Rheumatic Fever and Bacterial Endocarditis of the American Heart Association; and all participants in the Conference on Treatment of Infective Endocarditis. Susan White, my secretary at the University of Tennessee, and Sue Kaplan, administrative assistant for the Department of Medicine, devoted many hours to this project. The staff of the Word Processing Center, Division of Educational Development, The University of Tennessee Center for the Health Sciences, rendered invaluable assistance as did the editorial staff of Grune & Stratton, Inc. Finally, I would like to thank Dr. Gene H. Stollerman, my mentor in the field of infectious diseases, for many hours of productive discussions over the years on the topic of infective endocarditis.

PREFACE

The Committee on Rheumatic Fever and Bacterial Endocarditis of the American Heart Association has consistently played a leading role in providing guidance to the medical profession regarding optimal methods of prevention and diagnosis of the two diseases under its purview. The committee publishes official statements on "Prevention of Rheumatic Fever" and "Prevention of Bacterial Endocarditis" that are periodically revised and updated. In 1976, in preparation for its periodic revision of the statement on prevention of endocarditis, the committee convened a meeting of experts in infectious diseases and microbiology to review the current knowledge on this topic. The results were published in the form of an American Heart Association monograph edited by Drs. Edward L. Kaplan and Angelo V. Taranta.

The present volume emerged from a similar conference, focused this time on treatment of infective endocarditis, held at the Heart Association's National Center in Dallas, Texas, April 28–29, 1980.* Considerations of therapy are not entirely foreign to the Committee on Rheumatic Fever and Bacterial Endocarditis, because specific recommendations on treatment of streptococcal pharyngitis are incorporated in the statement on prevention of rheumatic fever. Nevertheless, the 1980 conference did represent a bit of a departure for the committee, one that was stimulated by the perceived need for placing in perspective the mass of data that had accumulated on this subject over the past four decades. These data included many case reports and retrospective clinical reviews; at least one controlled, randomized clinical trial (in endocarditis due to *Staphylococcus aureus*); and laboratory data consisting of experiments conducted both *in vitro* and in experimental animals. In particular, a considerable body of data had accumulated over the past decade using the rabbit model of infective endocarditis, and the potential

* Funding for this conference was provided by the National Institute of Allergy and Infectious Diseases, the National Heart, Lung and Blood Institute, and the American Heart Association. Additional sponsoring agencies included the National Institute of Child Health and Human Development, the National Institute on Aging, and the Fogarty International Center.

relevance of these experiments to treatment of endocarditis in humans has been a subject of lively debate.

Interest in the most appropriate treatment of endocarditis due to viridans streptococci has been particularly strong. These organisms remain the most common etiologic agents in infective endocarditis, and there also has been increasing recognition that a minority of cases of viridans streptococcal endocarditis is caused by so-called nutritionally deficient variants that may be more difficult to isolate and eradicate. Although a wide variety of treatment regimens has been proposed, most of which consist either of penicillin alone (in the non-allergic patient) or penicillin in combination with streptomycin, the relative cure rates and potential toxicities of these various regimens are much debated. Some centers have reported that the duration of therapy can be markedly shortened without compromising cure rates if a combination of penicillin and streptomycin is used. As a result of this interest in viridans streptococcal endocarditis, the conference considered in detail the relevant clinical and experimental data, and, immediately following the conference, an ad hoc subcommittee was appointed to formulate treatment recommendations. The resulting document is included here as Appendix II and has been adopted as an official statement of the American Heart Association.

The goal of both the conference and this book as a whole was to survey all aspects of the treatment of infective endocarditis and thus provide an assessment of the state of the art. Because time constraints prevented discussion of all relevant topics at the conference, additional papers were solicited for inclusion in this text. These are chapters on special problems by Drs. C. G. Cobbs, and W. K. Livingston, surgical treatment by Drs. B. A. Reitz, W. A. Baumgartner, P. E. Oyer, and E. B. Stinson, management of penicillin allergy in patients with bacterial endocarditis by Drs. J. E. Erffmeyer and P. Lieberman, and pediatric aspects by Dr. A. Rosenthal.

In editing this volume, I have tried to achieve some order but have not striven for slavish consistency. Thus, the reader may well find differences of opinion between contributors on a number of points relating to diagnosis, evaluation, and management of infective endocarditis. The last word has not been spoken on many of these points, and "clinical experience," which may differ significantly between individuals and medical centers, must still be our guide in many instances until definitive data are available.

Alan L. Bisno, M.D.
Chairman, Committee on Rheumatic
Fever and Bacterial Endocarditis
American Heart Association
1977 – 1980

CONTRIBUTORS

WILLIAM A. BAUMGARTNER, M.D., Assistant Professor of Cardiovascular Surgery, Stanford University School of Medicine, Stanford, California

ALAN L. BISNO, M.D., Professor of Medicine and Chief, Division of Infectious Diseases, The University of Tennessee Center for the Health Sciences, Memphis, Tennessee

C. GLENN COBBS, M.D., Professor of Medicine and Director, Division of Infectious Diseases, University of Alabama School of Medicine, Birmingham, Alabama

WILLIAM E. DISMUKES, M.D., Professor of Medicine, University of Alabama School of Medicine, Birmingham, Alabama

DAVID T. DURACK, M.B., D.Phil., Associate Professor of Medicine and Chief, Division of Infectious Diseases, Duke University Medical Center, Durham, North Carolina

JOHN E. ERFFMEYER, M.D., Fellow, Division of Allergy/Immunology, Department of Medicine, The University of Tennessee Center for the Health Sciences, Memphis, Tennessee

JOSEPH E. GERACI, M.D., Professor of Medicine, Mayo Graduate School of Medicine, Mayo Clinic, Rochester, Minnesota

ADOLF W. KARCHMER, M.D., Assistant Professor of Medicine, Harvard Medical School; Associate Physician, Massachusetts General Hospital, Boston, Massachusetts

DONALD KAYE, M.D., Professor and Chairman, Department of Medicine, The Medical College of Pennsylvania, Philadelphia, Pennsylvania

OKSANA M. KORZENIOWSKI, M.D., Assistant Professor of Medicine, The Medical College of Pennsylvania, Philadelphia, Pennsylvania

MATTHEW E. LEVISON, M.D., Professor of Medicine and Chief, Division of Infectious Diseases, The Medical College of Pennsylvania, Philadelphia, Pennsylvania

PHIL LIEBERMAN, M.D., Professor of Medicine and Chief, Division of Allergy/Immunology, The University of Tennessee Center for the Health Sciences, Memphis, Tennessee

WILEY K. LIVINGSTON, M.D., Fellow, Division of Infectious Diseases, Department of Medicine, University of Alabama School of Medicine, Birmingham, Alabama

ROBERT C. MOELLERING, JR., M.D., Shields Warren-Mallinckrodt Professor of Medicine, Harvard Medical School; Associate Physician, Massachusetts General Hospital; Physician-in-Chief, New England Deaconess Hospital, Boston, Massachusetts

PHILIP E. OYER, M.D., Ph.D., Assistant Professor of Cardiovascular Surgery, Stanford University School of Medicine, Stanford, California

JOHN P. PHAIR, M.D., Professor of Medicine and Chief, Infectious Disease Section, Northwestern University Medical School, Chicago, Illinois

JAMES J. RAHAL, JR., M.D., Chief, Infectious Disease Section, New York (Manhattan) V.A. Hospital; Associate Professor of Medicine, New York University School of Medicine, New York, New York

BORIS REISBERG, M.D., Assistant Professor of Medicine, Northwestern University Medical School, Chicago, Illinois

BRUCE A. REITZ, M.D., Assistant Professor of Cardiovascular Surgery, Stanford University School of Medicine, Stanford, California

L. BARTH RELLER, M.D., Associate Professor of Medicine, Director of Clinical Microbiology, University of Colorado School of Medicine, Denver, Colorado

AMNON ROSENTHAL, M.D., Director, Pediatric Cardiology, C. S. Mott Children's Hospital, University of Michigan, Ann Arbor, Michigan

MERLE A. SANDE, M.D., Professor of Medicine, University of California, San Francisco, California

MICHAEL S. SIMBERKOFF, M.D., Assistant Chief, Infectious Disease Section, New York (Manhattan) V.A. Hospital; Associate Professor of Medicine, New York University School of Medicine, New York, New York

EDWARD B. STINSON, M.D., Professor of Cardiovascular Surgery, Stanford University School of Medicine, Stanford, California

JAMES TAN, M.D., Professor of Medicine, Northeastern Ohio Universities College of Medicine, Akron, Ohio

FRANK VENEZIO, M.D., Fellow in Infectious Diseases, Department of Medicine, Northwestern University Medical School, Chicago, Illinois

CHATRCHAI WATANAKUNAKORN, M.D., Professor of Internal Medicine, Northeastern Ohio Universities College of Medicine, Akron, Ohio; Chief, Infectious Disease Section, St. Elizabeth Hospital Medical Center, Youngstown, Ohio

GRANT WESTENFELDER, M.D., Assistant Clinical Professor of Medicine, Northwestern University Medical School, Chicago, Illinois

WALTER R. WILSON, M.D., Associate Professor of Medicine, Mayo Graduate School of Medicine, Mayo Clinic, Rochester, Minnesota

Treatment of Infective Endocarditis

David T. Durack, M.B., D.Phil.

1

REVIEW OF EARLY EXPERIENCE IN TREATMENT OF BACTERIAL ENDOCARDITIS, 1940–1955

Forty years have passed since penicillin was first administered to a patient with endocarditis. Enough experience has now accumulated to allow development of a consensus on modern treatment of streptococcal endocarditis; it therefore seems timely to review the earliest experience with antimicrobial agents in treatment of this disease. Perhaps the lessons that our teachers learned 40 years ago will provide an informative background against which to discuss more recent experience.

This review will be confined largely to studies reported by the end of 1955. That date was chosen for three reasons: first, ten years had passed since penicillin became freely available, during which the principles of treatment had been firmly established; second, 1955 was the year of publication of Andrew Kerr's landmark monograph on subacute endocarditis,[1] and third, a full quarter century remains to be covered in subsequent chapters describing more modern experience.

It is common knowledge that in 1940 the outlook for patients with bacterial endocarditis (as, indeed, for the world in that year) was bleak. Lichtman reviewed the literature on spontaneous cures and showed that, even when a few doubtful cases were included, less than 1% of patients with endocarditis recovered without treatment.[2] After the introduction of prontosil in 1935, many patients with endocarditis received intensive therapeutic trials with sulfonamides. A small but significant proportion of cases was cured. In a few patients who received non–specific "adjuvants" such as heparin and typhoid vaccine, the cure rate with sulfonamides ranged as high as 15%.[3] Unfortunately, in other series it was often near zero.[2-6] This almost hopeless situation was succinctly summarized in a paper by Galbreath, Mathews and Hull, published in 1943: "During the four-year period covering the years 1938 to 1941. . . .67 proved cases of bacterial endocarditis were encountered in the Charity Hospital. One or more of the sulfonamides were used in the treatment of 42 cases. . . .All 67 of the patients died."[4]

The penicillin revolution began hesitatingly for bacterial endocarditis. The first 5 patients treated parenterally with penicillin prepared by Howard Florey and his team in the Sir William Dunn School of Pathology at Oxford and reported in 1941 did not include a case of endocarditis.[7] Mary Florey treated a single case of endocarditis in the Radcliffe Infirmary and reported an unfavorable outcome in March, 1943 in the second article from the Oxford team on results of penicillin treatment of human infections.[8] The patient was a 24 year old man with viridans streptococcal endocarditis. He received 4,670,000 units of penicillin over 30 days and showed symptomatic improvement, but relapsed and died after the supply of penicillin was exhausted. The Floreys commented "It would probably have been better to give very large doses initially but it may be admitted that this case does not give grounds for the belief that penicillin will cure subacute bacterial endocarditis."[8]

Six months later, in August, 1943, Chester Keefer's Committee on Chemotherapeutic and Other Agents published their report on 500 patients with various infections treated with penicillin in the United States.[9] The National Research Council had given this committee control over distribution of most of the limited supply of penicillin that was then available. Because Keefer and others already suspected that endocarditis might require higher doses of penicillin for cure than other common infections, this committee (which represented 22 centers, and included such well known names as William Altemeier, Henry Dawson, D.T. Smith, Wesley Spink, and Barry Wood) decided to limit the initial use of penicillin for endocarditis to 17 cases. Each of these patients received about 50,000 units of penicillin daily for 9—26 days. Again, the results were disappointing. Four patients died, ten were unchanged, three improved, and only one was cured.[9] This experience lead the committee to recommend that penicillin should be reserved for infections other than bacterial endocarditis until the supply improved.

While Keefer's committee was gaining general experience with penicillin, Dr. Henry Dawson (Figure 1) was already treating patients with endocarditis at the Presbyterian Hospital in New York. In fact, Dawson and his group occupy a very special place in the history of penicillin. The precise chronology of the first administration of parenteral penicillin is fascinating, and not widely known. In August, 1940, Karl Meyer, a biochemist working with Henry Dawson, read the report by Chain, Florey, and their team on the efficacy of penicillin *in vitro* and in

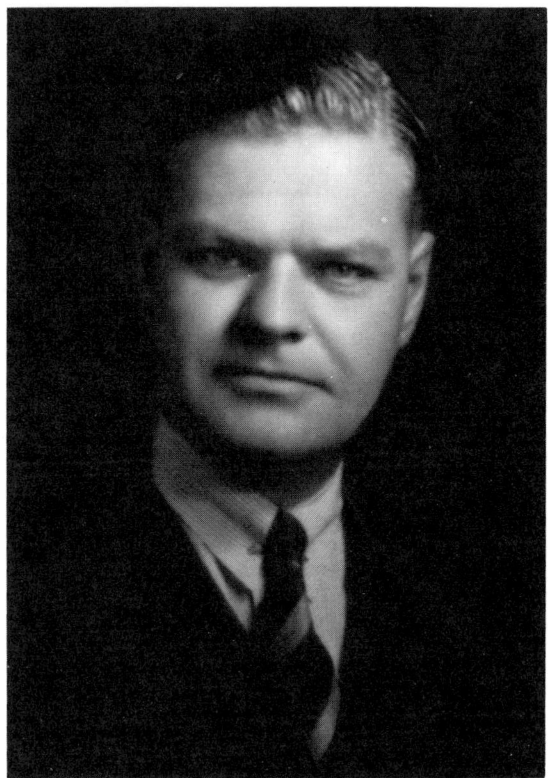

Figure 1: Martin Henry Dawson - first to administer penicillin parenterally to a patient, on October 16, 1940.

animals.[10] Meyer, who had done original work on lysozyme, was at that time somewhat incensed over a question of assignment of priority in one of Chain's own articles on lysozyme. He determined to undertake the purification of penicillin as quickly as possible, hoping to compete successfully with Chain (Meyer, K., personal communication). Under Dawson's direction he obtained Fleming's strain of *Penicillium notatum,* which had been brought to the United States some years before, and set to work. In less than three months he had prepared some partially purified penicillin.

Then occurred a series of historic events: on about October 15, 1940, Henry Dawson injected himself subcutaneously with a small quantity of the penicillin preparation, to test for toxicity. Shortly afterwards, on October 16 and 17, 1940, he injected penicillin subcutaneously into a young man with streptococcal endocarditis. The amount of penicillin available was very small, and it seemed obvious that the patient could not be cured by this short course of treatment. He was subsequently treated with sulfonamide and, remarkably enough, was cured. Three years later he again developed streptococcal endocarditis and again was cured, this time with a short course of low–dose penicillin, and heparin.

The historic importance of these events is obvious: this was not only the first patient in the United States to be treated with penicillin, but was also the first patient to receive parenteral penicillin anywhere in the world. This little-known fact is mentioned briefly in an article by Dawson and Hunter reporting treatment of 20 cases of endocarditis which appeared in 1945, [11] the year of Dawson's untimely death from myasthenia gravis. Dr. Tom Hunter had moved to Presbyterian Hospital as a resident in February, 1941; he then participated in Dawson's further trials of penicillin in patients with endocarditis, developing a life-long interest in the subject which led to his later work on penicillin-streptomycin synergy against viridans streptococci.[12–14] Incidentally, the young physician personally cared for his mentor during the last tragic months of Dawson's life (Hunter, T.H., personal communication).

The story of the early use of penicillin at Columbia was recently confirmed in a biography of Howard Florey by Macfarlane,[15] who notes that Dawson treated three cases of endocarditis with Meyer's preparations during 1940 and 1941. These cases were reported briefly in a paper presented before the American Society for Clinical Investigation at Atlantic City in 1941.[16] Dr. Gladys Hobby was the microbiologist who worked with Dawson and Meyer; she is presently preparing a book detailing these events (Hobby, G.L., personal communication).

Thus, at the end of 1943, initial results had been disappointing and penicillin did not appear to be a panacea for endocarditis. One month later the situation had changed dramatically; in January, 1944, Leo Loewe and his colleagues reported their small series of seven cases, all treated successfully with penicillin plus heparin.[17] This important paper first established the true potential of penicillin as a cure for streptococcal endocarditis. Within the next three years, enough patients had been treated and carefully recorded to establish that penicillin was dramatically effective when compared with sulfonamides.[3,5,11,18-20] Most authors reported cures in two-thirds to three-quarters of their patients, using low-dose and (frequently) short-term therapy (Table 1).

When recounting tales of the early days of penicillin, it is always fashionable to cite examples of cure with spectacularly low doses. For endocarditis, one example among many will suffice: Dawson and Hunter recorded the case of a young woman (M.L.) who was cured of streptococcal endocarditis with a grand *total* of 830,000 units of penicillin given over 10 days.[19] The point of emphasis is that by 1947, hundreds of patients had been cured by doses that were usually well below 300,000 units per day.[1,20] Subsequently, Cates and Christie in 1951 also recorded many cures with low doses of penicillin in their large series of 442 patients. However, they concluded that it was probably best to give a standard dose of 2,000,000 units daily in order to provide a wide margin of safety.[21]

Table 1: Summary of six early reports (1944—1947) on treatment of streptococcal endocarditis with penicillin. (Dosage listed in thousands of units per day.)

	reference	dose	duration	No. pts.	% cure
Loewe et al (1944)	17	56—229	14—51d	7	100%
Meads et al (1945)	18	215—340	13—19d	8	75%
White et al (1945)	5	100—288	14—28d	11	66%
Dawson & Hunter (1945)	11	62—258	10—103d	20	75%
Levy & McKrill (1946)	19	144—200	14—42d	11	73%
Seabury (1947)	3	154—304	14—73d	12	58%

It should be noted that failure to cure approximately one-third of the patients in these early series cannot be attributed solely to the low daily doses of penicillin that were usually employed. During that period, the necessary distinction between penicillin-sensitive viridans streptococci and enterococci was not yet appreciated, and techniques for supportive care were obviously less well developed than in later years. When these factors are taken into account, it seems likely that cure of about three-quarters of cases was actually fairly close to the "ceiling" that could be achieved in the 1940's. Of course, our "ceiling" today is much higher; this may be attributed largely to improvements in supportive care and cardiac surgery, in microbiologic techniques, and to the indefinable "practice effect" that comes with long experience, rather than to use of larger daily doses of penicillin.

To gather information on the optimal duration of treatment, Bloomfield, Armstrong, and Kirby studied the effects of long-term administration of penicillin. They used low doses (less than 300,000 units per day) but continued treatment for 42 to 69 days.[22] Their results were excellent, with ten bacteriologic cures and no relapses among ten cases. This important study, and subsequent experience showing the real need for long term therapy in *enterococcal* endocarditis, were probably the two leading factors that led to the entrenched clinical tradition, still often encountered, that streptococcal endocarditis requires treatment for six weeks.

King and co-workers reported the results of a very interesting and instructive experiment on treatment of endocarditis in 1949.[23] To test whether the disease could be cured by short-term, high dose penicillin therapy, they administered 14,000,000 units daily plus caronamide (an inhibitor of tubular secretion) to eight patients, for a total period of only ten days each. This was, of course, an extravagantly large dose of penicillin for that period, but even by today's standards the serum penicillin levels on this regimen were very high, ranging up to 240 units per milliliter of blood. The experiment was a dramatic failure; only one patient was cured, and seven relapsed. Notably, four of these seven patients were later cured with conventional doses of penicillin (less than

1,000,000 units per day) given for 34–56 days.[23] In the early 1950's Hunter showed that penicillin and streptomycin acted synergistically against penicillin-sensitive viridans streptococci, resulting in an increased rate of killing *in vitro*.[12–13] He[12] and Ernest Jawetz[24] first clearly stated the important principle (now almost axiomatic) that bactericidal drugs are necessary to cure most cases of endocarditis. This quotation from Jawetz's discussion [24] of a paper presented by Hunter [12] shows how well he appreciated all the fundamental principles of management of subacute endocarditis *by 1950:*

> "Adequate therapy in this disease is largely contingent on the recovery of the causative organism and its evaluation in the laboratory. Only 5 to 10 percent of cases fail to yield positive blood cultures in our hands. Once the causative organism is available, it should be tested for antibiotic sensitivity, the results of which can guide therapy. The treatment of subacute bacterial endocarditis does not require emergency measures. One is ordinarily justified to wait a week or two until the results of blood cultures and sensitivity tests are available . . . . It must be stressed, however, that only the *in vitro* killing action of the antibiotic should be considered, not its inhibitory effect. It seems likely that the failure of sulfonamide therapy in subacute bacterial endocarditis and the success of penicillin is probably based largely on the fact that the action of sulfonamides on bacteria is mainly bacteriostatic, whereas penicillin is rapidly bactericidal for streptococci of the viridans group. Enterococci are set apart from other streptococci by the fact that penicillin *in vitro* does not kill the entire exposed population but mainly inhibits it. This is paralleled by the clinical experience that enterococcic endocarditis is not cured by penicillin therapy. It can be cured frequently by the simultaneous administration of penicillin and streptomycin. In the test tube these two antibiotics have a clear cut synergistic effect, resulting in an increased bactericidal rate as well as the killing of the entire enterococcic population. These experiments support the hypothesis that rapid bactericidal action is a prerequisite of a drug or mixture of drugs capable of curing subacute bacterial endocarditis.[24]*

Because it had not yet become almost universally fashionable to treat endocarditis for six weeks, it is not surprising that Hunter and others chose short term regimens to test the efficacy of penicillin plus streptomycin in their patients. The results were uniformly good; Hunter cured five of five cases in only ten days with penicillin and streptomycin,[13] providing a sharp contrast to the failure of King's group to cure seven of eight cases with massive doses of penicillin alone for ten days.[23] Hunter,[14] Geraci[25-27] and others[28–31] subsequently reported a large number of cases treated with penicillin plus streptomycin for two weeks with very high rates of bacteriologic cure. At that time, overall

*Reprinted from discussion by Jawetz, E., in JAMA 144:533, 1950. Copyright 1950. American Medical Association.

relapse rates for two-week treatment with penicillin alone were 10—20%, while the relapse rate with penicillin plus streptomycin was usually less than 5 percent (Table 2). These findings may be further illustrated by combining a number of different studies and comparing the results of penicillin alone with those of penicillin plus streptomycin (Figure 2). Although there are obvious statistical objections to this crude combination of data, the trend of the curve provides a useful starting point for discussion of a vexing question: what are the merits of treatment with penicillin alone versus combined penicillin and streptomycin? The curves show a trend toward earlier cure for patients treated with various regimens combining penicillin plus streptomycin than

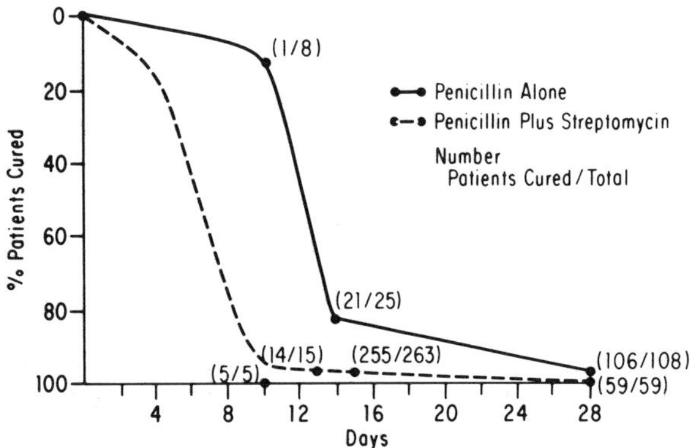

Figure 2: Crude curves to illustrate cure rate with time for penicillin sensitive streptococcal endocarditis, derived from the literature. The curve for treatment with various regimens containing penicillin plus streptomycin shows a trend towards earlier cure than for treatment with regimens employing penicillin alone. (Adapted from references 13, 14, 24—27, 29—35; number of cases shown in parentheses.)

with penicillin alone. It is noteworthy that 2 weeks is right "on the shoulder" before the curve for penicillin alone flattens out; a significant number of relapses occurs after two weeks' treatment, but few after four weeks. One further point should be clear from these curves: by four weeks, the rates of bacteriologic cure from *either* regimen are so high that it is futile to seek statistically significant differences between them. In a disease as variable in its course as subacute bacterial endocarditis, we should not expect, nor attempt, to show statistical differences between, say 96% cure for penicillin alone and 98% cure for penicillin plus streptomycin. The platitude "We need a good prospective, controlled

Table 2. Results of short-term therapy: summary of representative series of patients with viridans endocarditis treated for two weeks with various regimens using penicillin alone, or penicillin plus streptomycin.

		REFERENCE	No. PATIENTS	DURATION	RELAPSES	(%)
PENICILLIN ALONE	Meads et al., 1945	(18)	9	13—19 days	2	22%
	Hamburger & Stein, 1951	(32)	12	11—14 days	2	17%
	Tan et al., 1971	(30)	13	14 days	2	15%
	TOTAL		34		6	18%
PENICILLIN + STREPTOMYCIN	Hunter, 1952	(11)	5	10 days	0	0%
	Hall et al., 1955	(29)	13	10—17 days	1	8%
	Tompsett et al., 1958	(31)	35	10—18 days	3	10%
	Geraci, 1958	(27)	66	14 days	3	5%
	Hamburger et al., 1961	(28)	17	14—15 days	0	0%
	Tan et al., 1971	(30)	36	14 days	0	0%
	TOTAL		172		7	4%

study" is often heard, but it is not appropriate here; the choice between single versus combined therapy must be made on other grounds, such as toxicity and duration of hospitalization required to minimize the possibility of relapse. Because relapses occur occasionally after any treatment regimen, it would be worthwhile to study prospectively the incidence of *relapse* after combined short term therapy in larger numbers of patients than have been reported to date.

Once endocarditis could be cured, prognostic factors received attention. Cates and Christie's review of 442 cases identified the adverse prognostic factors that are now so familiar, especially heart failure, old age, acquired aortic valve disease, the general condition of the patient, and duration of infection before treatment.[21] The latter point deserves special attention in view of a recent report which raises the possibility that prolonged treatment regimens might be required for disease of long duration, in order to prevent relapse.[36] Cates and Christie[21] did find a significant, although not dramatic, correlation between duration of illness and mortality; six months after treatment, 27% of 357 patients with symptoms for less than ten weeks before treatment had died, while 50% of those with symptoms for 20 or more weeks were dead (Figure 3). However, these differences can be explained largely by the overwhelming prognostic significance of heart failure, which is naturally more likely to develop in cases of longer duration. When Cates' and Christie's cases were controlled for the effect of heart failure, the duration of illness before treatment carried relatively little prognostic significance (Figure 3). White and his colleagues also concluded that duration of infection was an unreliable indicator of prognosis, even though they did not control for the effect of heart failure.[5] They commented: "The opinion that the milder the infection and the earlier the treatment is instituted, the better the prognosis is only partially confirmed. Most of the patients who did recover gave histories of several month's duration and showed definite evidence of the disease, whereas other patients with shorter histories of infection and milder symptoms failed to recover."[5] Tompsett, referring to later experience with 63 patients treated with penicillin plus streptomycin, commented " . . . the results (of treatment) do not correlate with duration of the infection at all well. This has also been true . . . in some of the other large series. If one separates patients who have had symptoms one, two, three or four months or more, and then tabulates the end results, one does not find that the results are better in patients who have had symptoms for one or two months as opposed to three or four months."[37] Thus, while not entirely dismissing the possible prognostic significance of duration of infection before treatment, these extensive earlier experiences suggest that we should critically scrutinize any more recent evidence on this question before accepting the need to introduce a second level of treatment for cases of long duration.

During these early years, numerous attempts were made to cure endocarditis with two other new, powerful antibiotics -- aureomycin (chlortetracycline) and chloramphenicol.[38-40] Patients' symptoms often

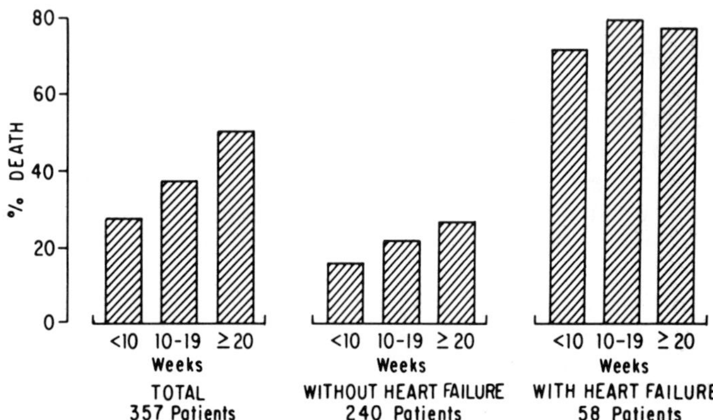

Figure 3: Influence of duration of symptoms before treatment on mortality, in a total of 357 patients, including 58 patients with, and 240 without, heart failure. (Adapted from Cates and Christie, 1951 [21].)

improved dramatically during treatment, but most relapsed promptly when it was discontinued. The results of this experience may be summarized simply: a few cases of bacterial endocarditis were undeniably cured by these bacteriostatic agents, but the failure rate compared to penicillin was far too high to allow their continued use.[38-40]

This review of early trials and successes in therapy of endocarditis caused by penicillin-sensitive viridans streptococci suggests the following conclusions:

1. *On the significance of duration of illness before treatment:* Review of cases reported by 1955 does not provide convincing evidence that disease of long duration has a strikingly worse prognosis *provided* that one controls for the *overwhelming prognostic influence of heart failure.* No evidence had accumulated to indicate that disease of long duration required escalated, or unusually prolonged, antibiotic treatment for cure, especially if combined treatment with penicillin plus streptomycin were used.
2. *On duration of therapy versus dosage*: Duration of treatment appeared to be more critical than dose, because ten days' treatment was too short, even with high dose, while many patients were cured by treatment for 14 days or longer. Further, many of these patients were cured with

less than 200,000 units of penicillin per day. No more than 2,000,000 units of penicillin daily was needed to cure most cases, *whether or not* streptomycin was added.

3. *On treatment with penicillin versus penicillin plus streptomycin*: It was clear by 1955 that penicillin alone cured *most* cases in 2 weeks, and *nearly all* in 4 weeks, while penicillin plus streptomycin cured *nearly all* cases in 2 weeks. Because both regimens give very high bacteriologic cure rates, it is futile to demand statistical demonstration of superior efficacy of one regimen over another. However, it should be stated clearly that by 1955, sufficient documentation of the efficacy and safety of two-week penicillin plus streptomycin regimens had already been provided to place the onus squarely on those requiring longer hospitalization to prove the necessity for it. The present enormous cost of hospitalization makes this conclusion even more relevant today than in 1955.

Certainly, a wealth of clinical experience and expertise in treatment of endocarditis had accumulated by 1955. Some of the controversies marking this field in later years inevitably bring to mind Santayana's epigram: "Those who cannot remember the past are condemned to repeat it."

This review of the early days of endocarditis treatment is respectfully dedicated to four men who made outstanding contributions to the field: Drs. Maxwell Finland, Joe Geraci, Tom Hunter, and Bill Kirby. Dr. Finland's first article on endocarditis[41] was published in 1928--fifty-three years ago!

REFERENCES

1. Kerr, A., Jr.: *Subacute Bacterial Endocarditis* (Springfield: Charles C. Thomas, 1955).
2. Lichtman, S.S.: Treatment of subacute bacterial endocarditis: current results, Ann. Intern. Med. 19:787, 1943.
3. Seabury, J.H.: Subacute bacterial endocarditis. Experiences during the past decade, Arch. Intern. Med. 79:1, 1947.
4. Galbreath, W.R., Mathews, D.W., and Hull, E.: Sulfonamide therapy of bacterial endocarditis; results in 42 cases, Ann. Intern. Med. 18:201, 1943.
5. White, P.D., Mathews, D.W., and Evans, E.: Notes on the treatment of subacute bacterial endocarditis encountered in 88 cases at the Massachusetts General Hospital during the six year period 1939 to 1944 (inclusive), Ann. Intern. Med. 22:61, 1945.

6. Schein, J., and Baehr, G.: Sulfonamide therapy of subacute bacterial endocarditis, Am. J. Med. 4:66, 1948.
7. Abraham, E.P., Chain, E., Fletcher, C.M., Florey, H.W., Gardner, D., Heatley, N.G., and Jennings, M.A.: Further observations on penicillin, Lancet, 2:177, 1941.
8. Florey, M.E., and Florey, H.W.: General and local administration of penicillin, Lancet 1:387, 1943.
9. Keefer, C.S., Blake, F.G., Marshall, E.K., Lockwood, H.S., and Wood, W.B.: Penicillin in the treatment of infections. A report of 500 cases, J.A.M.A. 122:1217, 1943.
10. Chain, E., Florey, H.W., Gardner, A.D., Heatley, N.G., Jennings, M.A., Orr-Ewing, J., and Sanders, A.G.: Penicillin as a chemotherapeutic agent, Lancet 2:226, 1940.
11. Dawson, M.H., and Hunter, T.H.: Treatment of subacute bacterial endocarditis with penicillin. Results in 20 cases, J.A.M.A. 127:129, 1945.
12. Hunter, T.H.: Speculations on the mechanism of cure of bacterial endocarditis, J.A.M.A. 144:524, 1950.
13. Hunter, T.H.: The treatment of some bacterial infections of the heart and pericardium, Bull. N.Y. Acad. Med. 28:213, 1952.
14. Hunter, T.H., and Paterson, P.Y.: Bacterial endocarditis, Disease-A-Month, November: 1956.
15. Macfarlane, R.G.: *Howard Florey: The Making of a Great Scientist* (Oxford: Oxford University Press, 1979).
16. Dawson, M.H., Hobby, G.L., Meyer, K., and Chaffee, E.: Penicillin as a chemotherapeutic agent, J. Clin. Invest. 20:434, 1941.
17. Loewe, L., Rosenblatt, P., Greene, H.J., and Russell, M.: Combined penicillin and heparin therapy of subacute bacterial endocarditis: Report of seven consecutive successfully treated patients, J.A.M.A. 124:144, 1944.
18. Meads, M., Harris, H.W., and Finland, M.: The treatment of bacterial endocarditis with penicillin. Experiences at the Boston City Hospital during 1944, New Engl. J. Med. 232:463, 1945.
19. Levy, L., and McKrill, N.: Results in the treatment of subacute bacterial endocarditis. Arch. Intern. Med. 77:367, 1946.
20. Anderson, D.G., and Keefer, C.S.: *The Therapeutic Value of Penicillin: A Study of 10,000 Cases* (Ann Arbor: Edwards Bros., 1948).
21. Cates, J.E., and Christie, R.V.: Subacute bacterial endocarditis, Quart. J. Med. 20:93, 1951.
22. Bloomfield, A.L., Armstrong, C.D., and Kirby, W.M.M.: The treatment of subacute bacterial endocarditis with penicillin, J. Clin. Invest. 24:251, 1945.

23. King, F.H., Schneierson, S.S., Sussman, M.L., Janowitz, H.D., and Stollerman, G.H.: Prolonged moderate dose therapy versus intensive short term therapy with penicillin and caronamide in subacute bacterial endocarditis, J. Mt. Sinai Hosp. 16:35, 1949.
24. Jawetz, E.: Abstract of discussion on papers by Drs. T.H. Hunter and C.K. Friedberg, J.A.M.A. 144:533, 1950.
25. Geraci, J.E., and Martin, W.J.: Antibiotic therapy of bacterial endocarditis IV. Successful short-term (two weeks) combined penicillin-dihydrostreptomycin therapy in subacute bacterial endocarditis caused by penicillin-sensitive streptococci, Circulation 8:494, 1953.
26. Geraci, J.E.: Further experiences with short-term (2 weeks) combined penicillin-streptomycin therapy for bacterial endocarditis caused by penicillin-sensitive streptococci, Proc. Staff Meet. Mayo Clin. 30:192, 1955.
27. Geraci, J.E.: The antibiotic therapy of bacterial endocarditis: Therapeutic data on 172 patients seen from 1951 through 1957. Additional observations on short-term therapy (two weeks) for penicillin-sensitive streptococcal endocarditis, Med. Clin. N. Am. 42:1101, 1958.
28. Hamburger, M., Kaplan, S., and Walker, W.F.: Subacute bacterial endocarditis caused by penicillin-sensitive streptococci, J.A.M.A. 175:554, 1961.
29. Hall, B., Dowling, H.F., and Kellow, W.: Successful short-term therapy of streptococcal endocarditis with penicillin and streptomycin, Am. J. Med. Sci. 230:73, 1955.
30. Tan, J.S., Terhune, C.A., Kaplan, S., Hamburger, M.: Successful two-week treatment schedule for penicillin-susceptible streptococcus viridans endocarditis, Lancet 2:1340, 1971.
31. Tompsett, R., Robbins, W.B., and Bernsten, C., Jr.: Short-term penicillin and dihydro-streptomycin therapy of streptococcal endocarditis, Am. J. Med. 24:57, 1958.
32. Hamburger, M., and Stein, L.: Streptococcus viridans subacute bacterial endocarditis. Two week treatment schedule with penicillin, J.A.M.A. 149:542, 1952.
33. Karchmer, A.W., Moellering, R.C., Maki, D.G., and Swartz, M.N.: Single-antibiotic therapy for streptococcal endocarditis, J.A.M.A. 241:1801, 1979.
34. Lerner, P.I., and Weinstein, L.: Infective endocarditis in the antibiotic era, New Engl. J. Med. 274:199, 259, 232, 388, 1966.
35. Wolfe, J.D., and Johnson, W.D.: Penicillin-sensitive streptococcal endocarditis. In vitro and clinical observations on penicillin-streptomycin therapy, Ann. Intern. Med. 81:178, 1974.
36. Malacoff, R.F., Frank, E., and Andriole, V.T.: Streptococcal endocarditis (non-enterococcal, non-group A). Single vs combination therapy, J.A.M.A. 241:1807, 1979.

37. Tompsett, R., and Hurst, M.L.: Bacterial endocarditis: selected aspects of treatment, Clin. Climatol. Assoc. 95:95, 1971.
38. Kane, L.W., and Finn, J.J.: The treatment of subacute bacterial endocarditis with aureomycin and chloromycetin, New Engl. J. Med. 244:623, 1951.
39. Spies, H.W., Dowling, H.F., Lepper, M.H., Wolfe, C.K., and Caldwell, E.R.: Aureomycin in the treatment of bacterial endocarditis. Report of nine cases together with a study of the synergistic action of aureomycin and penicillin in one case, Arch. Intern. Med. 87:66, 1951.
40. Friedberg, C.K.: Treatment of subacute bacterial endocarditis with aureomycin, J.A.M.A. 148:98, 1952.
41. Finland, M., and Davis, D.: An unusual distribution of peripheral gangrene in a case of subacute bacterial endocarditis, New Engl. J. Med. 199:1019, 1928.

Matthew E. Levison, M.D.

2

TREATMENT OF ENDOCARDITIS DUE TO VIRIDANS STREPTOCOCCI IN EXPERIMENTAL MODELS

Characteristics of the Viridans Group of Streptococci

The viridans streptococci are often referred to collectively as *Streptococcus viridans,* as if they were a single species. In fact, clinical isolates of viridans streptococci usually belong to one of six physiologically defined species: *S. sanguis I, S. sanguis II, S. salivarius, S. mitior* (or *mitis*), *S. mutans* and *S. MG-intermedius* (or *milleri*).[1] These micro-organisms give an alpha or non-hemolytic reaction on blood agar and do not have B or D antigen. *S. sanguis I* has been reported to be the most commonly isolated viridans streptococcus from patients with bacterial endocarditis (29% of isolates), followed by *S. sanguis II* (21%), *S. mutans* (18%) and *S.MG* (14%).[1]

In addition, viridans streptococci with specific nutritional growth requirements have been isolated from up to 5% of patients with endocarditis.[2] Some of these strains have been found to require increased concentration of thiol compounds or active forms of vitamin B_6 for optimal growth.

Model of Experimental Endocarditis

The effectiveness of antimicrobial therapy in endocarditis caused by viridans streptococci has been studied in a reproducible model of this disease in rabbits. This model, first developed by Garrison and Freedman[3,4], consists of a polyethylene catheter that is inserted into the right heart through the jugular vein or into the left heart through the right carotid artery. The presence of the catheter in the right or left side of the heart provokes rapid deposition of fibrin-platelet vegetations on the heart valves traumatized by the catheter. These sterile vegetations may then be infected either by filling the catheter with micro-organisms or by injecting them intravenously.[5] The micro-organisms in the vegetations rapidly enter the logarithmic phase of growth at a rate equivalent to unimpeded growth in broth cultures. The density of viridans streptococci within vegetations reaches 10^9 to 10^{10} bacteria/g which is greater than the maximum population densities achieved in broth.[6]

Pathologically, the vegetations are remarkably like those found in man. They consist of a relatively amorphous mass of fibrin, platelets, platelet debris, and bacteria. Leukocytes are scanty. Early in the infection organisms may be located on or just below the surface of the vegetation and later are found deep within the fibrin matrix isolated from host defense mechanisms.[7] Those micro-organisms deep within the vegetations are in a hypometabolic state and presumably more refractory to antibiotic action than bacteria more superfically located.[8]

On the right-side, infection with *Streptococcus sanguis* is infrequently fatal. On the left side of the heart, infection is progressive and death is almost invariable.[9] Rabbits with simultaneous left and right catheters have a bacterial density 300 times higher on the left than the right side.[10]

Nine studies have been published on the effectiveness of antibiotic therapy in the rabbit model of viridans streptococcal endocarditis.[2,6,11–17] In these studies, five different strains isolated from the blood of patients with endocarditis have been used: 2 strains of *S. sanguis*; 1 *S. mitis*, one unspeciated strain and one vitamin B_6-dependent strain of *S. mitis.* All except for the last were penicillin-sensitive [minimal inhibitory concentration (MIC) of ≤ 0.1 μg of penicillin/ml].

Antibiotic Susceptibility *In Vitro*

Eighty to 85% of strains of viridans streptococci isolated from the blood of patients with endocarditis are penicillin-sensitive (inhibited by $\leq$ 0.1 unit μg/ml).[18] The combination of penicillin plus streptomycin has been found to be more rapidly bactericidal *in vitro* against these penicillin-sensitive strains than penicillin alone. Wolfe and Johnson studied

48 strains of viridans streptococci isolated from the blood of patients with endocarditis *in vitro* for synergism to the combination of penicillin and streptomycin.[19] As shown in Figure 1, multiplication of organisms occurred in broth without antibiotics and in streptomycin alone. Despite relative penicillin-sensitivity (MIC $\leq$ 0.4 μg/ml), incubation for 48 hours

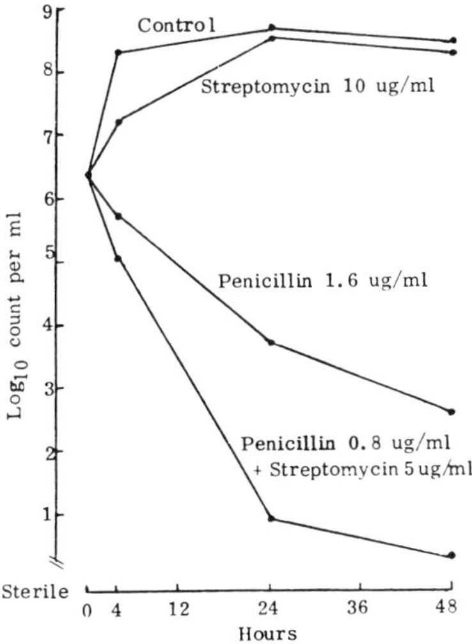

Figure 1: The geometric mean of the number of organisms recovered in synergism studies with 48 strains of viridans streptococci isolated from endocarditis patients between 1944 and 1947 and between 1967 and 1971. Wolfe and Johnson.[19]

in 1.6 μg of penicillin alone sterilized the inoculum of only one strain. In the other 47 strains, penicillin alone in a concentration of 1.6 μg/ml caused a 4 $\log_{10}$ fall in viable organisms at 48 hours. Between 10^2 to 10^3 CFU/ml persisted in penicillin at 48 hours. The rate or the completeness rate of killing was increased for 47 of the 48 strains by the addition of streptomycin to penicillin.[19]

The ability of antibiotic therapy to kill all organisms in vegetations is thought to be critical in endocarditis, and persistence of even a few viable bacteria may be sufficient to result in a relapse after discontinuation of therapy. From the *in vitro* data, if penicillin were used alone, prolonged dosing would probably be required to eliminate "persisting" organisms in vegetation. The enhanced rate and completeness of killing which occurs with penicillin plus streptomycin *in vitro* have suggested that therapy of endocarditis should consist of this combination, especially if a shortened course is planned, and possibly to prevent complications which may be related to duration of infection, such as valve destruction, congestive heart failure and need for valve replacement.

Effect of Antibiotic Therapy on Experimental Endocarditis

Carrizosa and Kaye[11] demonstrated the necessity of high doses of penicillin and also the importance of prolonged therapy required to cure viridians streptococcal endocarditis. In their studies, rabbits were infected on the left side of the heart with a strain of *S. mitis* and treatment was started 24 hours after infection, with the catheter remaining in place (Table 1). Separate groups of animals were treated for five, ten or twenty days. Regimens of 25 mg/kg/d of procaine penicillin or less, given every 6 hours for 5 to 10 days, were not sufficient to sterilize vegetations. A dose

Table 1. Therapy of Experimental Endocarditis

Procaine Dose (mg/kg/d)	Penicillin Frequency	Duration of Therapy (days) 5	10	20
25	6h	0/16*	0/4	
50	6h	10/20(1.7)+	3/5 (5/9)**	(1/8)**
100	6h	12/14	5/5 (0/5)**	(0/8)**
50	12h	4/11(4.5)+		

* No. Sterile Vegetations/No. Animals

\+ Log_{10} Colony Forming Units (CFU)/g Vegetation

** No. Relapsing/No. Rabbits

of 50 mg/kg/d of procaine penicillin every 6 hours for 5 days was effective in sterilizing only 50% of rabbits. At this dose, 20 days of therapy was required to prevent relapse in 7 of 8 rabbits. On 100 mg/kg/d, at 5 days, 12 of 14 rabbits had sterile vegetations, and at 10 or more days all vegetations were sterilized and no animals relapsed. Thus, 50 mg/kg/d was the lowest dose tested that cured most animals, but required at least 20 days, and 100 mg/kg/d was the lowest dose tested that cured all rabbits after at least 10 days of therapy. The dose of 50 mg/kg/d was significantly more effective when given every 6 hours than every 12 hours, i.e. log_{10} 1.7 CFU/g of vegetation for the former and 4.5 for the latter ($p < 0.01$).

Durack and Petersdorf[12] studied the effectiveness of single doses of antibiotic to prevent right-sided experimental *S. sanguis* endocarditis in rabbits. The antibiotics were either given 30 minutes prior to infection, or in some rabbits, 30 minutes after infection. The MIC of penicillin for this strain was 0.01 μg/ml, and the MIC of streptomycin was 8.0 μg/ml. The investigators believed this to be a model for treatment of very early endocarditis since seeding of the vegetation has been shown to occur less than 30 minutes after bacteria enter the circulation, at a time before antibiotic could be expected to have completed its antibacterial action. Their finding that a high dose of procaine penicillin (250 mg/kg) was equally effective in preventing endocarditis either when given 30 minutes before, or 30 minutes after, intravenous injection of streptococci is consistent with this concept (Table 2).

Table 2: Prevention and Therapy of Early Experimental Endocarditis in Rabbits

Therapy	Timing*	Dose (mg/kg)	Reciprocal Serum Inhibiting Dilution Peak/Trough (12h)	No. Infected/ No. Animals
Procaine penicillin	+ 30 min	250	1000/256	0/4
	- 30 min	250	1000/256	0/5
	- 30 min	50	1000/4	1/8
	- 30 min	10	64/2	8/8

* +, following injection of inoculum.
-, prior to injection of inoculum.

Modified From Durack, D.T., and Petersdorf, R.G.[12]

Although the strain of *S. sanguis* was highly sensitive to penicillin *in vitro,* and despite using doses of penicillin which resulted in high peak serum inhibiting activity, only single doses of 50 or 250 mg/kg which provided both a high peak level and a prolonged duration of inhibiting activity (as seen by the trough level) were successful (Table 2). Bacteriostatic agents such as tetracycline, erythromycin and clindamycin failed to prevent endocarditis. However, penicillin (or ampicillin), in doses which alone fail to prevent endocarditis, when combined with streptomycin uniformly prevent right-sided endocarditis (Table 3). The failure of some regimens of penicillin (and other bactericidal agents, such as ampicillin, cephalexin and cephaloridine) and of the bacteriostatic agents, and the effectiveness of the combination of penicillin plus streptomycin, suggest that completeness of kill is important, especially in short courses of antimicrobial agents which consisted in this case of a single dose.

Table 3: Prevention and Therapy of Early Experimental Endocarditis in Rabbits

Therapy	Timing*	Dose (mg/kg)	Reciprocal Serum Inhibiting Dilution Peak/Trough (12h)	No. Infected No. Animals
Penicillin G	- 30 min	150	16,000/2	19/21
Penicillin G	- 30 min	150	--	0/6
+ Streptomycin		15		

* -, prior to injection of inoculum.

Modified From Durack, D.T., and Petersdorf, R.G.[12]

In further experiments, Durack et al.[13] demonstrated increased refractoriness to antibiotic therapy when the strain of *S. sanguis* which had seeded the tricuspid vegetations was allowed 6 more hours of unimpeded growth, from a bacterial density of about 10^4 CFU/g at 30 minutes to about 10^8/g of vegetation, prior to initiation of therapy.

Single doses of procaine penicillin, 250 mg/kg intramuscularly, and vancomycin, 30 mg/kg intravenously, prevented endocarditis when given 30 minutes after infection. However, these same antibiotic dosages failed to prevent endocarditis when administered 6 hours after initiation of infection (Table 4).

Table 4. Prevention and Therapy of Early Experimental Endocarditis

Therapy	Dose (mg/kg)	Duration of Infection + 30 min	6h
Procaine penicillin	250	0/9	9/9
Vancomycin	30	0/11	11/14

* No. Infected/No. Animals

Modified From Durack, D.T., Pelletier, L.L., and Petersdorf, R.G.[13]

The enhanced activity of the combination of penicillin plus streptomycin was again demonstrated against a highly penicillin-sensitive strain in the 6 hour model (Table 5). While only 2 of 6 or 1 of 5 rabbits had sterilized aortic vegetations after treatment with either penicillin or streptomycin alone, when penicillin was combined with streptomycin, all vegetations were sterilized.

Table 5. Therapy of Early Experimental Endocarditis

Therapy	Dose (mg/kg)	Reciprocal Serum Cidal Dilution Peak/Trough (12h)	No. Infected/ No. Animals
Procaine penicillin	25 BID x 1d	512/$<$2	4/6*
Streptomycin	15 BID x 1d	2/$<$2	4/5*
Penicillin and Streptomycin	25 BID x 1d 15 BID	512/$<$2	0/8

* About $\log_{10}$ 3.0 CFU/g Vegetation vs $>$8.0 CFU/g in untreated controls.

Modified From Durack, D.T., Pelletier, L.L., and Petersdorf, R.G.[13]

Similar findings of enhanced *in vivo* activity against penicillin-sensitive viridans streptococci with penicillin plus an aminoglycoside have been reported by Sande and Irvin (Table 6).[6] Antibiotics in these studies were started after catheter removal, at a time when relatively large aortic vegetations with dense bacterial populations containing 10^9 to 10^{10} CFU/g were present.

Table 6. Therapy of Experimental Endocarditis in Rabbits

Therapy	Dose (mg/kg)	Log_{10} CFU/g Vegetation 3-5d		Relapse
Procaine penicillin	100 BID x 3-5d	6.3	(2)*	3/3
Procaine penicillin	100 BID			
+Streptomycin or	17.5 BID x 3-5d	<2	(2)	2/5
Gentamicin	or 5 BID			

*Number of Rabbits

Modified From Sande, M.A., and Irvin, R.G.[6]

Pelletier and Petersdorf[14] repeated these studies with larger numbers of rabbits after a 6-hour or a 48-hour delay in therapy and with and without the catheter remaining in place, in order to examine the effect of the age of infection prior to the initiation of therapy and the effect of the catheter on response to treatment with penicillin alone vs. penicillin plus streptomycin.

As in the previous experiments[13], these investigators found that 5 days of high dose procaine penicillin, 250 mg/kg/d, was required to cure all of the 6-hour model animals, but this regimen left 21 of 23 48-hour model rabbits with infected vegetations (Table 7). Procaine penicillin, 25 mg/kg, combined with streptomycin, 15 mg/kg, twice daily for 3 days cured all of the 6-hour model rabbits, but left 8 of 9 of the 48-hour model animals infected ($p < 0.05$). Even 5 days of combined low dose penicillin plus streptomycin therapy failed to cure the 48-hour model animals. Resistance of older vegetations to antibiotic therapy has been attributed to the fact that they are larger and contain deeply buried, denser populations of metabolically hypoactive bacteria which may be less accessible and less sensitivity to penicillin.

In rabbits with retained intracardiac catheters, a condition perhaps analogous to streptococcal prosthetic valve endocarditis in man, despite prolonged high dose therapy, penicillin alone only reduced the infection rate from 21 of 23 at 5 days to 6 of 18 rabbits at 10 days. Penicillin plus streptomycin on the other hand, cured 50% at 5 days and eradicated

Table 7. Therapy of Experimental Endocarditis

Therapy	Dose	Duration of Infection 6h	48h	
Procaine penicillin	250 (mg/kg/d) x5d	0/11*	21/23	$p < 0.01$
Procaine penicillin + Streptomycin	25 (mg/kg BID) x3d +15 (mg/kg BID)	0/6	8/9	$p < 0.01$
Procaine penicillin +Streptomycin	25 (mg/kg BID) x5d +15 (mg/kg BID)		4/4	

*Number Infected/Number Animals

Modified From Pelletier, L.L., and Petersdorf, R.G.[14]

streptococci from all vegetations in catheterized rabbits after 10 days of therapy (Table 8). Penicillin alone sterilized vegetations more rapidly in rabbits without catheters, but enhanced bactericidal activity in these rabbits treated with penicillin plus streptomycin was evident at 5 and 7 days. By 10 days, no significant difference was observed between penicillin-treated and penicillin plus streptomycin-treated rabbits without catheters. These experiments establish that penicillin plus streptomycin is significantly more effective than penicillin alone in eradicating penicillin-sensitive streptococci from vegetations. The catheter made the infection more refractory to therapy; thus, the therapeutic advantage of combined therapy was magnified in the presence of an intracardiac catheter. The larger vegetations found in association with retained catheters were thought to contribute to the resistance to treatment.[12]

Table 8. Therapy of Experimental Endocarditis

Therapy	Dose (mg/kg/d)	Catheter Retained Duration of Therapy (Days) 5	7	10	Catheter Removed Duration of Therapy (Days) 5	7	10
Procaine penicillin	250	21*/23	12/19	6/18	11/19	9/20	1/16
Procaine penicillin +Streptomycin	250 15	12/24	5/15	0/18	7/19	2/20	0/6

* Number infected/Number Animals

Modified From Pelletier, L.L., and Petersdorf, R.G.[14]

Effect of Warfarin on the Response to Antibiotic Therapy

Anticoagulants have been suggested to have a role in the therapy of infective endocarditis by reducing vegetation formation. Clinical experience has shown, however, that the use of anticoagulants may encourage the development of serious hemorrhagic complications. Problems concerning the use of anticoagulants in endocarditis still arise, usually in the setting of infective endocarditis complicating prosthetic valve replacement. Two reports describe the effect of anticoagulant on the response to antibiotic therapy in the rabbit model of viridans streptococcal endocarditis.[15,16] Hook and Sande[15] anticoagulated rabbits with warfarin 2 to 5 days prior to placement of left-heart catheters and infected these rabbits 4 to 5 days after catheterization. Pre-treatment with warfarin prevented fibrin deposition, but anticoagulated rabbits nevertheless developed valvular infection at the same rate after injection of bacteria as non-anticoagulated rabbits. Anticoagulation also decreased mean survival time from 12.7 days to 7 days. In anticoagulated rabbits, penicillin for 1 to 4 days lowered the bacterial population on valves from $\log_{10}$ 9.3 to 2.3 CFU/g and 3 of 4 valves were sterile, whereas in non-anticoagulated rabbits, penicillin lowered the bacterial population to 6.5 CFU/g of vegetation and none were sterile (Table 9). The significantly enhanced rate of bactericidal activity of penicillin in warfarin-treated rabbits was noted by Hook and Sande to be similar to the rate at which

Table 9. Effect of Penicillin Therapy in Warfarin-Treated Experimental Endocarditis

	Log_{10} CFU/g of Vegetation	
	Warfarin-Treated	Non-Warfarin-Treated
Days of Penicillin Therapy	Penicillin-Treated	Penicillin-Treated
0	9.3 (1)	9.5 (1)
1-4	2.3* (4)**	6.5 (4)

* 3/4 Vegetations were sterile (<2 CFU/g)

** Number of rabbits

Modified From Hook, E.W. III., and Sande, M.A.[15]

penicillin kills large numbers of viridans streptococci *in vitro.*[15] The investigators postulated that defective fibrin formation may allow the entire mass of bacteria to be more superficially located. The more superficial location may increase accessibility to antibiotic or may allow organisms to have greater metabolic activity and thus greater penicillin sensitivity.

In another study[16], left-heart catheters were placed in rabbits 48 hours before warfarin and the rabbits infected 24 hours after the start of warfarin. In this model, warfarin had no effect on the size of vegetation or on the susceptibility to infection but again shortened the mean survival from 15.5 days to less than 4 days. Early death in warfarin-treated rabbits was associated with rapidly increasing bacteremia, pulmonary edema and extensive lung hemorrhage. Early death of anticoagulated rabbits was not prevented with penicillin therapy despite sterile blood cultures and lowered bacterial populations in vegetations. This suggests that early death in these animals was not related to greater severity of infection alone. In addition, survival for at least a week in anticoagulated uninfected catheterized rabbits also excludes anticoagulation alone as the cause of early death, but implicates anticoagulation combined with infection.

Penicillin-Resistant Viridans Streptococcal Endocarditis

Carey et al.[2] reported on the treatment of tricuspid valve experimental endocarditis in rabbits caused by a strain of vitamin B_6-dependent viridans streptococcus. This organism had an MIC of 0.78 μg of penicillin/ml and was isolated from the blood of a patient with endocarditis who relapsed after a 4-week course of parenteral penicillin 10–20 million units/day, combined initially with streptomycin for 2 weeks. *In vitro* studies showed that both the rate of killing and the total number of organisms killed by penicillin were increased with the addition of streptomycin. Results of therapy of experimental endocarditis with this organism show that the combination of penicillin and streptomycin was synergistic against this vitamin B_6-dependent streptococcus resistant to penicillin (Table 10).

Table 10. Therapy of Penicillin-Resistant Viridans Streptococcal Experimental Endocarditis in Rabbits

Therapy (Intramuscular)	Dose (mg/kg)	Log_{10} CFU/g Vegetation at 12d	
Procaine penicillin	100 BID	4.3	(2)*
Streptomycin	10 BID	8.4	(3)
Penicillin + Streptomycin	100 + 10 BID	$<$ 2.0	(3)

* Number of Rabbits

Modified From Carey, R.B., Brause, B.D., and Roberts, R.B.[2]

Endocarditis Caused by Tolerant Viridans Streptococci

Tolerance is an *in vitro* phenomenom in which strains, although inhibited by low concentrations of penicillin G, are relatively resistant to its bactericidal action, i.e. the minimum bactericidal concentration (MBC) is many times ($\geq$ 10x) higher than the MIC as determined after 24 hours incubation in penicillin G. However, the MBC may be equal to be MIC at 48 hours *in vitro.* This finding is a reflection of the relatively slower rate of bactericidal action of penicillin G on these strains in comparison to the rate of killing of non-tolerant strains of the same species. Tolerance may be more common among viridans streptococci than is currently appreciated. Recently, Horne and Tomasz[20] have reported finding tolerance in all five strains tested of *S. sanguis* isolated from blood of patients with endocarditis. The effect of antibiotic therapy on response of endocarditis caused by tolerant viridans streptococci has been studied in the rabbit model. In these studies, penicillin therapy killed a tolerant strain of *S. sanguis* in cardiac vegetations more slowly than it killed a non-tolerant strain.[21]

In Vitro Tests

The effectiveness of *in vitro* tests to predict the response of bacterial populations in vegetations to antibiotic therapy has been studied in the experimental rabbit model. The more rapid rates and completeness of bactericidal activity of penicillin in combination with an aminoglycoside have been correlated with more rapid rates of eradication of viridans streptococci from vegetations *in vivo* in rabbits treated with this combination.[2,6,12,13] Conversely, in a study by Carrizosa et al.[17], the slower rate of bactericidal activity of penicillin when combined with chloramphenicol *in vitro* was associated with a slower eradication of viridans streptococci from vegetations *in vivo* in rabbits treated with penicillin preceded by chloramphenicol. In addition, the slower rate of *in vitro* bactericidal action of penicillin on a tolerant strain of viridans streptococcus was correlated with a slower rate of eradication of this strain from vegetations *in vivo* in rabbits treated with penicillin.[21]

However, others have not found this correlation. In a study of tolerant *Staphylococcus aureus,* Goldman and Petersdorf[22] have noted that despite the slower rate of bactericidal activity of methicillin against the tolerant strain *in vitro,* methicillin eradicated both a tolerant and non-tolerant strain from vegetations at identical rates, even though serum levels of the antibiotic were less than the MBC for the tolerant strain.

The rate of response to antibiotic *in vitro* does not necessarily predict the absolute rate of response of the same bacteria enmeshed in a fibrin-platelet vegetation. In a study in our laboratory, Carrizosa et al.[23] studied the fate of enterococci in vegetations when these vegetations were incubated in minimal concentrations of gentamicin combined with penicillin which resulted in relatively rapid bactericidal activity in broth cultures (Figure 2). For example, penicillin 20 μg/ml plus gentamicin 1.5 or 0.75 μg/ml sterilized a suspension of 10^8 enterococci/ml at 48 hours in broth. When vegetations infected with 10^8 enterococci/g were incubated in the presence of penicillin, 20 μg/ml and gentamicin, 1.5 μg/ml in broth,

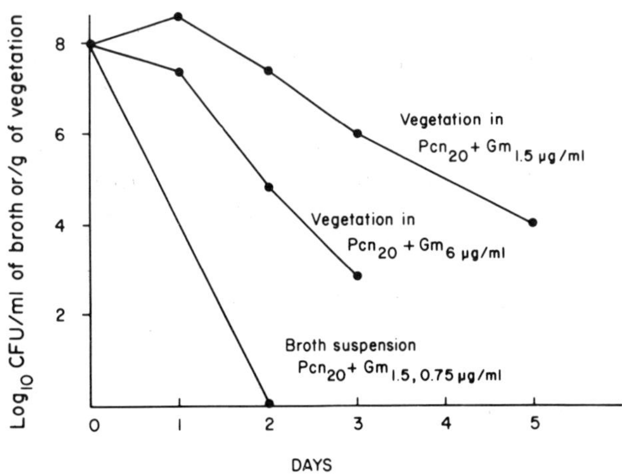

Figure 2: Effect of antibiotics on streptococci in vegetations vs. broth suspensions in vitro. Carrizosa et al.[23]

the bacterial population in the vegetation was $10^{8.6}$/g at 1 day and $10^{7.4}$ at 2 days and $10^{6.0}$ at 3 days. At 5 days, these vegetations still contained $10^{4.1}$ CFU/g. Only 2 of 10 vegetations were sterilized after 5 days in penicillin plus 1.5 μg of gentamicin/ml. To enhance the rate and completeness of kill in vegetations, a relatively high concentration of gentamicin *in vitro* was required. For example, penicillin plus gentamicin, 6 μg/ml, reduced the bacterial count in vegetations to $10^{2.8}$/g at 3 days and sterilized 4 of 6 vegetations. The slower rate of bactericidal activity in vegetations may be due to poor penetration of antibiotic or metabolic inactivity of bacteria buried deep within the vegetation.

The relation between serum bactericidal activity during therapy and the efficacy of treatment in endocarditis due to viridans streptococci have been studied in the experimental model, and the results are conflicting. In the study of Durack et al[13], streptomycin alone exerted substantial *in vivo* bactericidal activity in aortic vegetations infected with a strain of viridans streptococci, despite only low and transient serum bactericidal levels following administration of streptomycin consistent with its MBC of 8.0 μg/ml. On the other hand, studies of Carrizosa and Kaye[11] have shown good correlation between peak serum bactericidal levels and bacteriologic response to penicillin treatment of streptococcal endocarditis. In this study, regimens of procaine penicillin capable of sterilizing vegetations after 10 to 20 days of therapy gave peak maximal serum bactericidal dilutions of at least 1/8. In this study, when antibiotic was given every 6 hours, trough levels did not seem to be critical.

Summary

In vivo experiments in rabbits have documented that increased duration of valvular infection with viridans streptococci and the presence of a retained intracardiac foreign body are associated with increased resistance to antibiotic therapy. Bacteriostatic drugs, which may be effective in infections located in areas accessible to phagocytic defense mechanisms, are ineffective in curing infection in vegetations, where granulocytes are rarely found. Corresponding to *in vitro* results, penicillin has been found to eradicate viridans streptococci from vegetations at a relatively slow rate and cure requires prolonged therapy with high doses. The rate and completeness of sterilization of vegetations with penicillin is retarded when penicillin is combined with a bacteriostatic agent such as chloramphenicol, but is enhanced when penicillin is combined with an aminoglycoside. Enhanced activity *in vivo* has been demonstrated with penicillin-sensitive and a penicillin-resistant strain and was observed regardless of the age of the vegetation or the presence of intracardiac foreign body. If one assumes that complications such as congestive heart failure and valve perforation in man are related to the duration of infection, the more rapid the sterilization of the infection achieved with penicillin plus aminoglycoside, the less should be the risk of these complications and requirements of valve replacement. In addition, the combination of penicillin and an aminoglycoside could allow shortened courses of treatment. While anticoagulation has been demonstrated to increase the bactericidal action of penicillin *in vivo,* it fails to prevent left-sided endocarditis and results in early death. The rapidly fatal course in anticoagulated rabbits with bleeding is similar to the reported experience in man. Peak serum bactericidal activity of at least 1 to 8 dilutions is required, but information in this model is insufficient to draw firm conclusions about the effect of frequency of antibiotic administration or the predictive value of trough serum bactericidal activity. No data are available in the experimental model on possible differences in response to antibiotic therapy of left vs. right-sided vegetations. *In vitro* "tolerance" among viridans streptococci, which may be more common than currently appreciated, has been reported to be associated with a retarded eradication of organisms from vegetations in response to penicillin therapy in the rabbit model.

REFERENCES

1. Facklam, R.R.: Physiological differentiation of viridans streptococci. J Clin Microb 5:184–201, 1977.
2. Carey, R.B., Brause, B.D. and Roberts, R.B.: Antimicrobial therapy of vitamin B_6-dependent streptococcal endocarditis. Ann Intern Med 87:150–154, 1977.
3. Garrison, P.K. and Freedman, L.R.: Experimental endocarditis I. Staphylococcal endocarditis in rabbits resulting from placement of a polyethylene catheter in the right side of the heart. Yale J. Biol Med 42:394–410, 1970.
4. Perlman, B.B. and Freedman, L.R.: Experimental endocarditis II. Staphylococcal infection of the aortic valve following placement of a polyethylene catheter in the left side of the heart. Yale J. Biol Med 44:206–213, 1971.
5. Durack, D.T. and Beeson, P.B.: Experimental bacterial endocarditis I. Colonization of a sterile vegetation. Br J Exp Path 53:44-49, 1972.
6. Sande, M.A. and Irvin, R.G.: Penicillin-aminoglycoside synergy in experimental *Streptococcus viridans* endocarditis. J Infect Dis 129:572–576, 1974.
7. Durack, D.T.: Experimental bacterial endocartitis IV. Structure and evolution of very early lesions. J Path 115:81-89, 1975.
8. Durack, D.T. and Beeson, P.B.: Experimental bacterial endocarditis II. Survival of bacteria in endocardial vegetations. Br J Exp Path 53:50–53, 1972.
9. Durack . D.T., Beeson, P.B. and Petersdorf, R.G.: Experimental bacterial endocarditis III. Production and progress of the disease in rabbits. Br J Exp Path 54:142-151, 1973.
10. Freedman, L.R. and Valone, J. Jr.: Experimental infective endocarditis. Prog Cardiovasc Dis 22:169–180, 1979.
11. Carrizosa, J. and Kaye, D.: Antibiotic concentrations in serum, serum bactericidal activity, and results of therapy of streptococcal endocarditis in rabbits. Antimicrob Ag Chemother 12:479–483, 1977.
12. Durack, D.T. and Petersdorf, R.G.: Chemotherapy of experimental streptococcal endocarditis. I. Comparison of commonly recommended prophylactic regimens. J Clin Invest 52:592–598, 1973.
13. Durack, D.T., Pelletier, L.L. and Petersdorf, R.G.: Chemotherapy of experimental streptococcal endocarditis. II. Synergism between penicillin and streptomycin against penicillin sensitive streptococci. J Clin Invest 53:829–833, 1974.
14. Pelletier, L.L. Jr. and Petersdorf, R.G.: Chemotherapy of experimental streptococcal endocarditis. V. Effect of duration of infection and retained intracardiac catheter on response to treatment. J Lab Clin Med 87:692–702, 1976.

15. Hook, E.W. III and Sande, M.A.: Role of the vegetation in experimental *Streptococcus viridans* endocarditis. Infect Immun 10:1433–1438, 1974.
16. Thompson, J., Fulderink, F., Lemkes, H. and Furth, R.: Effect of warfarin on the induction and course of experimental endocarditis. Infect Immun 14:1284–1289, 1976.
17. Carrizosa, J., Kobasa, W.D. and Kaye, D.: Antagonism between chloramphenicol and penicillin in streptococcal endocarditis in rabbits. J Lab Clin Med 85:307–311, 1975.
18. Kaye, D., McCormack, R.C. and Hook, E.W.: Bacterial endocarditis: The changing pattern since the introduction of penicillin therapy In Antimicrobial Agents and Chemotherapy-- 1961. Maxwell Finland and George M. Savage (eds), American Society for Microbiology, Detroit, Mich., p. 37.
19. Wolfe, J.C. and Johnson, W.D. Jr.: Penicillin-sensitive streptococcal endocarditis. In-vitro and clinical observations on penicillin-streptomycin therapy. Ann Intern Med 81:178–181, 1974.
20. Horne, D. and Tomasz, A.: Lethal effect of a heterologous murein hydorlase on penicillin-treated *Streptococcus sanguis.* Antimicrob. Agents Chemother. 17:235–246, 1980.
21. Pulliam, L., Inokuchi, S., Hadley, W.K. and Mills, J.: Penicillin tolerance of viridans streptococci delays sterilization of vegetations in experimental endocarditis. Clin. Res. 28:45A, 1980.
22. Goldman, P.L. and Petersdorf, R.G.: Significance of methicillin tolerance in experimental staphylococcal endocarditis. Antimicrob Ag Chemother 15:802–806, 1979.
23. Carrizosa, J., Trestman, I.J. and Levison, M.E.: Minimal concentrations of gentamicin for synergy with penicillin in enterococcal endocarditis. Clin Res 27:341A, 1979.

Adolf W. Karchmer, M.D.

3

ISSUES IN THE TREATMENT OF ENDOCARDITIS CAUSED BY VIRIDANS STREPTOCOCCI

The vegetation in endocarditis serves as a protected environment wherein microorganisms are sheltered from the phagocytic cells and humoral defenses of the host. In part at least, as a consequence of the shielding of microorganisms from the defense mechanisms of the host, therapy with bacteriostatic antibiotics rarely sterilizes these vegetations and has been associated with high relapse rates and persistent infection. Effective therapy requires a bactericidal agent that can penetrate the vegetation. Penicillin and the related beta-lactam antibiotics are bactericidal, and their use has been associated with a low incidence of adverse side effects. Given these facts and the antibiotic susceptibility patterns of the bacteria which commonly cause endocarditis, the penicillins and cephalosporins have become the major agents used in the treatment of these infections. Although the optimal antibiotic regimen for endocarditis caused by penicillin-susceptible streptococci remains controversial, there is general agreement that penicillin or a bactericidal penicillin substitute is the antibiotic of choice.

While penicillin is the drug of choice for the treatment of endocarditis due to penicillin-susceptible streptococci [minimum inhibitory concentration (MIC) $\leq$ 0.1 μg/ml], the studies of the Medical Research Council in Great Britain demonstrated that the daily penicillin dose and the duration of therapy were critical determinants of outcome. In this series of trials the rate of relapse decreased as the duration of therapy and the daily intramuscular dose of penicillin increased.[1] Among patients receiving 1,000,000 units daily for 5 days, 83 percent relapsed; in those receiving 500,000 units daily for 10 days, 50 percent were not cured; but in the group receiving 250,000 units daily for 20 days, only 22 percent were not cured. In another study, patients were treated for a month with daily intramuscular penicillin doses of either 100,000 units, 250,000 units or 500,000 units; infection was not eradicated in 41 percent, 16 percent and 7 percent, respectively. Of 71 patients treated with 500,000 units daily for 28 days in a third trial, 14 (20 percent) remained infected. Finally, there were no therapeutic failures among 18 patients who received 2,000,000 units daily for between four and six weeks. Subsequently, Hamburger and Stein noted clinical and bacteriological relapse in only 2 (17 percent) of 12 patients with streptococcal endocarditis who received 15 to 16 million units of penicillin daily by the intramuscluar or intravenous route for two weeks. The second episodes of endocarditis in these two patients were cured by repeating the initial therapy.[2]

The observation of *in vitro* synergism between penicillin and streptomycin against a strain of viridans streptococci[3] resulted in the use of these two antibiotics in combination for the treatment of endocarditis caused by penicillin-susceptible streptococci. Hunter and Paterson reported a 6 percent rate of clinical or bacteriologic relapse in a pooled series of 146 patients who were treated for 2 weeks with 2 to 12 million units of penicillin and 2g of dihydrostreptomycin daily.[4] Using a similar 2 week regimen of penicillin and dihydrostreptomycin, Tompsett, et al noted bacteriologic relapse in 4 (11 percent) of 36 patients with streptococcal endocarditis.[5] Recent studies noted that the enhanced rate of killing of streptococci in nutrient broth by penicillin-aminoglycoside combinations was correlated with the rate of eradicating these organisms from vegetations of rabbits with experimental endocarditis.[6,7] Wolfe and Johnson demonstrated with penicillin-streptomycin combinations had a synergistic effect on most strains of viridans streptococci isolated from patients with endocarditis.[8]

These clinical and laboratory observations have given rise to the three major antibiotic regimens currently recommended for the treatment of endocarditis caused by non-group A, penicillin-susceptible streptococci: High-dose, parenteral aqueous penicillin for 4 weeks; parenteral aqueous or procaine penicillin and streptomycin for 2 weeks; concomitant parenteral penicillin and streptomycin for 2 weeks followed by parenteral penicillin for an additional 2 weeks. No prospective randomized trial has been done with these three regimens to compare their clinical efficacy, relapse rates, and toxicity. As a result, optimal therapy remains controversial. This chapter will review the clinical experience with the four week parenteral antibiotic regimens and other selected issues in the antimicrobial therapy of streptococcal endocarditis. Clinical experience with the two week regimen is evaluated in chapter four.

Streptococci Causing Endocarditis

Streptococci remain the most frequent cause of non-addict related infective endocarditis involving native valves.[9] Streptococci, excluding the enterococci, *Streptococcus pneumoniae* and *S. pyogenes,* accounted for 51 percent of all cases of endocarditis which were treated at the Massachusetts General Hosptial between 1944 and 1968,[10] and 45 and 46 percent of cases treated during the years 1958 to 1964[11] and 1964 to 1973,[12] respectively. Among cases classified as subacute endocarditis, streptococci caused 66 percent of these treated during the 1944 to 1958 period,[10] 74 percent of cases between 1958 and 1964,[11] and 71 percent of those occurring between 1964 and 1973.[12] At the New York Hosptial viridans streptococci have also remained the predominant organism causing infective endocarditis, accounting for 73 percent of cases from 1932 to 1943, 70 percent from 1944 to 1960, and 50 percent from 1970 to 1978.[13] In addition, streptococci are prominent causes of prosthetic valve endocarditis occurring 60 days or more after cardiac valve surgery.[14,15]

Although frequently considered together as viridans streptococci, the non-group A, nonenterococcal streptococci causing endocarditis are heterogenous. Of 125 strains isolated from patients with endocarditis at the Massachusetts General Hospital between 1964 and 1977, 52 were nongroupable, 8 were not studied, and 5 were indeterminate; the remainder were distributed between 9 Lancefield groups with most belonging to group D (*S. bovis*) or group H (Table 1). Roberts and colleagues at the New York Hospital have shown this heterogeniety

Table 1. Lancefield Grouping of Non-Group A, Non-Enterococcal Streptococci Causing Endocarditis

Group	Number of Isolates
Non-groupable	52
B	7
C	1
D *(S. bovis)*	22
G	8
H	15
K	2
L	2
M	2
0	1
Not grouped	8
Indeterminate*	5

*Shared group reactivity

through the speciation of 112 of 122 viridans streptococci (excluding *S. pneumoniae*) causing endocarditis between 1970 and 1978.[13] They noted the following distribution of strains: *S. mitior* accounted for 31 percent of isolates a pyridoxal-dependent variant of *S. mitior*, 5 percent; *S. sanguis*, 24 percent; *S. mutans*, 7 percent; *S. milleri*, 4 percent; *S. salivarius*, 1 percent; and *S. bovis*, 27 percent. This distribution of species differed from that noted among 92 viridans strains isolated at this same hospital between 1944 and 1955. During the earlier period *S. sanguis* was isolated more frequently (44 percent) and *S. bovis* less frequently (5 percent). The change in the frequency of isolating *S. sanguis* and *S. bovis* may relate indirectly to a shift in recent years from rheumatic to degenerative and congenital (particularly calcified bicuspid aortic valves) valvular lesions as the substrate for streptococcal endocarditis and a resultant increase in the age of patients with endocarditis.[11,16] Recent reviews have noted that the mean age of patients with endocarditis due to *S. bovis* is greater than that of patients with endocarditis due to other streptococci.[13,16,17] The increased age of patients with *S. bovis* endocaridits may reflect the association of *S. bovis* bacteremia with occult lesions of the gastrointestinal tract, particularly lower gastrointestinal tract malignancy, i.e. lesions which are more likely to be found among older persons.[18]

Despite the variety of species and Lancefield groups, the non-group A, nonenterococcal streptococci isolated from patients with endocarditis are generally susceptible to penicillin (Table 2). The MICs of penicillin for these isolates are usually very low with only 4 to 20 percent of isolates from various series having MICs that exceed 0.lμg of penicillin/ml, an arbitrarily selected breakpoint beyond which organisms are considered relatively penicillin-resistant. The frequency of resistance to penicillin among viridans streptococci causing endocarditis has remained relatively stable over an extended time at the New York Hospital. The MIC of penicillin was greater than 0.lμg/ml for 17 percent of the 112 strains studied since 1970, compared to 18 percent for isolates from 1944 to 1951 and 20 percent for those from 1952 to 1960.[13] For occasional strains tested during the most recent period MICs of penicillin were between 0.8 and 3.2μg/ml. The frequency of relative penicillin resistance was greater among *S. mitior*, including pyrodoxal-dependent strains, and *S. bovis* than among other species of viridans streptococci.[13] The antibiotic susceptibility of species of viridans streptococci from patients with endocarditis and bacteremia was also studied at the Mayo Clinic.[26] While 75 to 100 percent of most of the species studied were inhibited by 0.06μg of penicillin/ml, *S. mitis (mitior)* were again more resistant. Only 42 percent of strains of *S. mitis* were inhibited by that concentration of penicillin and 0.5 to 4.0μg/ml were required to inhibit the remaining strains (Figure 1). Cephalothin and cefamandol were less active than penicillin against these strains. Although 51 of the 63 strains studied required $<$1μg of penicillin/ml for killing, five strains of *S. mitis* and two of *S. sanguis* type II required from 2 to $>$8μg of penicillin/ml for killing.[26]

Table 2. Penicillin Susceptibility of Nonenterococcal Streptococci Isolated from Patients with Endocarditis

Source	Strain (No.)	Year Isolated	Method	Inoculum	%MIC ≥0.1 μg/ml	MIC range (median) μg/ml	MBC range (median)
Geraci[19]	viridans (36)	1953—57	plate dilution	--	11	0.03—0.3 (0.06)	--
Blount[20]	viridans (34)	1952—64	tube dilution	10^5	15	0.001—3.9 (0.06)	0.001—15.6 (0.12)
Karchmer, et al[21]	viridans - nonenterococcal (78)	1964—77	tube dilution	10^5	5	<0.005—1.6 (0.02)	--
Roberts, et al[13]	viridans (79)	1944—51	tube dilution	--	18	0.016—2.0	--
	viridans (45)	1952—60			20	0.016—0.25	--
	viridans (112)	1970—78			17	< 0.006—2.0	--
Wilson, et al[22]	nonenterococcal non-Group A or B (91)*	1972—79	tube dilution		4	≤0.09—.19 (0.09)	--
Baker and Thornsberry[23]	S. mutans (34)	--	microtiter	5×10^3	0	≤0.08—0.63 (<0.08)	<0.08—< 5.0 (<0.08)
Watanakunakorn and Glozbecker[24]	viridans (20)	--	agar dilution	2×10^3	--	0.016—0.125 (0.06)	--
Hoppes and Lerner[25]	viridans (20)	--	tube dilution	10^4	--	<0.007—0.12	≤0.007—0.25

*MIC not determined for 14 strains

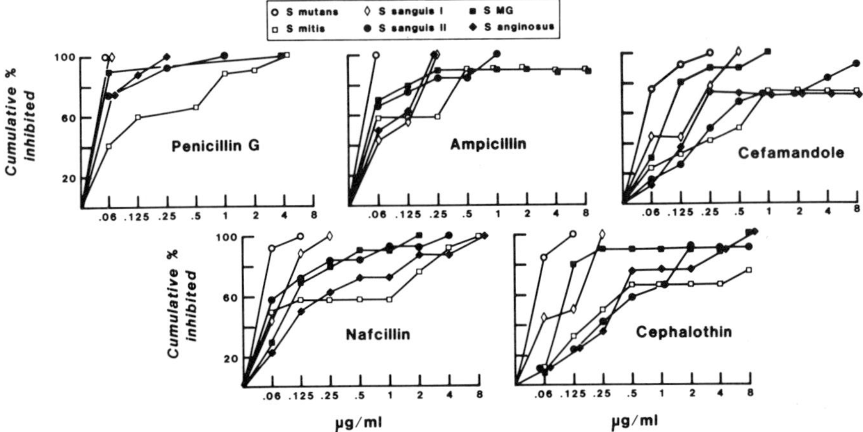

Figure 1: Cumulative percentage of species of viridans streptococci inhibited by five beta-lactam antibiotics. Twelve strains of *S. mutans*, 12 of *S. mitis*, 9 of *S. sanguis* type I, 12 of *S. sanguis*, type II, 10 of *S.* MG-*intermedius* and 8 of *S. anginosus-constellatus* were studied. Reprinted from Bourgault, A.M., Wilson, W.R., Washington, J.A., II. Antimicrobial Susceptibilities of Species of Viridans Streptococci. J. Inf. Disease *140*: 316, 1979 by permission of The University of Chicago Press. Copyright 1979 The University of Chicago Press 0022—1899/791/4003—0005$00.75.

The combination of a cell wall active antibiotic and an aminoglycoside is frequently synergistic against viridans streptococci. Wolfe and Johnson showed that the combination of penicillin and streptomycin had a synergistic effect on 47 of 48 strains of viridans streptococci which had been isolated from patients with endocarditis.[8] Although there was no significant correlation between the magnitude of the synergism demonstrated and the susceptibility of the organisms to either penicillin or streptomycin, all of the strains that were studied had MICs of <200µg of streptomycin/ml. Among enterococci, high level resistance to streptomycin (MIC >2000µ/ml) correlates with a lack of penicillin-streptomycin synergism.[27] High level streptomycin-resistance and its relationship to synergism has not been examined in viridans streptococci. The combination of cephalothin and streptomycin and vancomycin plus an aminoglycoside have also been shown to be synergistic against viridans streptococci and some strains of nonenterococcal group D streptococci.[8,28,29]

Treatment of Streptococcal Endocarditis: Massachusetts General Hospital

Between January 1964 and January 1977, 125 patients were treated for endocarditis caused by nonenterococcal streptococci. There were 99 patients treated with penicillin or a bactericidal penicllin substitute; these patients received no more than 3 days of concomitant aminoglycoside therapy.[21] Another 26 patients were treated with a combination of penicillin plus an aminoglycoside.[12] The aminoglycoside was given for 5 days or longer to these 26 patients. The MIC of penicillin was determined for 79 of the 125 strains causing endocarditis (Table 3). For 95 percent the MIC was 0.075μg of penicillin/ml or less, while all strains were inhibited by 0.63μg of penicillin/ml. There was no difference in the penicillin susceptibility of streptococci isolated from those cases treated with a single antibiotic compared with those treated by combination antibiotic therapy.

Table 3: Minimal Inhibitory Concentration of Penicillin* for Streptococcal Isolates From Endocarditis Patients, Massachusetts General Hospital, 1964—1977

Penicillin μg/ml	No. Inhibited	Cumulative Percent Inhibited
0.005	12	15
0.01	12	30
0.018	21	57
0.037	22	85
0.075	8	95
0.15	1	96
0.31	1	97
0.63	2	100

*Serial twofold tube dilution method[30] in dextrose phosphate broth, inoculum 10^5 organisms. For 17 strains, MIC was determined by agar dilution technique.[31]

Reprinted from Karchmer, A.W., Moellering, R.C., Jr., Maki, D.G., Swartz, M.N. Single Antibiotic Therapy for Streptococcal Endocarditis. JAMA 241:1801, 1979.

Although it is difficult to document precisely the onset of symptoms of endocarditis, the existence of untreated symptomatic endocarditis for greater than 3 months was related to the frequency of complications (new or worsening valvular dysfunction, congestive heart failure, and death). The duration of symptoms prior to therapy was recorded for 117 patients. Among 87 patients with symptoms for 3 months or less, 24 (28 percent) experienced complications as compared to 15 (50%) of 30 patients with symptoms for longer than 3 months ($p = .03$).

Single Antibiotic Therapy

Seventy-seven patients were treated with penicillin alone, two with cephalothin, two with vancomycin, and 18 with one or more of these agents in sequence. The patients ranged in age from 10 to 86 years (median, 54 years). During the treatment of endocarditis new or worsening murmurs of valvular regurgitation were noted in 16 patients and severe congestive heart failure developed in 25 patients. Prosthetic cardiac valves were inserted in 16 patients with severe congestive failure due to valve dysfunction. The frequency of valve destruction and congestive failure cannot be considered representative for single antibiotic therapy, however, because 16 of the patients with these complications were referred specifically for treatment of the complication.

Thirteen patients, 11 of whom were being treated with penicillin, died. Death was due to intractable congestive heart failure in 8 patients, major cerebrovascular accidents in two patients, and embolic myocardial infarction, pulmonary emboli and digitalis toxicity, each in one patient. In no case was death a direct result of uncontrolled infection in spite of therapy.

The antibiotic therapy of the 86 patients who survived enodcarditis is depicted in Figure 2. Among the 66 survivors who were treated primarily with penicillin, 48 received only intravenous (IV) aqueous penicillin. In addition to IV penicillin, seven patients were subsequently treated with procaine penicillin intramuscularly plus penicillin V orally. In another seven patients IV penicillin was followed by penicillin V, orally, and in four by erythromycin, orally. Those who received IV penicillin for 22 days or less were subsequently given penicillin intramuscularly and orally or orally. This non-intravenous therapy was administered for 14 days (except as noted in Figure 2). None of the survivors received parenteral penicillin for less than 24 days. The duration of IV antibiotic therapy among these 86 patients ranged from 7 to 60 days (mean, 30 days). Intravenous antibiotics were given to 60 of the survivors (70 percent) for 24 to 35 days and to 16 patients (19 percent) for 36 days or longer.

The daily dose of IV antibiotics varied. The 66 survivors treated with penicillin received daily IV dosages ranging from 8 to 30 million units. When used, procaine penicillin was given at a dose of 4 million units/day and penicillin V at 2 to 4 grams/day. Seventeen survivors received penicillin and/or penicillin substitutes sequentially. The dosages of penicillin given to these patients were similar to those noted above for patients treated primarily with penicillin. Cephalothin dosages were distributed almost equally between 8, 10, and 12g/day. Vancomycin was administered in daily dosages of 2g to 8 patients, 1.5g to three patients and lg to one patient.

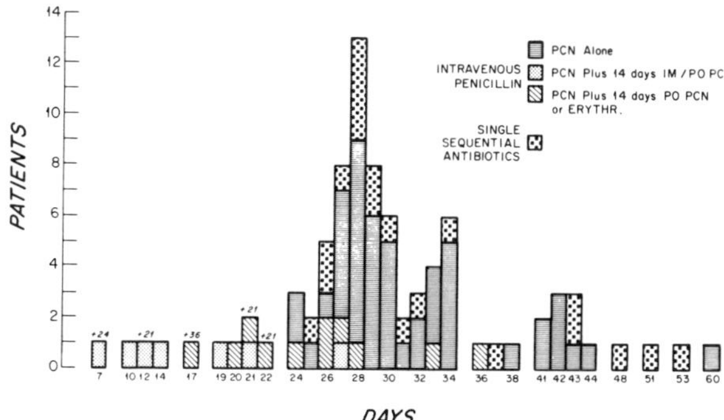

Figure 2: Duration of intravenous antimicrobial therapy for 86 survivors of streptococcal endocarditis. Numbers above bar (shaded or slashed) indicate total days of subsequent intramuscular and oral therapy received by that patient when total was greater than 14 days. Reprinted from Karchmer, A.W., Moellering, R.C., Jr., Maki, D.G., Swartz, M.N. Single Antibiotic Therapy for Streptococcal Endocarditis. J. Am. Med. Assoc. **241**:1801, 1979. Copyright 1979. American Medical Association.

To assess *in vivo* the efficacy of antibiotic therapy in 74 of the 99 patients, serum was collected at or near the expected nadir of the antibiotic concentration (trough) and was tested for bactericidal effect[38] against the causative organism of that patient's endocaridits (Table 4). The maximum serum dilution that remained bactericidal was at least 1:8 in 95 percent of these patients and was at least 1:128 and 54 percent. Serum from two patients receiving penicillin, 20 million units/day, remained bactericidal through a dilution of 1:16 when tested against streptococcal strains with MICs for penicillin of 0.16 and 0.63μg/ml.

Table 4: Serum Bactericidal Test in Seventy-four Patients*

Maximum Serum Dilution Which Is Bactericidal	Number Patients	Cumulative Percent
≥1:2048	6	11
1:1024	10	22
1:512	7	31
1:256	10	45
1:128	7	54
1:64	10	68
1:32	4	73
1:16	9	85
1:8	7	95
1:4	2	97
1:2	2	100

*Serum collected at or near expected nadir of antibiotic concentration

A second episode of endocarditis occurred among 6 (7 percent) of the 86 survivors (Table 5). In 4 patients (A,B,D, and E) the second episode was caused by a different streptococcus than that which caused the initial infection. In patient C the two infections were separated by 4 years. These 5 second episodes were reinfections rather than relapses. The strains of streptococci isolated from patient D were both group D streptococci; however, these strains differed from one another in a variety of morphologic and biochemical characteristics. Only patient F, with endocarditis symptomatic for 5 months prior to treatment, had a relapse. This occurred after treatment with IV penicillin, 20 million units daily for 7 days followed by vancomycin, 0.5g every 12 hours for 21 days. The MIC of penicillin for this strain was 0.08μg/ml initially and at the time of the relapse. Serum obtained 8 hours after vancomycin, 0.5g, was bactericidal at a 1:8 dilution. The second episode was successfully treated with cephalothin, 6 to 12g daily for 10 days followed by vancomycin, 2g daily for 27 days. Serum obtained 5 hours after vancomycin, 0.5g, was bactericidal at the 1:32 dilution.

Combination Antibiotic Therapy.

Among the 26 patients who received combination antibiotic therapy, 9 (35 percent) had new or worsening murmurs of valvular regurgitation and 7 (27 percent) had congestive heart failure. Prosthetic valve surgery was required by four patients (15 percent) during treatment of active endocarditis. Again, the frequency of these complications cannot be assumed to reflect their incidence during this mode of therapy, because the complications themselves had resulted in the referral to our hosptial of 4 of these patients. Four patients died. Death was due to complications following prosthetic valve surgery in three patients and to intractable congestive heart failure and a cerebral embolus in the fourth.

The duration of antibiotic therapy of the 22 patients who survived endocarditis is shown in Figure 3. Eighteen patients received intravenous penicillin throughout therapy; intravenous penicillin was followed by a parenteral cephalosporin in three and by vancomycin in one patient. Twenty patients received intravenous penicillin or a parenteral substitute for 25 days or longer. One patient received IV pencillin for 7 days followed by ampicillin, 6g/day orally, and probenecid; another received 21 days of IV penicillin followed by penicillin V, 4g/day orally. The daily dosage of penicillin ranged from 10 to 40 million units. Seventy-three percent of patients received 20 million units of penicillin or less per day. An aminoglycoside was given concomitantly with penicillin for periods ranging from 5 to 39 days. Combination therapy was given to 12 patients for eight days or less and to six for 20 to 39 days. Streptomycin was used predominantly; dailydosages were 1g in 11 patients, 1.5g in one, and 2g in three patients. Gentamicin, with dosages adjusted for renal function, was

Table 5: Recurrent Episodes of Streptococcal Endocarditis Among Survivors

Patient	Admission Date	Streptococcus Isolated	IV Therapy Antibiotic	Days	Outcome
A	10/11/66	Non-groupable	Penicillin	26	Cure
	10/02/69	group H	Penicillin	7***	Cure
B	4/10/68	group H	Penicillin	29	Cure
	2/27/73	Non-groupable	Cephalothin	29	Cure
C	6/18/70	Non-groupable	Penicillin	29	Cure
	6/20/74	Non-groupable	Vanco/Pen	25**	Cure
D	10/09/75	group D*	Ceph/Pen	26	Cure
	6/28/76	group D*	Vanco/Ceph	28	Died
E	8/06/76	Non-groupable	Penicillin	34	Cure
	1/19/77	group H	Penicillin	44	Cure
F	6/24/75	Indeterminate	Pen/Vanco	28	Relapse
	10/24/75	Indeterminate	Ceph/Vanco	37	Cure

* Different organisms by morphologic and biochemical characteristics
** 14 days supplemental intramuscular plus oral penicillin
*** 24 days supplemental intramuscular plus oral penicillin

IV = intravenous; Vanco = Vancomycin; Pen = Penicillin; Ceph = Cephalothin

Reprinted from Karchmer, A.W., Moellering, R.C., Jr., Maki, D.G., Swartz, M.N. Single Antibiotic Therapy for Streptococcal Endocarditis. JAMA 241:1801, 1979.

given to 7 patients. The 22 survivors were followed for at least one year or until death. Endocarditis did not relapse in these 22 patients.

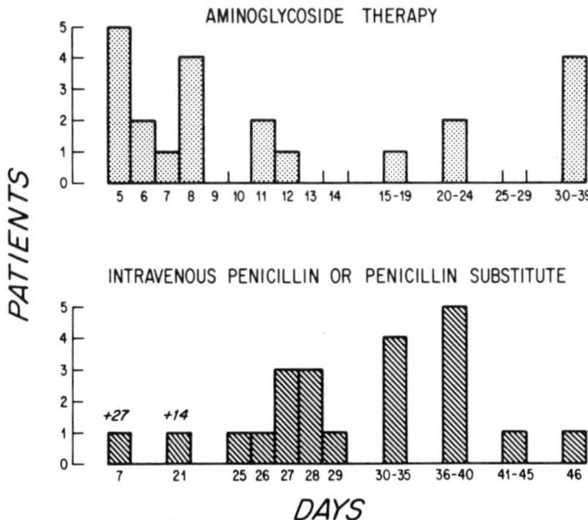

Figure 3: Duration of therapy with intravenous penicillin or a penicillin substitute and an aminoglycoside in 22 patients surviving streptococcal endocarditis. Numbers above bars indicate days of additional oral therapy with beta-lactam antibiotics (see text).

Additional Considerations Regarding Treatment

In the absence of randomized trials comparing the commonly recommended regimens for the treatment of endocarditis, decisions regarding therapy must be based upon the published retrospective experience with these regimens (Table 6). The problems of bias with retrospective studies are well known; furthermore, treatment programs reported from individual institutions are extremely heterogeneous and difficult to compare with those described elsewhere.

Many infectious disease specialists recommend four weeks of parenteral penicillin combined with streptomycin during the first two weeks as optimal therapy for endocarditis caused by penicillin-susceptible streptococci. This recommendation is based upon clinical experience as well as the observations of synergism between these two antibiotics *in vitro* and in animal models of endocarditis. Tompsett and Hurst treated 54 patients with 4 million units of penicillin daily for 4 weeks and streptomycin in a daily dose of 20 to 40mg/kg for the first 2 weeks; 4 patients (7 percent) died and there were no relapses among survivors.[37] Using a combination regimen (mean daily dose and duration: penicillin 11.4 million units for 30.4 days and streptomycin 1.2g for 13.4 days), Wolfe and Johnson described the successful treatment without relapse of 35 patients and commented that over 100 additional patients treated similarly had been cured without relapses.[38,8] Malacoff, et al using various combinations of penicillin and streptomycin, noted no relapses

Table 6. Outcome of Therapy for Endocarditis Caused by Penicillin Susceptible Streptococci

Source	Days Therapy	No. Treated	No. Deaths(%)	No. Relapses (%)
Penicillin or Penicillin substitute				
Lerner and Weinstein[33]	28	42	5 (12)	0
Hoppes, et al[34]	≥28	40	--	0
Karchmer, et al[21]*	≥28	99	13 (13)	1 (1)
Malacoff, et al[35]*	7–50	49	3 (6)	2 (4)
	≤ 21	9	--	2 (22)
	22–50	37	--	0
Phair and Tan[36]	11–17	13	--	2 (15)
	>21	8	--	1 (12)
Penicillin and Aminoglycoside**				
Tompsett and Hurst[37]	P,28: SM * *, 14	54	4 (7)	0
Wolfe and Johnson[8]	P,30: SM 13	35	--	0
Johnson, W.D., Jr.[38]	P,28: SM 14	>100	--	0
Phair and Tan[36]	P,11–17: SM≥11	39	--	0
	P,≥21: SM≥12	25	--	3 (12)
Malacoff, et al[35]	P,14–42: SM5–28	19	1 (5)	0
Wilson, et al[22]	P 14: SM 14	91	2 (2)	0
Karchmer, et al[12]	P 25–>46: SM5–>30	26	4 (15)	0

*Streptomycin given for ≤3 days to some patients
**Streptomycin, dihydrostreptomycin, or gentamicin
P = penicillin

among 18 patients.[35] Treatment with penicillin and an aminoglycoside at the Massachusetts General Hospital has yielded a 15 percent mortality rate and no relapses among the 22 patients who were cured. In a selected group of 91 patients treated for two weeks with the combination of procaine penicillin, 4.8 million units daily, and streptomycin lg daily, Wilson et al noted 2 deaths and no relapses.[22] In spite of these successes, treatment with penicillin and an aminoglycoside has not been entirely free of relapse. Phair and Tan noted three relapses (5 percent) among 64 patients receiving combination antibiotic therapy for endocarditis due to penicillin-susceptible streptococci.[36] Although one of these relapses followed somewhat abbreviated treatment (#1: penicillin G 2.4 to 3.6 million units/day plus streptomycin 1g/day for 12 days then penicillin V lg/day orally for 18 days), the other two relapses occurred after more prolonged treatment (#2: penicillin G 6 million units and streptomycin lg, daily for 18 days, then penicillin V 625mg every 4 hours orally for nine days; #3: procaine penicillin 3 to 4 million units/day for 30 days and streptomycin 1g/day for 21 days).

A 5 to 10 percent relapse rate has been attributed to treatment programs for streptococcal endocarditis which utilize parenteral penicillin for 4 weeks. In this regard, the experience of Lerner and Weinstein is often cited.[33] These authors, in fact, reported the treatment of 42 patients with nonenterococcal streptococcal endocarditis; five of their patients (12 percent) died but no survivors experienced a relapse. One patient who died was said to have uncontrolled infective endocarditis in spite of treatment with penicillin and streptomycin. Hoppes et al[34] noted no relapses among 40 patients treated with single antibiotic therapy for 28 days or longer. Similarly, at the Massachusetts General Hospital, we have noted only one relapse among 86 patients surviving endocarditis with single antibiotic therapy for 28 days or longer.[21] Malacoff et al reported 2 relapses among 46 surviving patients treated with a single antibiotic regimen.[35] Of particular note, however, was the occurrence of both relapses among 9 patients who received antibiotics for 15 to 21 days and none among 37 patients treated for 22 to 50 days. One relapse followed a relatively low-dose penicillin regimen, i.e. penicillin G 12 million units/day for 7 days followed by procaine penicillin 2.4 million units/day for 14 days. Phair and Tan observed 3 relapses among patients treated with penicillin for streptococcal endocarditis.[36] Again, however, 2 occurred after two week penicillin regimens and the third after relatively low dosage treatment, penicillin G 4 to 6 million units daily for 23 days. Notably all but one of the 6 relapses in these 193 cases followed less than 4 weeks of a single antibiotic therapy.[21,34–36]

Malacoff et al[35] and Phair and Tan[36] have suggested that duration of symptoms for longer than three months prior to treatment was a significant risk factor in the development of bacteriologic relapse. (See also chapter five of this volume.) Although there are inherent risks in combining data from recent reviews,[21,35,36] by doing this it is possible to examine the frequency of relapse following antibiotic treatment in relation to the duration of disease prior to therapy (Table 7). Among patients receiving single antibiotic therapy relapse was noted in 6 (15 percent) of 39 with symptoms in excess of 3 months compared with none of 106 with shorter duration disease ($p=<.001$). However, in the single antibiotic group the major risk of relapse was among those patients with longer duration disease who recieved therapy for 21 days or less. These patients experienced more frequent relapses than similarly treated patients with shorter duration disease ($p = .03$) and than patients with longer duration disease who were treated for more than 21 days ($p=.03$). Duration of disease did not clearly increase the risk of relapse in patients receiving single antibiotic therapy for more than 21 days. Although the frequency of relapse approaches significance ($p=.054$), one of the two relapses noted in this group was treated with a low dose of penicillin G (4 to 6 million units/d) for only 23 days. It does not seem justified to condemn the regimen as less effective for the treatment of endocarditis with symptoms for more than 3 months on the basis of relapse in this atypically treated patient. These data then suggest that single antibiotic

Table 7. Relationship of Relapse to Antibiotic Therapy and Duration of Endocarditis***

Duration of Therapy	Duration of Symptoms No. Relapses/No. Treated ≤3 Months	>3 Months	Total
Single antibiotic therapy*			
≤21 days+	0/12	‡4/10	4/22
>21 days++	0/94	2/29	2/123
	0/106	6/39	
Combined antibiotic therapy**			
≤21 days	0/35	0/9	0/44
>21 days @	1/46	2/13	3/59
	@1/81	2/22	

+p = .03

++p = .054

‡p = .03

@p = .12

*Parenteral penicillin or penicillin substitute with 3 or less days of an aminoglycoside
**Parenteral penicillin plus an aminoglycoside for >5 days
***From Malacoff, et al,[35] Karchmer, et al, [21] and Phair and Tan[36]

therapy for 21 days or less is not adequate for longer duration disease, that therapy for more than 21 days is effective for shorter duration disease and may be effective for longer duration streptococcal endocarditis, although the experience in the latter group is limited.

Treatment with both short and long combination antibiotic regimens appeared equally effective for endocarditis regardless of duration of symptoms. However, the numbers of patients treated with combined therapy were small and differences could have been missed. Even with the addition of Wilson's patients (treated for 2 weeks),[22] the differences in relapse rates are not significant: 1 among 152 short duration patients and 2 of 43 long duration patients relapsed (p=.11).

If the reports of single drug therapy for 21 days or more were combined, 2(1.2 percent) of 171 patients relapsed.[21,34,36] Among patients receiving penicillin for 4 weeks and an aminoglycoside for the initial 2 weeks, 3 (1.2 percent) of 250 patients relapsed.[8,12,35–38] All three relapses were reported by Phair and Tan.[36] One relapse might justifiably be excluded from consideration because low penicillin doses were used (penicillin V 1g/day for the last 18 days of treatment). The adjusted relapse rate (2/249,0.8%) remains similar to that for single drug therapy.

Several features of the successful experience with single antibiotic therapy of streptococcal endocarditis at the Massachusetts General Hospital were potentially important. Antibiotics were given in large doses at frequent intervals, and serum antibiotic concentrations were likely to have greatly exceeded those required for killing throughout the interval between doses. In 95 percent of our patients, serum which was obtained at the end of the interval between antibiotic doses was bactericidal at a dilution of 1:8 or greater. Given our bolus form of intravenous administration, the 1:8 level implied even greater bactericidal activity in serum at earlier times during this interval. In addition, careful attention was directed to duration of therapy. All of our patients received at least 24 days of parenteral antibiotics and 89 percent received intravenous therapy for 24 days or more.

The studies of penicillin dosage for streptococcal endocarditis in the rabbit model by Carrizosa and Kaye indicate that dose and duration of antibiotics are important.[39] The frequency of sterilizing vegetations was directly related to the dose of penicillin. Those doses providing peak median serum bactericidal dilutions of 1:16 or greater were most effective. However, the frequency of valve sterilization by moderately effective dosing schedules was increased when treatment was prolonged. Although the duration of bactericidal activity was not studied specifically, it was noted that the serum bactericidal activity at the trough time, while not universally present, was higher in those regimens which were more effective. Furthermore, for a given daily dose of penicillin, shortening the interval between doses reduced the bacterial titers in the infected vegetations. These observations suggest that, in addition to the importance of antibiotic dose and duration of therapy, the persistence of serum bactericidal activity between doses may be significant. Studies of experimental staphylococcal endocarditis by Scheld, VanNess, and Sande[40] demonstrated that persistant serum bactericidal titers of 1:2 or greater for at least 50 percent of the treatment interval correlate more closely with eradication of bacteria from vegetations than do peak serum bactericidal titers. In the light of these studies, generous penicillin doses for 28 days or more with trough serum bactericidal dilutions of 1:8 or greater may be the features which accounted for successful single antibiotic therapy in recent studies.

Several additional factors should be considered in a discussion of recommended antibiotic regimens for streptococcal endocarditis. Streptomycin ototoxicity, although a small risk, is significant. Among 91 patients treated with a 2 week penicillin-streptomycin regimen, Wilson noted mild vestibular toxicity in two elderly patients (78 and 82 years old), one of whom had renal insufficiency.[22] Wolfe and Johnson observed ataxia in 2 of 35 patients receiving penicillin-streptomycin therapy.[8] One patient (age 50) received streptomycin 13g in 13 days; the other patient (age 39) received 48g in 24 days. These reports and past experience with streptomycin indicate a significant risk of ototoxicity for those who are elderly or who have prior impairment of renal or vestibular function. Also, visual impairment limiting the ability to compensate for vestibular toxicity is an argument against streptomycin therapy. In addition, the pharmacokinetics of aminoglycosides are better understood now than when the combined antibiotic regimens for streptococcal endocarditis were originally formulated. Given the similar pharmacokinetics of streptomycin and amikacin,[41] a more appropriate streptomycin dose is 7.5mg/kg lean body weight, every twelve hours. Peak streptomycin serum concentrations should be maintained between 15 and 25μg/ml. Adjustments should be made for renal impairment by using nomograms designed for amikacin and measurements of serum streptomycin concentration.

The prior comparison of the recommended antibiotic regimens has considered toxicity and relapse rate. The clinical significance of the time required to sterilize an infected valve and difference in the rapidity of sterilizing vegetations with single versus combination therapy cannot be assessed. It is possible to speculate that more rapid sterilization of vegetations by combination therapy, as suggested by animal model studies, would reduce the risks of complications such as valve damage, congestive heart failure, and immune complex glomerulonephritis. However, data are not available to support this contention. Most authorities accept a 10–15 percent mortality rate for streptococcal endocarditis regardless of the antibiotic regimen.[42]

Other Issues of Antibiotic Therapy

Penicillin Hypersensitivity

Treatment of the patient with nonenterococcal streptococcal endocarditis who has severe penicillin hypersensitivity has required a choice between attempted desensitization (Chapter 14) and penicillin treatment, vancomycin, and treatment with a bacteriostatic agent such as erythromycin or clindamycin. The risks of allergic reactions during desensitization or subsequently during therapy with penicillin are significant.[36] Cephalosporins are effective agents for treating endocarditis due to viridans streptococci and have been used successfully in treating endocarditis in patients with penicillin allergy that is not an immediate type of hypersensitivity.[21,43] Their use in patients with immediate type hypersensitivity to penicillins is controversial because of potential cross-allergenicity; cephalosporins are avoided generally in this setting. Recent experience with bacteriostatic antibiotics in the treatment of streptococcal endocarditis is limited and therapy with these agents is not recommended.[42] Viridans and nonenterococcal group D streptococci are, in general, highly susceptible to vancomycin. For occasional strains, however, the MICs of vancomycin are relatively high, although still at concentrations easily achieved in serum with standard doses (Table 8).[23–25,48–51] Vancomycin used alone or as the predominant antibiotic

Table 8. Vancomycin Susceptibility of Viridans Streptococci Isolated from Patients with Endocarditis

Source	No. Strains	Inoculum	MIC µg/ml range (median)	MBC µg/ml range (median)
Watanakunakorn & Glotzbecker[24]	16	2×10^3	0.5 (0.5)+	--
Hoppes & Lerner[25]	16	10^4	0.39—1.56*	0.39—50
Baker & Thornsberry[23]	34	5×10^3	0.63—>5.0 (1.3)**	0.63—>5.0 (10.0)
Geraci, etal[40]	12	--	≤0.31—1.25 (0.625)*	≤0.31—>10.0 (2.5)
Harder, etal[41]	6	--	1.0—5.0 (5.0)+	--

+agar dilution   *tube dilution   **microtiter

has been effective in the treatment of 17 patients with streptococcal endocarditis (Table 9). Given a susceptible streptococcus, vancomycin is the antibiotic of choice for the treatment of streptococcal endocarditis in a patient with marked penicillin hypersensitivity.

Relative Penicillin-Resistance (MIC>0.lμg penicillin/ml).

Effective therapy for endocarditis caused by relatively penicillin-resistant, nonenterococcal streptococci may require more vigorous antibiotic therapy, including the use of synergistic antibiotic combinations. It is often recommended that these patients be treated with the very intensive penicillin-aminoglycoside combinations designed for enterococcal endocarditis.[42] However, it is important to recognize that these strains are usually not as resistant to penicillin as the enterococci. Furthermore, enterococci are typically highly resistant to the killing effect of penicillin, such resistance often extending beyond penicillin concentrations achieved clinically. In contrast, the relatively penicillin-resistant nonenterococcal strains do not usually exhibit large discrepancies between penicillin concentrations required for inhibition and killing. In fact, penicillin concentrations well in excess of those required to kill these viridans strains may often be obtained clinically.

The therapeutic dilemma posed by endocarditis due to relatively penicillin-resistant streptococci is illustrated by two patients described by Parrillo, et al.[52] While receiving oral penicillin prophylaxis, which has been associated with a high prevalence of penicillin-resistant bacteria in the gingival flora, these pateints acquired endocarditis due to relatively penicillin-resistant streptococci. In case #1 symptomatic endocarditis of 5 months duration was caused by *S. mitis* (MIC and MBC: 4μg of penicillin/ml). Initial treatment with penicillin G, 8 million units daily given intravenously for 3 weeks, was followed promptly by a relapse of endocarditis. Repeat treatment for 3 weeks using a similar dose of penicillin combined with streptomycin lg daily was unsuccessful. A third treatment, using penicillin G 36 million units and gentamicin 260mg daily for 6 weeks, eradicated the infection. The second patient had endocarditis due to *S. sanguis* (MIC and MBC: lμg penicillin/ml) and was successfully treated with a seven week regimen combining penicillin 24 million units and gentamicin 150mg daily. These two streptococci were studied for antibiotic synergism. Combinations of penicillin and streptomycin or gentamicin produced synergism against the *S. mitis* only when the concentration of penicillin was at or just below the MIC of the strain. Penicillin alone at concentrations equivalent to the MIC and higher was rapidly bactericidal and the addition of an aminoglycoside did not enhance killing. In studies with the *S. sanguis,* a concentration of penicillin in excess of the MIC was required before the addition of streptomycin or gentamicin resulted in synergism. At this concentration

Table 9. Vancomycin Therapy of Non-enterococcal Streptococcal Endocarditis

Streptococci Source	Strain	Vancomycin MIC/MBC μg/ml	Maximum serum bactericidal dilution (trough)	Vancomycin gram/d (days)	Other antibiotics Units or grams/d (days)	Outcome
Karchmer, et al[12]						
#66	viridans	0.5/0.5	1:8	2 (22)	++Eryth 3g (10)	Cured
#68	viridans	--	1:16	2 (29)	--	Cured
#71	Group H	0.5/0.5	1:8	1.5 (28)	--	Cured
#88	Non-enterococcal, D	--	--	2 (21)	++Ceph 8g (8)	Died-CHF
#111	indeter.	--	1:8	2 (21)	+Pen 15MU (7)	Cured
#119	indeter.	--	1:8	1 (21)	+Pen 20MU (7)	Relapsed
#120	indeter.	--	1:32	2 (27)	+Ceph 6–12g (10)	Cured
PVE–78	viridans	--	--	2–1.2 (42)	+Pen 24MU (9)	Cured
PVE–44	Group M	0.25/0.25	--	1.5–1.0 (30)	++Eryth lg (17)	Cured
Friedberg, et al[48]						
	viridans	--	--	3 (7) +2 (21)	--	Cured
	viridans	<5/–	--	2 (20)	+Pen 20MU + Strep 2 (8)	Cured
Cook, et al[49]						
	S. bovis	0.1/0.1	1:64	2 (28)	*Strep (14)	Cured
	viridans	0.4/0.4	1:8	2 (42)	*Genta 240mg (24)	Cured
	Group B	0.15/0.3	1:32	2 (24)	+Pen 4MU+Strep (5) +Clinda 2.4g (15)	Cured
Hoppes, et al[34]						
	viridans	--	--	2g (42)	--	Cured
Hoppes, et al[25]						
	S. bovis	--	--	1 or 2 (19)	+Linco 4g (5) ++Clinda 0.9g (14)	Cured
Kirby, et al[50]						
	viridans	--	--	— (14)	--	Cured
Hook & Johnson[51]						
	viridans	1.6/1.6	--	2 (14)	*Cephalothin (28) *Strep (28)	
	viridans	1.6/1.6	--	2.(21) and 1.4 (7)	--	Cured

Genta = gentamicin, Eryth = erythromycin, Linco = lincomycin, Strep = streptomycin, Clinda = clindamycin, Pen = penicillin G, Ceph = cephalothin, PVE = prosthetic valve

*Given concomitantly with vancomycin

+Given before vancomycin

Indeter. = indeterminate

++Given after vancomycin

penicillin alone was also highly bactericidal. As noted by the authors, given the high doses of penicillin used in treating these patients, it was difficult to know whether the addition of gentamicin played an important role in therapy. Although both patients were cured by intensive combination antibiotic therapy, neither was treated with high dose penicillin alone. In view of the *in vitro* bactericidal effect of high concentrations of penicillin, high-dose penicillin therapy alone might have been effective, in spite of the relapse following a lower penicillin dose for 21 days in case #1.

Antibiotic regimens recommended for endocarditis due to penicillin-susceptible streptococci (MIC $<0.1\mu g/ml$) have been used to treat patients with infection due to relatively penicillin-resistant strains (Table 10). Although this experience has not been large, it demonstrated the successful treatment of endocarditis due to these relatively penicillin-resistant strains with therapy that was less intensive than that recommended for enterococcal endocarditis. It is important to spare patients the risk of ototoxicity and nephrotoxicity associated with aminoglycoside therapy as given for enterococcal endocarditis whenever feasible. Optimum therapy of these patients requires further study.

The inhibition of growth of viridans streptococci by penicillin and other cell wall active antibiotics without lysis or major loss of viability, i.e. antibiotic tolerance, has been reported.[53,54] With the exception of the enterococci, the frequency and clinical significance of this observation is unknown. Goldman and Petersdorf found that methicillin had the same activity against experimental endocarditis caused by tolerant and non-tolerant strains of *Staphylococcus aureus*.[55] Gopal, et al, however, reported a case of endocarditis due to a strain of *S. aureus* with antibiotic susceptibility features suggesting tolerance.[56] Antibiotic therapy was not effective in this patient until gentamicin was added to the treatment with methicillin and vancomyicn. Savitch, et al have reported two patients with infective endocarditis caused by *S. bovis* strains which were relatively resistant to the *in vitro* killing effect of cell wall active antibiotics (penicillin, cefazolin, and vancomycin).[57] The clinical course described for these two patients, however, did not clearly demonstrate that the organisms were tolerant to the killing effect of cefazolin and penicillin. It is important to note that the minimum bactericidal concentration (MBC) of an antibiotic is very dependent upon definition of the end-point and methodology. The clinical significance of antibiotic tolerance awaits a more precise and method-independent definition as well as clinical experience. In the interim, given the possibility of penicillin-resistant viridans and nonenterococcal streptococci, all strains causing endocarditis should be tested by dilution techniques and, where necessary, adjustments in therapy be made based upon clinical response, *in vitro* antibiotic inhibition and killing, and serum bactericidal activity.

Table 10 Antibiotic Treatment of Endocarditis Caused by Streptococci with Relative Penicillin Resistance (MIC $>$ 0.1 μg/ml)

Source	MIC of Penicillin μg/ml	Treatment Antibiotic, daily dose (days)	Total days Treatment	Outcome
Tompsett, et al[5]				
Case 2St.	0.19	Pen 2.4MU+SM 2g (14)	14	Cured
Case 6Fa.	0.25	Pen 6MU+SM 2g (16)	16	Cured
Case 17Ha.	0.25	Pen 6 MU+SM 2g (14)	14	Cured
Hoppes, et al[34]				
	0.2	Pen 20MU (28)+SM 1.5g (10)	28	Cured
	0.25	Pen 12—16MU (30)+20MU (7)	30	Cured
	0.2	Pen 20MU (42) +SM 1g (7)	42	Cured
	0.2	Pen 8MU (30)	30	Cured
	0.4	Pen 20MU (42) +SM 1.5g 14/lg (7)	42	Cured
Wilson, et al[22]				
4 cases	0.19	Procaine Pen 4.8MU+SM lg (14)	14	Cured
2 cases	0.78	Procaine Pen 4.8MU+SM lg (14)	14	Cured
Karchmer, et al[12]				
Case 31	0.63	Pen 20MU (6)+Ceph 10g (13) + Vanco 2g (9)	28	Cured
Case 46	0.19	Amp 6g(9)+Pen 20MU(24)	33	Cured
Case 57	0.31	Oxa 10g+Genta (3)+Pen 12MU (31)	34	Cured

*Pen = penicillin; SM = streptomycin or dihydrostreptomycin
Amp = ampicillin; Ceph = cephalothin; Oxa = oxacillin;
Genta = gentamicin; MU = million units

Endocarditis Due to Nonenterococcal Group D Strains.

The group D streptococci include not only the enterococci *(S. faecalis, S. faecium,* and *S. durans*) but also the nonenterococcal species *S. equinus* and *S. bovis..* The latter organism, a common cause of endocarditis, may be confused with enterococci by clinical laboratories which rely on growth in bile-esculin media or serologic grouping as the sole methods of identifying group D streptococci. These tests do not differentiate *S. bovis* from the enterococci. The distinction can be made, however, by growth in 6.5 percent salt broth, starch hydrolysis and arginine hydrolysis. In addition, the antibiotic susceptibility patterns of the enterococci and nonenterococcal group D streptococci can be useful in tentatively distinguishing these species. *S. bovis* is usually susceptible by standard disc tests to both methicillin and clindamycin; enterococci, in contrast, are usually resistant to these two antibiotics.[47] Strains of *S. bovis* are susceptible to penicillin *in vitro* and have an antibiotic susceptibility profile similar to viridans streptococci rather than enterococci[25,47,58] (Table 11). Patients with endocarditis caused by *S. bovis* can be treated with the antibiotic regimens formulated for penicillin-susceptible streptococcal endocarditis; the potentially more toxic combination regimens used to treat enterococcal endocarditis are not required.[21,22,25,47,58]

Therapeutic Recommendations of the American Heart Association.

The data presented in this chapter, and in other chapters of this volume, have recently been reviewed in detail by an *ad hoc* subcommittee of the American Heart Association (AHA) Committee on Rheumatic Fever and Bacterial Endocarditis. The subcommittee's report, outlining specific regimens currently recommended by the AHA for treatment of endocarditis due to viridans streptococci, is contained in Appendix II of this volume.

SUMMARY

Streptococci excluding enterococci, *S. pneumoniae,* and *S. pyogenes* remain the most common cause of infective endocarditis, particularly of endocarditis which is subacute in its presentation. While often "lumped" together as viridans streptococci, these are heterogenous strains belonging to multiple species and Lancefield groups. A common feature of these streptococci, however, is marked susceptibility to penicillin. More than 85 percent of strains are susceptible to 0.1μg of penicillin/ml, with only rare isolates having significant penicillin resistance.

Although penicillin is the drug of choice for treating nonenterococcal streptococcal endocarditis, clinical and laboratory experience indicate that the dose of penicillin and duration of therapy are important determinants

Table 11. Antibiotic Susceptibility of *Streptococcus Bovis* Strains Isolated from Patients with Endocarditis

Source	No. Strains	MIC μg/ml range (median)	% MIC >0.1 μg/ml	MBC μg/ml range (median)
Penicillin				
Thornsberry, et al[46]	72	≤0.04–1.25 (≤0.04)**	3	≤0.08–5 (≤0.08)
Hoppes & Lerner[25]	13	0.015–0.12*		0.03–0.12
Watanakunakorn & Glotzbecker[24]	10	0.03–0.06(0.046)+	—	--
Moellering, et al[47]	13	0.01–0.12(0.06)*		0.03–62.0)0.06)
Cephalothin				
Thornsberry, et al[46]	74	≤0.04–>5.0(0.31)**	63	0.16–>5.0(1.3)
Hoppes & Lerner[25]	13	0.1–0.78*		0.2–0.78
Watanakunakorn & Glotzbecker[24]	10	0.125 (0.125)+	—	--
Vancomycin				
Thornsberry, et al[46]	74	0.31–>5.0(0.63)**	—	0.63–>5.0 (>5.0)
Hoppes & Lerner[25]	13	0.39–1.56*	—	0.39–12.5
Watanakunakorn & Glotzbecker[24]	10	0.25–0.5(0.5)+	—	--

*tube dilution **microtiter +agar dilution

of outcome. The recognition of synergism between penicillin and aminoglycosides against nonenterococcal streptococci has influenced the way in which endocarditis is treated. Clinical experience at several centers has indicated that treatment of streptococcal endocarditis with high dosages of penicillin parenterally for 4 weeks or with parenteral penicillin for 4 weeks and concomitant streptomycin during the first two weeks is extremely effective. Survival rates approached 85 to 90 percent with death due to cardiovascualr complications rather than uncontrolled infection. Relapse was noted in only one percent of surviving patients. Recent experience has suggested that a two week regimen combining procaine penicillin and streptomycin may be equally effective. The potential for aminoglycoside ototoxicity and nephrotoxicity, especially the increased risks of these in the elderly and those with prior renal or vestibular disease, must be considered before regimens employing aminoglycosides are begun.

While the treatment of endocarditis is highly successful, many important gaps remain in our understanding of antibiotic therapy for this infection. The optimal treatment of endocarditis caused by relatively penicillin-resistant strains of streptococci is not known. Although regimens designed for enterococcal endocarditis are frequently recommended in this setting, the data suggest that they may not be required. In addition, the clinical significance of antibiotic tolerant streptococci is also unknown. Clarification of the relationship between the magnitude and duration of antibiotic bactericidal activity and the eradication of bacteria from vegetations will allow more precisely designed therapeutic programs. Furthermore, knowledge of the effect of the rate of sterilizing vegetations upon the prevention of complications and morbidity due to endocarditis could profoundly alter our concepts of treatment. It is incumbent upon us to continue the careful study of patients with endocarditis, the infecting streptococcus, and the response to therapy. This coupled with the creative use of the rabbit endocarditis model should provide new insights into the treatment of this challenging disease.

REFERENCES

1. Cates, J.E., and Christie, R.V.: Subacute bacterial endocarditis. Quart. J. Med. 20:93, 1950.
2. Hamburger, M., and Stein, L.: *Streptococcus viridans* subacute bacterial endocarditis. JAMA 149:542, 1952.
3. Hunter, T.H.: Treatment of some bacterial infections of heart and pericardium. Bull. N.Y. Acad. Med. 28:213, 1952.
4. Hunter, R.H., and Paterson, P.Y.: Bacterial endocarditis. DM 1:1–48, 1956.

5. Tompsett, R., Robbins, W.C., and Berntsen, C., Jr.: Short-term penicillin and dihydrostreptomycin therapy of streptococcal endocarditis. Am. J. Med. 24:57, 1958.
6. Durack, D.T., Pelletier, L.L., Petersdorf, R.G.: Chemotherapy of experimental streptococcal endocarditis: II. Synergism between penicillin and streptomycin against penicillin-sensitive streptococci. J. Clin. Invest. 53:829, 1974.
7. Sande, M.A., and Irvin, R.G.: Penicillin-aminoglycoside synergy in experimental *Streptococcus viridans* endocarditis. J. Inf. Dis. 129:572, 1974.
8. Wolfe, J.C., and Johnson, W.D., Jr.: Penicillin-sensitive streptococcal endocarditis: *In-vitro* and clinical observations on penicillin-streptomycin therapy. Ann. Int. Med. 81:178, 1974.
9. Durack, D.T. and Petersdorf, R.G.: "Changes in the epidemiology of endocarditis," *In:* E.L. Kaplan and A.V. Taranta, editors, Infective Endocarditis--An American Heart Association Symposium, American Heart Association, Dallas, 1977, p 3.
10. Morgan, W.L. and Bland, E.F.: Bacterial endocarditis in antibiotic era. Circulation 19:753, 1959.
11. Uwaydah, M.M., and Weinberg, A.N.: Bacterial endocarditis--A changing pattern. New Engl. J. Med. 273:1231, 1965.
12. Karchmer, A.W., Moellering, R.C., Jr., Maki, D.G., Swartz, M.N.: unpublished data.
13. Roberts, R.B., Krieger, A.G., Schiller, N.L., and Gross, K.C.: Viridans streptococcal endocarditis: The role of various species, including pyridoxal-dependent streptococci. Rev. Inf. Dis. 1:955, 1979.
14. Karchmer, A.W., Dismukes, W.E., Buckley, M.J., Austen, W.G.: Late prosthetic valve endocarditis: clinical features influencing therapy. Am. J. Med. 64:199, 1978.
15. Watanakunakorn, C: Prosthetic valve infective endocarditis. Prog. Cardiovasc. Dis. 22:181, 1979.
16. Garvey, G.J., and New, H.C.: Infective endocarditis--an evolving disease: A review of endocarditis at the Columbia-Presbyterian Medical Center, 1968–1973. Medicine 57:105, 1978.
17. Wannamaker, L.W., and Parker, M.T.: "Microbiology of bacteria often responsible for infective endocarditis," *In*: E.L. Kaplan and A.V. Taranta, editors, Infective endocarditis--An American Heart Association Symposium, American Heart Association, Dallas, 1977, p 9.
18. Klein, R.S., Catalano, M.T., Edberg, S.C., et al: *Streptococcus bovis* septicemia and carcinoma of the colon. Ann. Int. Med. 91:560, 1979.
19. Geraci, J.E.: The antibiotic therapy of bacterial endocarditis. Med. Clin. N. Am. 42:1101, 1958.

20. Bount, J.G.: Bacterial endocarditis. Am. J. Med. 38:909, 1965.
21. Karchmer, A.W., Moellering, R.C., Jr., Maki, D.G., and Swartz, M.N.: Single antibiotic therapy for streptococcal endocarditis. JAMA 241:1801, 1979.
22. Wilson, W.R., Thompson, R.L. Wilkowske, C.J. et al: Short-term therapy for streptococcal infective endocarditis: combined intramuscluar administration of penicillin and streptomycin. JAMA 245:360–363, 1981.
23. Baker, C.N., and Thornsberry, C.: Antimicrobial susceptibility of *Streptococcus mutans* isolated from patients with endocarditis. Antimicrob. Ag. Chemoth. 5:268, 1974.
24. Watanakunakorn, C., and Glotzbecker, C.: Synergism with aminoglycosides of penicillin, ampicillin, and vancomycin against nonenterococcal group D streptococci and viridans streptococci. J. Med. Microbiol. 10:133, 1977.
25. Hoppes, W.L., and Lerner, P.I.: Nonenterococcal group D streptococcal endocarditis caused by *Streptococcus bovis.* Ann. Int. Med. 81:588, 1974.
26. Bourgault, A.M., Wilson, W.R., and Washington, J.A., II: Antimicrobial susceptibilities of species of viridans streptococci. J. Inf. Dis. 140:316, 1979.
27. Moellering, R.C., Jr., Wennersten, C., Medrek, T., Weinberg, A.N.: Prevalence of high level resistance to aminoglycosides in clinical isolates of enterococci. Antimicrob. Ag. Chemoth. - 1970. G.L. Hobby, editor. American Society for Microbiology, Bethesda, 1971, p 35.
28. Herrell, W.E., Balows, A., Becker, J.: Bactericidal effect of the combination of cephalothin and streptomycin against viridans group stretococci. Antimicrob. Ag. Chemoth., J. Sylvester editor, American Society for Microbiology, 1964, p 350.
29. Wilkowske, C.J., Facklam, R.R., Washington, J.A., II, Geraci, J.E.: Antibiotic synergism: enhanced susceptibility of group D streptococci to certain antibiotic combinations. Antimicrob. Ag. Chemother., G.L. Hobby, editor, American Society for Microbiology, 1970, p 195.
30. Anderson, T.G.: Testing of susceptibility to antimicrobial agents in body fluids, *In*: J.E. Blair, E.H. Lennette, J.P. Truant editors. Manual of Clinical Microbiology. American Society for Microbiology, Bethesda, 1970, Chapter 37.
31. Karchmer, A.W., Moellering, R.C., Jr., Watson, B.K.: Susceptibility of various serogroups of streptococci to clindamycin and lincomycin. Antimicrob. Ag. Chemoth. 7:164, 1975.
32. Schlicter, J.G., MacLean, H., Milzer, A.: Effective penicillin therapy in subacute bacterial endocarditis and other chronic infections. Am. J. Med. Sci. 217S:600, 1949.

33. Lerner, P.I., and Weinstein, L.: Infective endocarditis in the antibiotic era. N. Engl. J. Med. 247:199, 1966.
34. Hoppes, W.L., Smith, J.W., Lerner, P.I., White, A.: Treatment of penicillin-sensitive streptococcal endocarditis. Abstract #239. 17th Interscience Conference on Antimicrobial Agents and Chemotherapy, New York, October, 1977.
35. Malacoff, R.F., Frank, E., Andriole, V.T. Streptococcal endocarditis (nonenterococcal, non-group A): Single vs. combination therapy. JAMA 241:1807, 1979.
36. Phair, J.P., and Tan, J.S.: "Therapy of *Streptococcus viridians* endocarditis," *In*: E.L. Laplan and A.V. Taranta, editors, Infective Indocarditis--An American Heart Association Symposium, American Heart Association, Dallas, 1977, p 55.
37. Tompsett, R., and Hurst, M.L. Bacterial endocarditis: selected aspects of treatment. Clin. Climat. Assoc. 95:95, 1971.
38. Johnson, W.D., Jr.: Unpublished data.
39. Carrizosa, J., and Kaye, D.: Antibiotic concentrations in serum, serum bactericidal activity, and results of therapy of streptococcal endocarditis in rabbits. Antimicrob. Ag. Chemoth. 12:479, 1977.
40. Scheld, M.A., VanNess, M.M., Sande, M.A.: "Therapy of experimental *Staphylococcus aureus* endocarditis: relative importance of serum bactericidal activity," *In*: Current Chemotherapy and Infectious Disease, J.D. Nelson & C. Grossi, editors, American Society for Microbiology, Washington, 1980, p 309.
41. Barza, M., and Sciefe, R.T.: Antimicrobial spectrum, pharmacology and therapeutic use; IV aminoglycosides. Am. J. Hosp. Pharm. 34:723, 1977.
42. Hook, E.N., and Guerrant, R.L.: "Therapy of infective endocarditis," *In:* D. Kaye, editor, Infective Endocarditis, University Park Press, Baltimore, 1976, p 167.
43. Rahal J.J., Meyers B.R., Weinstein L., Treatment of bacterial endocaridits with cephalothin. New Engl. J. Med. 279:1305, 1968.
44. Geraci, J.E., Heilman, F.R., Nichols, D.R., et al: Some laboratory and clinical experiences with a new antibiotic vancomycin. Proc. Staff Mayo Clin. 31:564, 1956.
45. Harder, E.J., Wilkowske, C.J., Washington, J.A., II, Geraci, J.E.: *Streptococcus mutans* endocarditis. Ann. Int. Med. 80:364, 1974.
46. Thornsberry, C., Baker, C.N., Facklam, R.R.: Antibiotic susceptibility of *Streptococcus bovis* and other group D streptococci causing endocarditis. Antimicrob. Ag. Chemoth. 5:228, 1974.
47. Moellering, R.C., Jr., Watson, B.K., Kunz, L.J.: Endocarditis due to group D streptococci: comparison of disease caused by *Streptococcus bovis* with that produced by the enterococci. Am. J. Med. 57:239, 1974.

48. Friedberg, C.K., Rosen, K.M., Beinstock, P.A.: Vancomyicn therapy for enterococcal and *Streptococcus viridans* endocarditis. Arch. Int. Med. 122:134, 1968.
49. Cook, F.V., Coddington, C.C., Wadland, W.C., and Farrar, W.E., Jr.: Treatment of bacterial endocarditis with vancomycin. Am. J. Med. Sci. 276:153, 1978.
50. Kirby, W.M.M., Perry, D.M., Lane, J.L.: Present status of vancomycin therapy of staphylococcal and streptococcal infections. Antibiotics Annaul 1958–1959:580, 1959.
51. Hook, E.W., III, and Johnson, W.D., Jr.: Vancomycin therapy of bacterial endocaridits. Am. J. Med. 65:411, 1978.
52. Parrillo, J.R., Borst, G.C., Mazur, M.H., et al: Endocarditis due to resistant viridans streptococci during oral penicillin chemoprophylaxis. New Engl. J. Med. 300:296, 1979.
53. Horne, D., and Tomasz, A.: Tolerant response of *Streptococcus sanguis* to beta-lactams and other cell wall inhibitors. Antimicrob. Ag. Chemoth. 11:888, 1977.
54. Horne, D., and Tomasz, A.: Lethal effect of a heterologous murein hydrolase on penicillin-treated *Streptococcus sanguis.* Antimicrob. Ag. Chemoth. 17:235, 1980.
55. Goldman, P.L., and Petersdorf, R.G.: Significance of methicillin tolerance in experimental staphylococcal endocarditis. Antimicrob. Ag. Chemoth. 15:802, 1979.
56. Gopal, V., Bisno, A.L., Silberblatt, F.J.: Failure of vancomycin treatment in *Staphylococcus aureus* endocarditis. JAMA 236:1604, 1976.
57. Savitch, C.B., Barry, A.L., Hoeprich, P.D.: Infective endocarditis caused by *Streptococcus bovis* resistant to the lethal effects of penicillin G. Arch. Int. Med. 138:931, 1978.
58. Ravreby, N.D., Bottone, E.J., and Keusch, G.T.: Group D streptococcal bacteremia, with emphasis on the incidence and presentation of infections due to *Streptococcus bovis.* New Engl. J. Med 289:1400, 1974.

Walter R. Wilson, M.D.
Joseph E. Geraci, M.D.

4

ANTIMICROBIAL THERAPY FOR PENICILLIN-SENSITIVE STREPTOCOCCAL INFECTIVE ENDOCARDITIS: TWO-WEEK REGIMENS

Penicillin-susceptible streptococci are the most common cause of infective endocarditis (IE). The antimicrobial therapy of these infections is controversial. Intravenous penicillin administered alone for four weeks or in combination with streptomycin for the first two weeks has been considered conventional therapy.[1-8] The use of short-term (two weeks) combined penicillin and streptomycin therapy for IE caused by penicillin-susceptible streptococci was suggested more than 25 years ago,[1 3,9] but has not gained wide acceptance, probably because of the relatively high relapse rates reported in earlier studies and because of the risk of streptomycin-associated toxicity. If the two-week regimen were equivalent in therapeutic efficacy to four weeks of antimicrobial therapy without an increase in toxicity, substantial cost savings could result from reduced periods of hospitalization.

In this chapter, we will review previously published reports of the use of two-week regimens and describe our experience with 104 patients with penicillin-susceptible streptococcal IE treated for two weeks with intramuscular procaine penicillin and streptomycin. Sixty-eight of these patients were reported earlier.[10]

Previously Reported Studies of Two-Week Regimens for Penicillin-Susceptible Streptococcal Infective Endocarditis

At least 45 percent of all cases of IE are caused by penicillin-sensitive viridans streptococci and *Streptococcus bovis* (minimum inhibitory concentration penicillin $\leqslant$0.2 mgm/ml).[11–15] In early clinical trials, more than 50 percent of patients receiving 500,000 to 1,000,000 units of penicillin per day for less than two weeks were treatment failures.[16,17] Increase of the dosage of penicillin to 14 to 16 million units/day for 10 to 14 days was still associated with an unacceptably high relapse rate of 15 percent.[18]

Based on *in vitro* studies demonstrating synergy between penicillin and streptomycin against viridans streptococci, Hunter[9] originally suggested the use of short-term combined penicillin-streptomycin therapy for patients with IE caused by these microorganisms. In 1956 in a survey of the collected experience of 23 investigators, Hunter and Paterson[18] reported a relapse rate of 6 percent among 146 patients with penicillin-sensitive IE treated for approximately two weeks with variable doses of penicillin and streptomycin.

Recent studies have demonstrated conclusively that penicillin and streptomycin act synergistically *in vitro* against viridans streptococci.[19,20] That the combination of penicillin and streptomycin may be superior to penicillin alone is supported by data obtained from studies of experimental endocarditis in animals. Combined penicillin and streptomycin were more effective than penicillin alone in preventing experimental streptococcal endocarditis[20,21] and in treating established infections[22,23] (Chapters 17 and 2).

Table 1 summarizes the results of previously published studies of two-week combined penicillin-streptomycin therapy for penicillin-sensitive IE and includes experience with this regimen in 104 patients treated at Mayo Clinic. A combined total of 257 patients were reported in these studies with a relapse rate of 2 percent. Since the report of Tompsett and associates[24] in 1958, we were unable to find a single published case of relapse of penicillin-susceptible IE following treatment with combined penicillin-streptomycin administered for two weeks. These data suggest that the two-week regimen is at least as effective as four weeks of parenteral therapy for the majority of patients with penicillin-sensitive streptococcal IE. There is no readily apparent explanation for the descrepancy between the relapse rates encountered in earlier studies compared with recent reports utilizing two-week combined penicillin-streptomycin therapy. Dihydrostreptomycin was utilized in earlier studies, while streptomycin was administered to patients in our study and in the report by Tan, et al.[5] The dosages of penicillin were similar in early and current studies.

Table 1. Results of treatment of penicillin-susceptible streptococcal infective endocarditis for two weeks with combined penicillin-streptomycin* therapy.

Series, Date Published	Number of Patients	Penicillin Dosage and Route of Administration	Relapses %	Streptomycin Toxicity (%)	DEATHS			
					Heart Failure	Embolic	Other	Total %
Geraci and Martin 1953 (1) Geraci 1955 (2) Geraci 1958 (3)	82	1.2 — 2.4 M units parenterally or 4 — 9 M units orally (10 pts)	1(1)	3(4)	10	4	2	16(20)
Tompsett et al 1958 (25)	35	1.6 — 6 M units parenterally	4(11)	0	1	0	0	1(3)
Tan et al 1971 (5)	36	3.6 — 4.5 grams orally or 2.4 — 12 M units parenterally (9 pts)	0	0	2	0	0	2(6)
Wilson et al+	104	4.8 M units parenterally	0	2(2)	1	0	1	2(2)
TOTAL	257		5(2)	5(2)				21(8)

* All patients received streptomycin or dihydrostreptomycin or both 1—2 grams per day.

\+ Sixty-eight of these patients were reported previously (Wilson, W.R. et al: 18th Interscience Conference on Antimicrobial Agents and Chemotherapy, October 1—4, 1978. Abstract No. 268.)

Among these 257 patients the frequency of streptomycin-associated toxicity was low -- 2 percent. The overall mortality was 8 percent. However, the majority of deaths were reported in the earlier studies and most of these were associated with heart failure. The lower mortality reported in more recent studies probably reflects advances in techniques of cardiac valve replacement and in supportive care of seriously ill patients.

Mayo Clinic Experience with Two-Week Combined Penicillin-Streptomycin Therapy for Penicillin-Sensitive Infective Endocarditis

From January, 1972, through December, 1979, penicillin-susceptible streptococcal IE occurred in 153 patients. Of these, 104 patients (68 percent) were impaneled in our study. The remaining 49 patients (32 percent) were excluded from our protocol (Table 2). Of the 16 patients excluded because of treatment with other antimicrobials, 12 received other antimicrobial agents before the diagnosis of IE was made or before the patient could be enrolled in the protocol. The remaining four patients had suspected intracranial mycotic aneurysm or cerebritis and treatment was initiated with intravenous penicillin instead of intramuscular penicillin. Patients with shock and decreased peripheral perfusion were excluded from our protocol because of presumed reduced absorption of penicillin administered intramuscularly.

Antimicrobial therapy in the 104 patients included in our study was procaine penicillin G, 1.2 million units every six hours, and streptomycin, 500 mg every twelve hours given intramuscularly for fourteen days. The

Table 2. Patients Excluded From Study

Reason for exclusion	No. of patients
Treatment with other antibiotics	16
Allergy to penicillin	14
Prosthetic valve endocarditis	11
Shock with decreased peripheral perfusion	3
Thrombocytopenia	2
Nutritionally dependent streptococci	1
Self-dismissal against medical advice	1
Presence of carcinoma	1
Total	49

injections of procaine penicillin and streptomycin were administered simultaneously. Of the 104 patients, 67 (64 percent) were male and 37 (36 percent) were female. The mean age was 58.7 years (range 14 to 84) (Table 3).

Table 3. Age of Patients, by Decades

Decade	No. of patients
10–19	1
20–29	6
30–39	7
40–49	9
50–59	21
60–69	34
≥70	26
Total	104

The mitral valve alone was affected in 56 patients (54 percent), the aortic valve alone in 45 patients (43 percent), and 3 patients (3 percent) had infection involving multiple cardiac valves. Forty-three (96 percent) patients with aortic valve IE had murmurs of aortic insufficiency; all patients with mitral valve IE had murmurs of mitral incompetence.

Eighty-one patients (78 percent) had infections caused by viridans streptococci. *Streptococcus bovis* was isolated from 23 patients (22 percent). Fourteen of these 23 patients (61 percent) were identified as having colonic disease (Table 4).

Table 4. Colonic disease among 23 patients with *S. bovis* infection

Colonic disease	No. patients (%)*
Inflammatory bowel disease	5 (22)
Colonic polyps	3 (13)
Bleeding diverticula	3 (13)
Villous adenoma	2 (9)
Carcinoma of colon	1 (4)
Total	14 (61%)

*Percent of 23 patients with *S. bovis* infection

Symptoms of IE greater than 3 months in duration were present in 21 patients (20 percent). Fourteen of the 56 patients (25 percent) with mitral valve infections and 7 of the 45 patients (16 percent) with aortic valve disease had symptoms for longer than 3 months. Five of the 23 patients (22 percent) with *S. bovis* IE had symptoms for at least 3 months in duration.

Agar dilution minimum inhibitory concentration (MIC) values for penicillin were determined in all 104 isolates. In 100 cases (96 percent), MIC was 0.1 mcg/ml or less; in the remaining 4 cases, MIC was 0.5 mcg/ml in 3 and 0.2 mcg/ml in 1 case. Broth dilution MIC values for penicillin were 0.09 mcg/ml or less in 83 patients (80 percent), 0.19 mcg/ml in 4 (4 percent), 0.78 mcg/ml in 2 (2 percent), and indeterminate in 15 (14 percent). Broth dilution MIC could not be determined in these 15 patients because no bacterial growth occurred in the control tubes that did not contain penicillin.

Blood samples were obtained for determination of the peak serum bactericidal titer (SBT) one hour after the simultaneous administration of penicillin and streptomycin. SBT was 1:8 or more in 90 patients (87 percent) and 1:4 in 6 (6 percent). SBT was indeterminate in 8 patients (8 percent). In the 8 indeterminate cases, the isolate exhibited no growth in the control tubes that contain no penicillin. One of the cases with an SBT of 1:4 had a viridans streptococcal infection with an MIC of 0.78 mcg/ml and a minimum bactericidal concentration (MBC) of more than 100 mcg/ml. Another patient with an SBT of 1:4 had viridans streptococcal IE and MIC of 0.09 mcg/ml or less and an MBC of 12.5 mcg/ml. The remaining 4 patients with SBT of 1:4 had streptococci with MIC of 0.09 mcg/ml or less and MBC of 0.19 mcg/ml.

One patient had mitral valve infection caused by a nutritionally-dependent streptococcus.[25,26] Its MIC was 0.78 mcg/ml, MBC 1.56 mcg/ml. The SBT could not be determined with this microorganism.

Table 5. Class of functional heart failure and valve replacement

Class	No. patients (% of total pts.)	Valve replacement No. (% of pts. in functional class)
≤II	70 (67)	0
III	13 (13)	11 (85)
IV	21 (20)	21 (100)
Total	104	32

Table 5 lists patients catagorized according to functional class of heart failure according to the New York Heart Association criteria[27] present at the completion of antimicrobial therapy. Eleven of 13 (85 percent) with functional class III heart failure and all 21 patients with functional class IV heart failure underwent cardiac valve replacement. Twenty-one of these patients had aortic or multiple valve involvement. Eleven patients underwent mitral valve replacement. None of the 21 patients with aortic valve disease had sudden onset severe aortic incompetence. All patients had evidence of previous IE at the time of surgery. Gram's stained smears and cultures of the excised valves were negative in all cases.

Audiograms and tests of vestibular function were performed in all patients on at least two separate occasions. The majority of patients had

VIIIth cranial nerve function tests performed at the beginning of treatment, during, and at the completion of treatment. Two patients (2 percent) developed mild vestibular toxicity. One was a 78-year-old male with mild renal insufficiency; the other episode occurred in an 82-year-old female.

Two patients (2 percent) died. One of these died elsewhere three weeks after completing antimicrobial therapy for mitral valve viridans streptococcal IE. MIC was 0.09 mcg/ml or less, MBC 3.12 mcg/ml, and SBT 1:8. Because of functional class III heart failure, mitral valve replacement was suggested. The patient declined and returned home. Her heart failure worsened, she had a cardiac arrest and died. Antemortem blood cultures were reportedly negative. Postmortem examination performed elsewhere did not reveal evidence of active IE and postmortem cultures of the mitral valve were reportedly negative. The second death occurred in a 64-year-old male with aortic valve IE. MIC was 0.09 mcg/ml or less, MBC 0.19 mcg/ml, and SBT 1:64. Because of functional class IV heart failure, aortic valve replacement was performed two days after completion of antimicrobial therapy. The patient's immediate postoperative course was uncomplicated. Five days postoperatively the patient died unexpectedly from cardiac arrest presumably caused by dysrhythmia. No evidence of prosthetic valve endocarditis (PVE) or valve dehiscence was noted at postmortem examination. Cultures and Gram's stained smears of the prosthetic valve and surrounding tissue were negative.

Follow-up of the remaining 102 patients ranged from 2 years to 7 years and 3 months. Blood cultures were negative at 1- and 2-month intervals after completion of antimicrobial therapy in all 102 patients. None had clinical or laboratory signs of relapse of IE.

The mortality among the 49 patients excluded from our study was six times higher (12 percent) than that of the 104 patients included in our protocol (Table 6). Cerebral angiography was performed on four patients excluded who had clinical signs suggesting mycotic aneurysm. Three of these 4 had intracranial mycotic aneurysms and 2 of these 3 died from rupture of the aneurysm. The 3 patients with shock and decreased peripheral perfusion had sudden-onset, severe aortic insufficiency and 2 of these patients died of severe heart failure. The single death which occurred among patients with PVE was a 57-year-old male who died 11 days after aortic valve replacement from cardiac arrest caused by a dysrhythmia. Among the 31 other patients excluded, one patient died following completion of antimicrobial therapy from acute myocardial infarction and cardiac arrest. Postmortem cultures and Gram's stain of cardiac valve tissue were negative in all 6 cases. The 6 deaths were the result of vascular or hemodynamic consequences which may occur in patients with IE rather than failure of antimicrobial therapy to sterilize infected valve vegetations.

Table 6. Mortality among patients excluded

Condition	No. patients	No. deaths
Suspected mycotic aneurysm or cerebritis	4	2
Shock	3	2
Prosthetic valve endocarditis	11	1
Other	31	1
Total	49	6 (12%)

Among the 43 surviving patients excluded, adequate follow-up was available in 37. Two of these 37 patients relapsed; both patients had PVE treated for two weeks with intramuscular procaine penicillin and streptomycin and relapse occurred 11 and 22 days, respectively, after completion of antimicrobial therapy. Both patients were cured following retreatment with aqueous penicillin 20 million units/day administered intravenously for four weeks plus streptomycin 500 mg twice daily for the first two weeks of therapy. One other patient with prosthetic valve endocarditis was cured of infection with two weeks of combined intramuscular procaine penicillin and streptomycin therapy.

Additional Considerations Regarding Two-Week Regimens

The *in vitro* susceptibility data of penicillin-susceptible streptococci are difficult to interpret because this is a heterogeneous group of bacteria with varying growth characteristics and CO_2 requirements. *In vitro* susceptibility data may reflect interspecies differences and as yet incompletely studied intraspecies differences.[28] Only 5 of our 104 patients had infections caused by microorganisms with MIC greater than 0.2 mcg/ml. The significance of relative penicillin resistance among viridans streptococci is not clear. Some investigators believe that when MIC values for viridans streptococci exceed 0.2 mcg/ml, patients should receive antimicrobial therapy identical for that for enterococcal IE.[29] Parillo, et al.[30] described two patients with IE caused by relatively resistant streptococci (MIC's 1 and 4 mcg/ml, respectively). Both patients had received long-term oral penicillin prophylaxis for rheumatic fever. One patient relapsed after penicillin therapy alone or in combination with streptomycin. The other patient relapsed after prolonged penicillin therapy (supplemented with 14 days of doxycycline therapy). Both patients were cured with four weeks of combined penicillin-gentamicin therapy. We are unaware of data comparing cure rates in patients with IE caused by relatively penicillin-resistant streptococci. The number of patients reported previously and in our study with relatively penicillin-resistant streptococci is too small to permit one to conclude that these patients may be treated successfully with two weeks of combined penicillin-streptomycin therapy. Until more data are available, we suggest that patients with IE caused by streptococci with MIC greater than 0.2 mcg/ml be treated with high-dose penicillin administered intravenously for four weeks combined with streptomycin administered for the first two weeks of therapy. Wolfe and Johnson[8] encountered no relapses among 35 patients treated with this regimen and, in unpublished data, these authors cite in excess of 100 additional patients treated successfully without relapse. Tompsett and Hurst[7] encountered no relapses among 55 surviving patients treated with a regimen similar to that of Wolfe and Johnson.

Some authors suggest that patients who have had symptoms of IE longer than three months prior to initiation of therapy may be at high risk of relapse and that therapy should be prolonged in these patients[31] (Chapter 5). In the report by Phair and Tan,[32] however, more intensive or longer therapy did not result in a lower relapse rate among patients who had been ill for more than three months. Moreover, 4 of 5 patients in that report who had symptoms for more than three months whose infection relapsed were cured after antimicrobial retreatment for 17 days or less. Twenty percent of our 104 patients had symptoms of IE longer than three months in duration; none relapsed. Until more data are available, we suggest that patients with symptoms of IE for longer than three months prior to initiation of antimicrobial therapy be treated with the regimen described by Wolfe and Johnson above.

The low vestibular toxicity rate (2 percent) observed in our patients is similar to that reported by Tompsett and Hurst.[7] Vestibular toxicity is more likely to occur in the elderly, in association with renal failure, and in patients with preexisting vestibular dysfunction. These patients should be treated with high-dose penicillin G therapy alone administered intravenously for four weeks. In patients receiving streptomycin, we suggest that audiograms and caloric determinations be obtained prior to therapy and at least once during treatment or at the completion of treatment and that physical examination of patients be performed frequently during treatment. If signs of vestibular dysfunction develop, streptomycin should be discontinued and high-dose penicillin therapy should be administered intravenously.

The low mortality among our patients in part reflects patient selection for inclusion in our study. The high mortality observed in the patients excluded from study was likely related to deaths caused by vascular or hemodynamic complications of IE rather than to failure of antimicrobial therapy to sterilize cardiac valve vegetations. We suggest that patients with shock, cerebritis, or intracranial mycotic aneurysm be treated with intravenous penicillin with or without streptomycin. The relatively low serum and cerebrospinal fluid concentration achieved with intramuscular procaine penicillin may not be sufficient to treat these patients successfully.

One of the two deaths among our 104 patients resulted from severe worsening of preexisting functional class III heart failure. In patients with severe heart failure caused by IE, cardiac valve replacement should be considered (Chapter 13). Ninety-four percent of our patients with functional class III or IV heart failure required cardiac valve replacement. The operative risk of cardiac valve replacement in these patients is related not to the presence of IE but rather to the degree of heart failure present at the time of surgery, and patients with class IV heart failure have a significantly higher operative mortality risk than those with functional class II heart failure.[33]

Two week combined penicillin-streptomycin therapy should not be used to treat patients with PVE. We suggest that patients with PVE caused by penicillin-sensitive streptococci be treated with penicillin administered intravenously for four weeks combined with streptomycin for the first two weeks of therapy (Chapter 12).

Among patients allergic to penicillin, we have treated 11 patients successfully with combined clindamycin and streptomycin administered parenterally for two weeks. Five patients were treated for two weeks with vancomycin and streptomycin. None of these 16 patients relapsed. The number of penicillin-allergic patients treated with these two short-term regimens is too small to conclude that these regimens are effective alternatives to the use of conventional treatment with penicillin alone or in combination with streptomycin. We suggest that penicillin-allergic patients with penicillin-susceptible streptococcal IE be treated for four weeks with vancomycin or, alternatively, with a cephalosporin (provided that the isolate is susceptible *in vitro* to cephalosporins).

We do not have data on the use of two weeks of intravenous penicillin combined with streptomycin for the treatment of patients with penicillin-susceptible streptococcal IE. Presumably, the administration of penicillin intravenously in these patients would be equally effective as penicillin administered intramuscularly. In patients with a small muscle mass, thrombocytopenia or decreased peripheral perfusion, or those who complain of frequent intramuscular injections, we advise the use of 10 to 20 million units of penicillin per day administered intravenously combined with intramuscular streptomycin.

In conclusion, we believe that short-term combined therapy with intramuscular procaine penicillin and streptomycin is effective, safe therapy for the large majority of patients with penicillin-susceptible streptococcal IE.[34] For these patients, this form of therapy appears to be roughly as effective as four weeks of intravenous penicillin alone or in combination with streptomycin. The principal advantage of two-week over four-week therapy is that two-week therapy is more cost effective and there is a more efficient use of hospital facilities and personnel. The possible disadvantages of two-week intramuscular therapy are the small risk of streptomycin-associated vestibular toxicity (this risk would be presumably the same with four-week regimens that include streptomycin) and the frequent intramuscular injections. The tolerance of patients to intramuscular injections was enhanced when patients understood that with this form of therapy their mobility in hospital would be increased and the period of hospitalization would be decreased.

We do not recommend two-week therapy for patients with symptoms of illness greater than three months in duration, prosthetic valve endocarditis, mycotic aneurysm, cerebritis, shock, abnormal renal function, or preexisting vestibular dysfunction, or for patients with infections caused by nutritionally-dependent streptococci or streptococci with penicillin MIC greater than 0.2 mcg/ml. For the large majority of patients with penicillin-susceptible streptococcal IE who do not have these complications, two-week combined penicillin-streptomycin therapy is effective.

REFERENCES

1. Geraci, J.E., Martin, W.J.: Antibiotic therapy of bacterial endocarditis. IV. Successful short-term (two-weeks) combined penicillin-dihydrostreptomycin therapy in subacute bacterial endocarditis caused by penicillin-sensitive streptococci. Circulation 8:494–509, 1953.
2. Geraci, J.E.: Further experiences with short-term (two weeks) combined penicillin-streptomycin therapy for bacterial endocarditis caused by penicillin-sensitive streptococci. Proc. Staff Meet. Mayo Clin. 30:192–200, 1955.
3. Geraci, J.E.: The antibiotic therapy of bacterial endocarditis: therapeutic data on 172 patients seen from 1951 through 1957; additional observations on short-term therapy (two weeks) for penicillin-sensitive streptococcal endocarditis. Med. Clin. North Am. July 1958:1101.
4. Kaye, D.: Changes in the spectrum, diagnosis and management of bacterial and fungal endocarditis. Med. Clin. North Am. 57:941, 1957.
5. Tan, J.S., Terhune, C.A., Jr., Kaplan, S., Hamburger, M.: Successful two-week treatment schedule for penicillin-susceptible *Streptococcus viridans* endocarditis. Lancet 2:1340, 1971.
6. Hoeprich, P.D.: Infectious Diseases: A guide to the understanding and management of infectious processes. Hagerstown: Harper & Rowe, Publishers; 1972:1056.
7. Tompsett, R., Hurst, M.L.: Bacterial endocarditis: selected aspects of treatment. Trans. Am. Clin. Climatol. Assoc. 83:95, 1971.

8. Wolfe, J.C., Johnson, W.D., Jr.: Penicillin-sensitive streptococcal endocarditis: in-vitro and clinical observations on penicillin-streptomycin therapy. Ann. Intern. Med. 81:178, 1974.
9. Hunter, T.H.: The treatment of some bacterial infections of the heart and pericardium. Bull N.Y. Acad. Med. 28:213, 1952.
10. Wilson, W.R., Geraci, J.E., Thompson R.L., Wilkowske, C.J., Giuliani, E.R.: Treatment of penicillin-sensitive streptococcal infective endocarditis (PSSIE) with short-term intramuscular (IM) procaine penicillin and streptomycin (PP&S). 18th Interscience Conference on Antimicrobial Agents and Chemotherapy, October 1–4, 1978, Abstract No. 276.
11. Lerner, P.I., Weinstein, L.: Infective endocarditis in the antibiotic era. NEJM 274:199, 259, 323, 388, 1966.
12. Tompsett, R.: Bacterial endocarditis: changes in the clinical spectrum. Arch. Intern. Med. 119:329, 1967.
13. Shinebourne, E.A., Cripps, C.M., Hayward, G.W., Shooter, R.A.: Bacterial endocarditis 1956–1965: analysis of clinical features and treatment in relation to prognosis and mortality. Br. Heart J. 31:536, 1969.
14. Wilson, W.R., Washington, J.A. II: Infective endocarditis--a changing spectrum? (Editorial) Mayo Clin. Proc. 52:254, 1977.
15. Cates, J.E., Christie, R.V.: Subacute bacterial endocarditis: a review of 442 patients treated in 14 centers appointed by the Penicillin Trials Committee of the Medical Research Council. Q. J. Med. ns 20:93, 1951.
16. Christie, R.V.: Subacute bacterial endocarditis. Br. Med. J. 2:438, 1953.
17. Hamburger, M., Stein, L.: *Streptococcus viridans* subacute bacterial endocarditis: two week treatment schedule with penicillin. JAMA 149:542, 1952.
18. Hunter, T.H., Paterson, P.Y.: Bacterial endocarditis. D.M. November, 1956, pp 1-48.
19. Duperval, R., Bill, N.J., Geraci, J.E., Washington, J.A. II: Bactericidal activity of combinations of penicillin or clindamycin with gentamicin or streptomycin against species of viridans streptococci. Antimicrob. Agents Chemother. 8:673, 1975.
20. Durack, D.T., Petersdorf, R.G.: Chemotherapy of experimental streptococcal endocarditis. I. Comparison of commonly recommended prophylactic regimens. J. Clin. Invest. 52:592, 1973.
21. Pelletier, L.L., Jr., Petersdorf, R.G.: Chemotherapy of experimental streptococcal endocarditis. V. Effect of duration of infection and retained intracardiac catheter on response to treatment. J. Lab. Clin. Med. 87:692, 1976.
22. Sande, M.A., Irvin, R.G.: Penicillin-aminoglycoside synergy in experimental *Streptococcus viridans* endocarditis. J. Infect. Dis. 129:572, 1974.

23. Durack, D.T., Pelletier, L.L., Petersdorf, R.G.: Chemotherapy of experimental streptococcal endocarditis. II. Synergism between penicillin and streptomycin against penicillin-sensitive streptococci. J. Clin. Invest. 53:829, 1974.
24. Tompsett, R., Robbins, W.C., Berntsen, C., Jr.: Short-term penicillin and dihydrostreptomycin therapy of streptococcal endocarditis: results of the treatment of thirty-five patients. Am. J. Med. 24:57, 1958.
25. Carey, R.B., Gross, K.C., Roberts, R.B.: Vitamin B_6-dependent *Streptococcus mitior (mitis)* isolated from patients with systemic infections. J. Infect. Dis. 131:722, 1975.
26. Carey, R.B., Brause, B.D., Roberts, R.B.: Antimicrobial therapy of vitamin B_6-dependent streptococcal endocarditis. Ann. Intern. Med. 87:150, 1977.
27. Friedberg, C.K.: Diseases of the heart. Vol 1. Third Edition. Philadelphia: W.B. Saunders Company; 1966:242.
28. Bourgault A–M, Wilson, W.R., Washington, J.A. II: Antimicrobial susceptibilities of species of viridans streptococci. J. Infect. Dis. 140:316, Sept. 1979.
29. Hook, E.W., Guerrant, R.L.: Therapy of infective endocarditis. In: Kaye D, ed. Infective Endocarditis. Baltimore: University Park Press, 1976, pp 169, 172 173.
30. Parrillo, J.E., Borst, G.C., Mazur, M.H., et al.: Endocarditis due to resistant viridans streptococci during oral penicillin chemoprophylaxis, NEJM 300:296, 1979.
31. Malacoff, R.F., Frank E., Andriole, V.T.: Streptococcal endocarditis (nonenterococcal, non–group A): single vs combination therapy. JAMA 241:1807, 1979.
32. Phair, J.P., Tan, J.S.: Therapy of *Streptococcus viridans* endocarditis. In: Kaplan E.L., Taranta, A.V., eds. Infective Endocarditis. Dallas, American Heart Association, 1977, pp 55–7.
33. Wilson, W.R., Danielson, G.K., Guiliani, E.R., Washington, J.A., II, Jaumin, P.M., Geraci, J.E.: Cardiac valve replacement in congestive heart failure due to infective endocarditis. Mayo Clin. Proc. 54:223, 1979.
34. Wilson, W.R., Thompson, R.L., Wilkowske, C.J., Washington, J.A., II, Giuliani, E.R., Geraci, J.E.: Short-term treatment for streptococcal infective endocarditis: combined intramuscular administration of penicillin and streptomycin. JAMA 245:360, 1981.

J.P. Phair, M.D.
J. Tan, M.D.
F. Venezio, M.D.
G. Westenfelder, M.D.
B. Reisberg, M.D.

5

THERAPY OF INFECTIVE ENDOCARDITIS DUE TO PENICILLIN-SUSCEPTIBLE STREPTOCOCCI: DURATION OF DISEASE IS A MAJOR DETERMINANT OF OUTCOME

The treatment of infective endocarditis due to penicillin susceptible streptococci remains controversial. Reports advocating efficacy and safety of penicillin for four weeks or more,[1] penicillin for four weeks plus an aminoglycoside for two weeks[2] or two weeks of combined therapy[3,4] have been published. In a previous retrospective analysis, we identified a "high risk" group of patients, who, in spite of "optimal therapy", relapsed. Such patients had been ill for three months or longer before treatment was instituted. Five of 25 patients with a prolonged illness, as opposed to 1 of 60 with an illness shorter than three months, relapsed after completing therapy.[5] We have recently analyzed the outcome of 50 courses of therapy in 48 additional patients with endocarditis due to penicillin susceptible streptococci (minimal inhibitory concentration, 0.2 μgm/ml or less) seen in the last four years at Northwestern Memorial Hospital, Evanston Hospital and Akron City Hospital. Results of therapy were correlated with duration of disease and the treatment regimen utilized. In addition, results of M. mode echocardiography were correlated with the duration of illness and the outcome of therapy in 18 patients in whom such data were available.

Four treatment regimens were used:

Group I: Penicillin alone 24 to 32 days; 5 courses

Group II: Alternate antibiotic with or without an aminoglycoside, 24 to 32 days; 3 courses

Group III: Penicillin, 24 to 32 days, plus an aminoglycoside for the initial 12 to 16 days; 25 courses

Group IV: Penicillin plus an aminoglycoside for 12 to 16 days; 17 courses.

Eleven of the 48 patients had infection on a prosthetic or porcine valve, three had a congenital cardiac lesion, the remainder had infection on the aortic, mitral or tricuspid valve. None were addicted to intravenous drugs. Thirty-nine patients were cured, 37 with the initial course and two after a second course of therapy required for treatment of a relapse. Eight patients died while receiving treatment. One patient was apparently cured but lost to follow-up.

The patients with prosthetic valve endocarditis had late infections, occurring longer than six months after surgery. Ten of the 11 survived, all received four weeks of penicillin or an alternate drug plus two weeks of an aminoglycoside. The one death was due to a cerebral embolus which occurred during treatment. None of the surviving 10 patients with prosthetic valve endocarditis required surgery to eradicate the infection or to correct a valvular dysfunction.

The remaining seven early deaths were due to cerebral embolism,[1] cerebral hemorrhage,[2] congestive failure and/or arrhythmia[3] or pulmonary emboli[1] which occurred in an 87 year-old gentleman with right-sided endocarditis.

In addition four late deaths occurred six months or longer after completing therapy. Three were due to an unrelated illness, and one patient died during cardiac surgery which was undertaken to correct valvular dysfunction resulting from the endocarditis.

The results of therapy according to treatment regimen are presented in Table 1. Patients dying during therapy or lost to follow-up are excluded

Table 1: Treatment Regimen and Outcome[1]

Regimen	Cure	Relapse
Penicillin, 24—32 days	3 (3)[2]	0
Penicillin, 24—32 days plus aminoglycoside, 12—16 days	17 (13)	0
Penicillin, 12—16 days plus aminoglycoside, 12—16 days	15 (9)	2
Other	3 (1)	0
TOTALS	38 (26)	2

1. Early deaths and patients lost to follow-up excluded

2. Number of patients ill for less than 2 months

from this tabulation. Thirty-nine patients completed therapy (41 courses) and were available for follow-up. All thirty–nine patients were cured. The length of follow-up averaged 23 months. No bacterologic relapses were noted. Two clinical relapses occurred within one month of completion of an initial two week course of therapy. Both patients had been ill for longer than two months before initiation of the original therapy. The patients were retreated because of recurrent persistent fever; blood cultures were sterile. One patient developed a positive rheumatoid factor during the interval between the first and second treatment course. A second course of penicillin (four weeks) plus an aminoglycoside (two weeks) resulted in clearing of fever and a return to the previous state of health in both patients.

Overall, the outcome of the infection was related to the duration of symptomalogy (Table 2). Twenty-nine patients (27 first episode, 2 relapses) were ill for less than two months when diagnosed, two died during therapy and one was lost to follow-up. The death and relapse rate among the 21 patients ill for two months or longer was significantly higher (38.2% vs. 7.2%) ($x^2 = 5.30$, $p < 0.05 > 0.02$).

Table 2: Duration of Symptoms Before Therapy and Outcome

Duration	Cure	Relapse	Death[1]	Lost	Total
<2 mo.	26	0	2	1	29
≥2 mo.	13	2	6	0	21

1. Death during treatment

The finding of a vegetation by echocardiography correlated directly with the duration of symptoms (Table 3) and inversely with outcome. None of the 9 patients with symptoms for less than two months had a vegetation demonstrated by M-mode echocardiography. In contrast six of nine with a prolonged course had positive findings. Of the 12 patients with a negative study 10 were cured with medical management, one died during treatment and one was lost to follow-up. Two of the six patients with a vegetation demonstrable by echocardiography died during treatment, three required surgery because of severe valvular regurgitation and one was cured by antibiotic therapy alone.

Table 3: Echocardographic Results Related to Duration of Symptoms

Duration	Vegetation	No Vegetation
<2 mo.	0	9
≥2 mo.	6	3

This analysis extends our previous findings.[5] Duration of illness appears to be a highly relevant determinant of survival, six of eight early deaths occurred in patients with infection for eight weeks or longer. In addition, the two clinical relapses occurred in patients with a prolonged history of illness. There appears to be no advantage of one treatment regimen over another among patients receiving therapy shortly (within two months) after the onset of symptoms. All 9 patients receiving two weeks of combined therapy and 13 of 14 receiving penicillin for four weeks and an aminoglycoside for two weeks were cured; and the fourteenth patient was lost to follow-up.

Determination of the onset of endocarditis can be difficult in individual patients. Symptoms can be vague and confused with other minor infections by the patients. However, an indication of the duration of the disease can be ascertained with attention to history and specific tests. The onset commonly occurs within two weeks of a procedure associated with bacteremia.[6] A positive test for serum antiglobulins indicates prolonged illness. Previous studies have reported that positive tests for rheumatoid factor are found in 50% of patients with infective endocarditis and are associated with disease of six weeks duration and hypergammaglobulinemia.[7] Finally, our data demonstrate a correlation of duration of disease with the finding of vegetation by echocardiography.

In summary, appropriate antibiotic therapy should be initiated without delay in patients with a prolonged history consistent with infective endocarditis. An echocardiogram should be obtained. If a vegetation is demonstrated, consideration should be given to early surgical intervention.[8] If no vegetation is found medical management will probably be curative but antibiotic therapy should be given for a minimum of four weeks. If the apparent duration of symptoms is short, and the echocardiogram does not demonstrate a vegetation, two weeks of combined therapy, penicillin plus an aminoglycoside, is sufficient.

REFERENCES

1. Karchmer, A.W., Moellering, R.C., Maki, D.G. and Swartz, N.M.: Single antibiotic therapy for streptococcal endocarditis. J.A.M.A. 241: 1801, 1979.
2. Wolfe, J.C. and Johnson, W.D., Jr.: ,Penicillin-sensitive streptococcal endocarditis. Ann. Int. Med. 81: 178, 1974.
3. Wilson, W.R., Geraci, J.E., Wilkowske, C.J. and Washington, J.A.: Short term intramuscular therapy with procaine penicillin plus streptomycin for infective endocarditis due to Viridans Streptococcus. Circulation 57: 1158, 1978.

4. Tan, J.S., Terhune, C.A., Kaplan, S. and Hamburger, M.: Successful two week treatment schedule for penicillin-susceptible Streptococcus Viridans endocarditis. Lancet 2: 1340, 1971.
5. Phair, J.P. and Tan, J.S.: Therapy of Streptococcus Viridans endocarditis in Kaplan, E.L. Taranta, A.V. (eds) Infective Endocarditis, An American Heart Association Symposium, Dallas American Heart Association, 1977, p. 55.
6. Starkebaum, M., Durack, D., and Beeson, P.: The "incubation period" of subacute bacterial endocarditis. Yale J. Biol. and Med. 50: 49, 1977.
7. Messner, R.P., Laxdal, T., Quie, P.G. and Williams, R.C.: Rheumatoid factors in subacute bacterial endocarditis-bacteremia, duration of disease or genetic predisposition. Ann. Int. Md. 68: 746, 1968.
8. Mintz, G.S., Kotler, M.N., Segal, B.L., and Parry, W.R.: Survival patients with aortic valve endocarditis. The prognostic implications of the echocardiogram. Arch. Int. Med. 139: 862, 1979.

Robert C. Moellering, Jr., M.D.

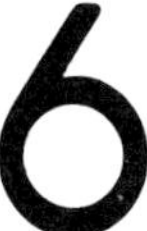

ANTIMICROBIAL SUSCEPTIBILITY OF ENTEROCOCCI: IN VITRO STUDIES OF THE ACTION OF ANTIBIOTICS ALONE AND IN COMBINATION

The enterococci consist of several species of group D streptococci.[1] In the United States, *S. faecalis* (including *S. faecalis* var. *zymogenes* and *S. faecalis* var. *liquefaciens*) account for the majority of organisms isolated from patients with bacterial endocarditis[2] and likely account for the majority of organisms from all clinical sources. *S. faecium* are the next most frequently isolated species, while *S. durans* are rarely found among strains causing human infections in the U.S.A. Several investigators have found significant differences in antimicrobial susceptibility patterns among the various species of enterococci.[3,4] In addition, there are also major differences between the susceptibility patterns of the enterococci and non-enterococcal group D streptococci such as *S. bovis* and *S. equinus*.[5,6,7,8,9] Enterococci are unique among all streptococci in their resistance to a wide range of antimicrobial agents; indeed, single agents are rarely bactericidal against these organisms *in vitro.*[10] It is because of the above facts that special considerations are required for the appropriate choice of antimicrobial agents to treat enterococcal endocarditis and other severe infections caused by these resistant microorganisms.

Compared with other streptococci, enterococci exhibit decreased susceptibility to virtually all classes of antimicrobial agents.[10] This may be observed in Table 1, which gives the median and range of minimal inhibitory concentrations (MIC's) of 34 antimicrobial agents against enterococci.

Table 1. Antimicrobial Susceptibility of Enterococci

Antibiotic	Range	Median
Amikacin	62 — 1000	500
Amoxycillin	0.2 — 1.0	.5
Ampicillin	0.4 — 12.5	1.0
Bacitracin	25 — >100	>100
Carbenicillin	32 — 256	50
Cefazolin	1.0 — >32	32
Cephalexin	100 — >100	≥100
Cephaloridine	12.5 — 50	12.5
Cephalothin	6 — 500	20
Chloramphenicol	≤1.9 — >100	25
Clindamycin	1.6 — >100*	25
Cloxacillin	50 — >100	>100
Cycloserine	100 — 200	——
Demeclocycline	3.1 — >100	50
Dicloxacillin	16 — >64	——
Doxycycline	.8 — >100	25
Erythromycin	0.4 — >100	6.2
Gentamicin	1.9 — 125	31
Kanamycin	16 — >2000	125
Lincomycin	12.5 — >100*	50
Methicillin	25 — >200	64
Minocycline	0.2 — >100	25
Nafcillin	3.2 — 50	12.5
Netilmicin	16 — 500	32
Novobiocin	12.5 — >100	25
Oxacillin	8 — 250	32
Penicillin	0.8 — 25.0	2.0
Polymyxin B	Resistant	——
Rifampin	0.4 — 6.25	0.8
Sisomicin	16 — 1000	64
Streptomycin	31 — >2000	312
Tetracycline	≤1.9 — >100	100
Tobramycin	31 — >2000	125
Vancomycin	0.78 — 12.5	3.0

Data derived from a composite of published studies (3,6,8,9,11—22)

*MIC's of clindamycin and lincomycin for some strains of *S. durans* may be lower. (27)

Relative resistance to the penicillins and cephalosporins appears to be an intrinsic feature of enterococci. The fact that serial studies have shown no change in penicillin susceptibility of enterococci with the passage of time[3] and the observation that the MIC's of penicillin for enterococci isolated from the stools of natives from antibiotic-virgin populations (such as the Solomon Islanders) are similar to those presently isolated in the United States and Europe are consistent with this concept.[10] Of the currently available penicillins, benzylpenicillin, ampicillin, and amoxycillin are the most active (in increasing order of effectiveness) against enterococci (Table 1;[3,14,23]).

Several studies have demonstrated that the MIC's of the penicillins and cephalosporins for *S. faecium* are even higher than those for *S. faecalis*.[3,4] Even more striking, however, is the large discrepancy between the MIC and the minimal bactericidal concentration (MBC) of the penicillins and cephalosporins against most strains of *S. faecalis* and *S. faecium*.[6,10,23] This phenomenon has been noted when enterococci are exposed *in vitro* to virtually any agent which inhibits cell wall synthesis, including cycloserine, bacitracin, and vancomycin.[13,16,18,21,24] Thus it appears that most antimicrobial agents which inhibit bacterial cell wall synthesis as their primary mode of action are poorly or only slowly bactericidal against enterococci, and in many instances, their effect is clearly only bacteriostatic. The mechanism of intrinsic resistance to the penicillins and cephalosporins (and to other agents which inhibit cell wall synthesis) in enterococci has not been defined, but there is no evidence that production of an extracellular beta-lactamase is involved.[20]

Low-level resistance (MIC $\leqslant$ 250–500 μg/ml) to various aminoglycosidic aminocyclitols is found in virtually all strains of enterococci.[3,10,17] This type of resistance is characteristic of strains isolated from antibiotic-free populations as well as of those currently isolated in the United States[10]; there is evidence that it is due to impermeability or to decreased uptake via transport mechanisms for aminoglycosidic aminocyclitols.[25,26] The cell wall and/or closely related structures appear to play an important role in this resistance since exposure of enterococci to agents which impair cell wall formation at any point in the synthetic pathway results in increased aminoglycoside uptake and enhanced susceptibility.[25,26]

Low-level resistance to lincomycin and clindamycin is also a characteristic feature of certain species of enterococci *(S. faecalis* and *S. faecium*) and probably represents another example of intrinsic resistance.[27] Such resistance to clindamycin has consistently been observed even among strains of *S. faecalis* and *S. faecium* from populations which have never been exposed to these drugs.[10] Thirty-one of 32 strains of enterococci from stool cultures of Solomon Islanders were shown to be resistant to clindamycin in a recent survey.[10] The molecular basis for low-level resistance to lincomycin and clindamycin among enterococci is currently unknown.

As is the case with most gram positive bacteria, enterococci are resistant to the polymyxins. On the other hand, almost all strains are susceptible *in vitro* to nitrofurantoin (Table 2).

Resistance to erythromycin among enterococci appears to be an acquired characteristic and is not found among all strains. Indeed, among Solomon Islanders who had had no previous exposure to erythromycin, we were able to discover no erythromycin-resistant strains of enterococci in 1972.[10] Toala et al noted that strains of enterococci isolated at the Boston City Hospital in 1968–1969 were considerably more resistant to erythromycin than those from 1952. A similar trend has been seen at the Massachusetts General Hospital (Table 2) where presently only half of the strains of enterococci are susceptible to erythromycin.

The molecular basis for erythromycin resistance has received considerable attention recently and in a number of strains of enterococci this resistance has been shown to be mediated by plasmids of varying molecular weights (4.5 – 50 x 10^6), the larger of which are transferable from resistant donor strains to susceptible recepient strains which acquire part or all of the resistance patterns of the donor.[10,28,29,30,31,32,33] Direct cell-cell contact is required for transfer of plasmids to take place. Recent electron microscopic studies suggest that this process in enterococci does not require sex pili or other appendages such as are found among gram negative bacilli.[34] Clewell et al have demonstrated the production of sex pheromones in enterococci which produce clumping and presumably aid in bringing about the cell-cell contact necessary for conjugation.[35] The mechanism by which plasmids render their host strains of enterococci resistant to erythromycin is presently unknown. In many instances, the plasmids which are associated with erythromycin resistance in enterococci also mediate resistance to other antimicrobials, including lincomycin (high-level), tetracycline, aminoglycosides (high-level), pristinamycin factor I, virginiamycin factor S, and/or streptogramin B.[10,28,29,30,31,32,33]

Plasmid-mediated resistance to chloramphenicol and tetracycline also occurs in enterococci.[31,33,36,37] The plasmids mediating chloramphenicol resistance which have been characterized have had molecular weights between 26 x 10^6 and 76 x 10^6 and in some instances, have been shown to code for the production of chloramphenicol acetyltransferase which appears to account for the resistance to chloramphenicol in the cells which contain such plasmids.[37,38] At present approximately one-fifth of the strains of enterococci isolated from patients at the Massachusetts General Hospital are resistant to chloramphenicol (Table 2).

Resistance to tetracycline is much more prevalent; approximately 80% of strains at the Massachusetts General Hospital are not inhibited by this antibiotic or its closely related cogeners (Table 2). Several different plasmids (molecular weights 6 x 10^6 to 50 x 10^6) mediating tetracycline resistance have been demonstrated in enterococci.[28,33,39,40] Yagi and

Table 2. Antimicrobial Susceptibility of Enterococci - Massachusetts General Hospital 1971 — 1979

Year	No. of Isolates	Percent of Organisms Susceptible to: PEN	METH	ERYT	CEPH	TETR	CHLR	CLIN	NITR
1971 (Jul-Dec.)	1101	28	5	79	29	23	79	--	97
1972	2317	23	3	81	32	23	81	4	97
1973	2624	21	0	70	19	20	78	1	96
1974	3056	19	0	51	11	16	78	2	95
1975	2782	33	0	49	16	18	79	2	92
1976	2430	38	0	46	9	15	76	2	94
1977	2120	25	0	54	8	18	76	2	94
1978	2178	35	0	52	15	18	78	2	96
1979	1833	32	0	49	27	22	78	2	95

Abbreviations: CEPH = cephalothin; CHLR = chloramphenicol; CLIN = clindamycin; ERYT = erythromycin; METH = methicillin; NITR = nitrofurantoin; PEN = penicillin; TETR = tetracycline.

Data collected in collaboration with Dr. L.J. Kunz.

Clewell have described increases in tetracycline resistance which can be induced by growth of enterococci containing certain 6 megadalton plasmids in subinhibitory concentrations of tetracycline. This results in the formation of plasmids which are increased in size because of the inclusion of repeated units of a 2.65 megadalton segment of DNA containing the tetracycline resistance determinant.[40] This gene amplification results in a 3-fold increase in tetracycline resistance, but the mechanism by which amplified (or unamplified) plasmids produce tetracycline resistance in enterococci has not been determined.

The majority of strains of enterococci tested thus far have been susceptible to rifampin.[15] However, *in vitro* resistance to rifampin occurs readily on exposure to the drug.[15,32,41] Therefore, the use of rifampin as a single agent to treat infections may result in therapeutic failures due to the development of resistance. Combining rifampin with ampicillin *in vitro* to prevent resistance resulted in bactericidal antagonism.[15] More studies will be needed to define the potential therapeutic utility of rifampin for enterococcal infections.

Although ampicillin-rifampin combinations may demonstrate *in vitro* antagonism, the combination of penicillins and aminoglycosides often produces striking synergistic killing of enterococci. Numerous investigators have confirmed this fact since the initial studies of Hunter[42] and of Jawetz et al.[43] This is particularly important since penicillins (and other agents which inhibit cell wall synthesis) are usually not bactericidal against enterococci (or kill them at a very slow rate). Thus these agents are often ineffective when utilized alone for the treatment of infections such as endocarditis which require bactericidal therapy.

All agents which impair bacterial cell wall synthesis including cycloserine[24], bacitracin[24] vancomycin[16,24,47,48] benzylpenicillin [4,17,22,23,42,43,44,45,47,49,50,51,52,53,54,55], ampicillin[15,23,44,45,47,51,55,56], amoxycillin[45,55], carbenicillin[18,56], the semisynthetic penicillinase-resistant penicillins[11,12,13], and the cephalosporins[19,20,21,44,51] have been shown to produce synergistic killing of enterococci when combined with aminoglycosides such as streptomycin, neomycin, kanamycin, gentamicin, tobramycin, amikacin, sisomicin, netilmicin, dibekacin, and others[17,22,24,45,46,47,48,49,50,51,52,53,54,55,56]. Combinations of aminoglycosides with agents which primarily act on the cell membrane, such as the polymyxins, or which inhibit protein synthesis, such as chloramphenicol, the macrolides and the tetracyclines, fail to produce synergism against enterococci.[24,25,44]

The bactericidal synergy which results from combining antimicrobials which inhibit cell wall synthesis with certain aminoglycosidic aminocyclitols is most easily demonstrated by time-kill curves[57] (Figure 1). Although synergy may also be demonstrated by isobolograms derived from checkerboard broth titrations[11,47,56], our experience suggests that this method is less reliable, even when bactericidal endpoints are determined.

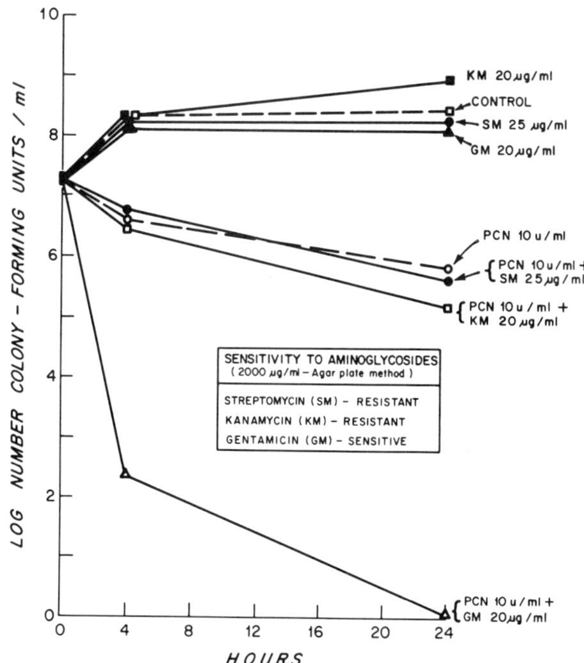

Figure 1: Effect of penicillin (PCN), kanamycin (KM), streptomycin (SM), and gentamicin (GM) alone and in combination against a strain of enterococcus which has high-level resistance to both SM and KM but not GM.

Several recent studies have been carried out in an attempt to determine the minimal concentrations of antimicrobials (especially aminoglycosides) necessary for *in vitro* synergism against enterococci. Matsumoto et al found that concentrations of streptomycin of $\geqslant$ 10 µg/ml and of gentamicin of $\geqslant$3 µg/ml in combination with penicillin where required to produce synergism against at least 20–30% of "synergistic" strains of enterococci.[58] Our studies confirm that maximum clinically achievable doses of aminoglycosides may be required for synergism against certain strains.[22,53,54] Using different techniques, Soriano and Greenwood have recently demonstrated that bactericidal synergism did not occur against the Hook strain of *S. faecalis* unless both the penicillin and aminoglycoside were present in concentrations equal to or exceeding the minimum active concentration (MAC)*, which was 1 µg/ml for penicillin and 2 µg/ml for gentamicin.[59]

---

* The minimal active concentration is defined as the lowest concentration of antibiotic which exerts any detectable suppressive effect on the growth of the microorganism.

Although the semisynthetic penicillinase-resistant penicillins and cephalosporins produce syngergism with aminoglycosides against enterococci *in vitro*[11,12,13,19,20,21,44,51], such combinations are often ineffective *in vivo* The reasons for this are not fully understood, but presently available data suggest a number of factors, including the lack of intrinsic activity of these drugs (high MAC's and MIC's); this, in turn, is accentuated by the high degree of binding of many of these analogs to serum proteins, which may further decrease their activity.[60] Finally, for some of the cephalosporins, *in vivo* desacetylation results in the formation of metabolites with diminished activity.[20]

The mechanism of penicillin-aminoglycoside synergism against enterococci has been extensively investigated and is now at least partially understood. It is clear from a number of studies[24,59,61] that penicillin and the aminoglycoside must be simultaneously present in order for effective synergistic killing of enterococci to occur. This makes it unlikely that the production of enterococcal spheroplasts in the presence of penicillin, followed by the subsequent killing of these spheroplasts by an aminoglycoside[62] is the entire explanation for synergism, although this phenomenon could be a contributor to the overall lethal effects of penicillin-aminoglycoside combinations.

Studies utilizing ^{14}C-labelled streptomycin[25], tobramycin and gentamicin[26], have demonstrated that significant aminoglycoside uptake does not occur in enterococci exposed to clinically achievable concentrations of aminoglycosides alone. However, in the presence of penicillin (or any agent which inhibits cell wall synthesis) there is a marked enhancement of aminoglycoside uptake which coincides with killing of the organism. Only agents which produce synergy in combination with aminoglycosides produce enhanced uptake. Agents such as erythromycin, chloramphenicol, tetracycline, and colistin, which fail to synergize with aminoglycosides, also fail to enhance aminoglycoside uptake.[25] It thus appears that killing of enterococci is primarily due to the action of the aminoglycoside.[25,59] Since agents which inhibit cell wall synthesis by different mechanisms all produce synergism with aminoglycosides, it appears that the cell wall (or a closely related structure) is the barrier to effective aminoglycoside uptake in enterococci.[25] Breaching the barrier results in killing of enterococci by aminoglycosides, the phenomenon which seems to correspond with bactericidal synergy.

Unfortunately, not all enterococci are killed synergistically by penicillin-aminoglycoside combinations. In the case of penicillin-streptomycin and penicillin-kanamycin (or penicillin-neomycin) combinations, failure of synergism is seen in those isolates which exhibit high-level resistance (MIC $\geqslant$ 1000–2000 μg/ml) to the aminoglycoside *in vitro*.[17,48,63,64] At present, the prevalence of enterococci with such high-level resistance to streptomycin and kanamycin is 54% and 49%

respectively among blood isolates from the clinical microbiology laboratory at the Massachusetts General Hospital .[17] Similar (25–50%) prevalences of high-level resistance to these aminoglycosides among enterococci have been reported from a number of other geographic areas, including Los Angeles[46], Denver[15], Seattle[63], and London.[65] The prevalence of isolates resistant to penicillin-streptomycin and penicillin-kanamycin synergism appears to be increasing.[17] That this phenomenon may be due to the selective pressure which results from the heavy clinical usage of aminoglycosides is strongly suggested by the fact that a survey of enterococci from a population of Solomon Islanders with minimal antibiotic exposure in 1972 reveal that only one of 43 strains of enterococci exhibited high-level resistance to streptomycin and none to kanamycin.[10]

There appear to be at least two different mechanisms involved in high-level aminoglycoside resistance and in resistance to synergism in highly resistant organisms. Alterations in the 30S subunit of enterococcal ribosomes can result in ribosomal resistance to streptomycin.[66] Strains of enterococci with this type of resistance are not killed synergistically by penicillin plus streptomycin.[66] Although the prevalence of ribosomal resistance among clinical isolates of enterococci has not been determined, preliminary studies would suggest that it only infrequently accounts for high-level resistance to streptomycin among clinical isolates (R.C. Moellering, Jr. and B.E. Murray, unpublished data). It appears that in most instances, high-level resistance to streptomycin and kanamycin and resistance to penicillin-streptomycin and penicillin-kanamycin synergism (as well as to penicillin-amikacin synergism) is due to the presence of plasmid-mediated aminoglycoside modifying enzymes.[67,68] Such resistant strains have been shown to contain conjugative plasmids with a molecular weight of 45 x 10^6. The high-level resistance to streptomycin and resistance to penicillin-streptomycin synergism is due to the production of a plasmid-mediated adenylyltransferase with activity against streptomycin but not spectinomycin[37,67], while resistance to penicillin-kanamycin, penicillin-neomycin, and penicillin-amikacin synergism is related to the production of a 3′ phosphotransferase (APH) (3′)) with activity against kanamycin, neomycin, and amikacin (as well as butirosin, ribostamycin, and lividomycin A).[37,67,68] Studies in which enzyme preparations from these organisms have been used to phosphorylate amikacin clearly demonstrate that phosphorylated aminoglycosides are not capable of producing synergism in the presence of penicillin .[67] Thus these enzymes seem to be responsible for resistance to antimicrobial synergy.

To date we have found no strains of enterococci with high-level resistance (MIC $\geqslant$ 2000 μg/mg) to gentamicin although we have found a single strain which was resistant to penicillin-gentamicin synergism but was killed by penicillin-tobramycin and penicillin-kanamycin combinations. This organism, which grew as a small-colony variant, exhibited an apparent defect in uptake of gentamicin (but not tobramycin) in the presence of penicillin.[26] Such strains presently appear to be rare, but the recent isolation in France of three strains of enterococci with transmissible high-level resistance to gentamicin raises the possibility that high-level gentamicin resistance may also become a problem with which to reckon.[69] The mechanism of resistance to gentamicin in the French strains was not determined by the authors, but they cited unpublished data suggesting that the high-level aminoglycoside resistance was associated with the presence of two aminoglycoside-modifying enzymes: a 6′ acetyltransferase (AAC (6′)) and a 2″ phosphotransferase (APH (2″)).

Unlike *S. faecalis, S. faecium* appear to be consistently resistant to synergistic killing by combinations of penicillin with kanamycin, tobramycin, sisomicin, and netilmicin.[4,70] This resistance to synergism appears to be related to the production of a 6′ acetyltransferase (AAC (6′)) which is capable of inactivating the above aminoglycosides.[70] The genetic basis for the production of this enzyme has not yet been defined, since it does not appear to be easily transferable by conjugation.[70]

Figure 2 provides a summary of the presently known mechanisms of resistance of penicillin-aminoglycoside synergism in enterococci. It is very likely that this figure will soon be obsolete as more data are accumulated concerning the mechanisms of antibiotic interaction and the mechanisms of resistance to such interaction among enterococci.

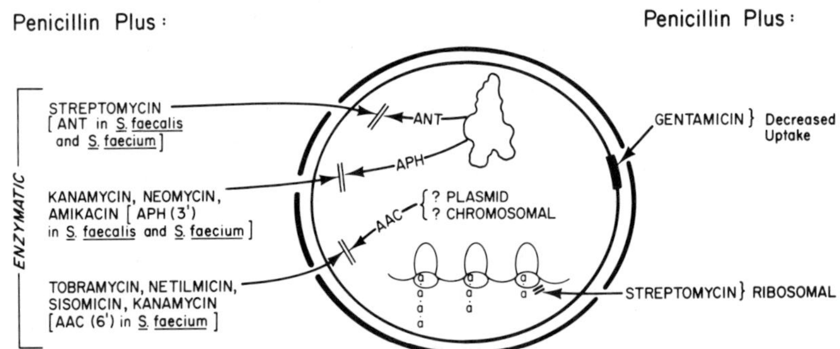

Figure 2: Presently known mechanisms of resistance to antimicrobial synergism in enterococci. ANT, adenylytransferase; APH, phosphotransferase; AAC, acetyltransferase. Reproduced with permission from Holloway, W.J., ed., Infectious Disease Reviews, 6:11, 1981.

REFERENCES

1. Deibel, R.H.: The group D streptococci. *Bacteriol. Rev.* 28:330–366, 1964.
2. Facklam, R.R.: Recognition of group D streptococcal species of human origin by biochemical and physiological tests. *Appl. Microbiol.* 23: 1131–1139, 1972.
3. Toala, P., McDonald, A., Wilcox, C., and Finland, M.: Susceptibility of group D streptococcus (enterococcus) to 21 antibiotics in vitro, with special reference to species differences. *Am. J. Med. Sci.* 258:416–430, 1969.
4. Moellering, R.C., Jr., Korzeniowski, O.M., Sande, M.A., and Wennersten, C.B.: Species-specific resistance to antimicrobial synergism in *Streptococcus faecium* and *Streptococcus faecalis.* J. Inf. Dis. 140:203–208, 1979.
5. Raverby, W.D., Bottone, E.J., and Keusch, G.T.: Group D streptococcal bacteremia, with emphasis on the incidence and presentation of infection due to *Streptococcus bovis. N. Engl. J. Med.* 289:1400–1403, 1973.
6. Moellering, R.C., Jr., Watson, B.K., and Kunz, L.J.: Endocarditis due to group D streptococci: comparison of disease caused by *Streptococcus bovis* with that produced by the enterococci. *Am. J. Med.* 57:239–250, 1974.
7. Watanakunakorn, C.: *Streptococcus bovis* endocarditis. *Am. J. Med.* 56:256–260, 1974.
8. Thornsberry, C., Baker, C.N., and Facklam, R.R.: Antibiotic susceptibility of *Streptococcus bovis* and other group D streptococci causing endocarditis. Antimicrob. Agents Chemother. 5:228–233, 1974.
9. Hoppes, W.L., and Lerner, P.I.: Nonenterococcal group D streptoccal endocarditis caused by *Streptococcus bovis. Ann. Intern. Med.* 81:588–593, 1974.
10. Moellering, R.C., Jr., and Krogstad, D.J.: Antibiotic resistance in enterococci. *Microbiology* 1979:293–298, 1979.
11. Marier, R.L., Joyce, N., and Andriole, V.T.: Synergism of oxacillin and gentamicin against enterococci. *Antimicrob. Agents Chemother.* 8:571–573, 1975.
12. Watanakunakorn, C., and Glotzbecker, C.: Comparative in vitro activity of nafcillin, oxacillin and methicillin in combination with gentamicin and tobramycin against enterococci. *Antimicrob. Agents Chemother.* 11:88–91, 1977.
13. Glew, R.H., Moellering, R.C., Jr., and Wennersten, C.: Comparative synergistic activity of nafcillin, oxacillin, and methicillin in combination with gentamicin against enterococci. *Antimicrob. Agents Chemother.* 7:828–832, 1975.

14. Basker, M.J., Slocombe, B., and Sutherland, R.: Aminoglycoside-resistant enterococci. *J. Clin. Path.* 30:375–380, 1977.
15. Iannini, P.B., Ehret, J., and Eickhoff, T.C.: Effect of ampicillin-amikacin and ampicillin-rifampin on enterococci. *Antimicrob. Agents Chemother.* 9:448–451, 1976.
16. Mandell, G.L., Lindsey, E., and Hook, E.W.: Synergism of vancomycin and streptomycin for enterococci. *Am. J. Med. Sci.* 259:346–349, 1970.
17. Calderwood, S.A., Wennersten, C., Moellering, R.C., Jr., Kunz, L.J., and Krogstad, D.J.: Resistance to six aminoglycosidic aminocyclitol antibiotics among enterococci: Prevalence, evolution, and relationship to synergism with penicillin. *Antimicrob. Agents Chemother.* 12:401–405, 1977.
18. Libke, R.D., Regamey, C., Clarke, J.T., and Kirby, W.M.M.: Synergism of carbenicillin and gentamicin against enterococci. *Antimicrob. Agents Chemother.* 5:564–568, 1973.
19. Fekety, F.R., Jr., and Weiss, P.: Antibiotic synergism: Enhanced susceptibility of enterococci to combinations of streptomycin and penicillins or cephalosporins. *Antimicrob. Agents Chemother.* 1966:156–164, 1967.
20. Weinstein, A.J., and Moellering, R.C., Jr.: Studies of cephalothin: aminoglycoside synergism against enterococci. *Antimicrob. Agents Chemother.* 7:522–529, 1975.
21. Bourque, M., Quintiliani, R., and Tilton, R.C.: Synergism of cefazolin-gentamicin against enterococci. *Antimicrob. Agents Chemother.* 10:157–163, 1976.
22. Korzeniowski, O.M., Wennersten, C., Moellering, R.C., Jr., and Sande, M.A.: Penicillin-netilmicin synergism against *Streptococcus faecalis. Antimicrob. Agents Chemother.* 13:430–434, 1978.
23. Sonne, M., and Jawetz, E.: Comparison of the action of ampicillin and benzylpenicillin on enterococci in vitro. *Appl. Microbiol.* 16:645–648, 1968.
24. Moellering, R.C., Jr.,Wennersten, C., and Weinberg, A.N. Studies on antibiotic synergism against enterococci. I. Bacteriologic studies. *J. Lab. Clin. Med.* 77:821–828, 1971.
25. Moellering, R.C., Jr., and Weinberg, A.N.: Studies on antibiotic synergism against enterococci. II. Effect of various antibiotics on the uptake of ^{14}C–labeled streptomycin by enterococci. *J. Clin. Invest.* 50:2580–2584, 1971.
26. Moellering, R.C., Jr., Murray, B.E., Schoenbaum, S.C., Adler, J., and Wennersten, C.B.: A novel mechanism of resistance to penicillin-gentamicin synergism in *S. faecalis. J. Inf. Dis.* 141:81–96, 1980.
27. Karchmer, A.W., Moellering, R.C., Jr., and Watson B.K.: Susceptibility of various serogroups of streptococci to clindamycin and lincomycin. *Antimicrob. Agents Chemother.* 7:164–167, 1975.

28. Courvalin, P.M., Carlier, C., and Chabbert, Y.A.: Plasmid-linked tetracycline and erythromycin resistance in group D "streptococcus". *Ann. Inst. Pasteur Paris* 123:755–759, 1972.
29. Clewell, D.B., Yagi, Y., Dunny, G.M., and Schultz, S.K.: Characterization of three plasmid deoxyribonucleic acid molecules in a strain of *Streptococcus faecalis:* identification of a plasmid determining erythromycin resistance. *J. Bacteriol.* 117:283–289, 1974.
30. Yagi, Y., Franke, A.E., and Clewell, D.B. Plasmid-determined resistance to erythromycin: comparison of strains of *Streptococcus faecalis* and *Streptococcus pyogenes* with regard to plasmid homology and resistance inducibility. *Antimicrob. Agents Chemother.* 7:871–873, 1975.
31. Marder, H.P., and Kayser, F.H.: Transferable plasmids mediating multiple-antibiotic resistance in *Streptococcus faecalis* subsp. *liquefaciens. Antimicrob. Agents Chemother.* 12:261–269, 1977.
32. Jacob, A.E., and Hobbs, S.J.: Conjugal transfer of plasmid-borne multiple antibiotic resistance in *Streptococcus faecalis* var. *zymogenes J. Bacteriol.* 117:360–372, 1974.
33. Van Embden, J.D.A., Engel, H.W.B., and Van Klingeren, B.: Drug resistance in group D streptococci of clinical and non-clinical origin: prevalence transferability and plasmid properties. *Antimicrob. Agents Chemother.* 11:925–932, 1977.
34. Krogstad, D.J., Smith, R.M., Moellering, R.C., Jr., and Parquette, A.R.: Visualization of cell-cell contact during conjugation in *Streptococcus faecalis. J. Bacteriol.* 141:963–967, 1980.
35. Dunny, G.M., Brown, B.L., and Clewell, D.B.: Induced cell aggregation and mating in *Streptococcus faecalis:* evidence for a bacterial sex pheromone. *Proc. Natl. Acad. Sci. U.S.A.* 75:3479–3483, 1978.
36. Raycroft, R.E., and Zimmerman, L.N.: New mode of genetic transfer in *Streptococcus faecalis* var. *liquefaciens.J. Bacteriol.* 87:799-801, 1964.
37. Courvalin, P.M., Shaw, W.V., and Jacob, A.E.: Plasmid-mediated mechanisms of resistance to aminoglycoside-aminocyclitol antibiotics and to chloramphenicol in group D streptococci. *Antimicrob. Agents Chemother.* 13:716-725, 1978.
38. Miyamura, S.E., Ochiai, H., Nitahara, Y., Nakagawa, Y., and Terao, M.: Resistance mechanism of chloramphenicol in *Streptococcus haemolyticus, Streptococcus pneumoniae* and *Streptococcus faecalis. Microbiol. Immunol.* 21:69-76, 1977.
39. Dunny, G.M., and Clewell, D.B.: Transmissible toxin (hemolysin) plasmid in *Streptococcus faecalis* and its mobilization of a noninfectious drug resistance plasmid. *J. Bacteriol.* 124:784-790, 1975.

40. Yagi, Y., and Clewell, D.B.: Plasmide-determined tetracycline resistance in *Streptococcus faecalis:* tandemly repeated resistance determinants in amplified forms of pAMα1 DNA. *J. Mol. Biol.* 102:583-600, 1976.
41. Krogstad, D.J., Korfhagen, T.R., Moellering, R.C., Jr., Wennersten, C., and Swartz, M.N.: Plasmid-mediated resistance to antibiotic synergism in enterococci. *J. Clin. Invest.* 61:1645-1653, 1978.
42. Hunter, T.H.: Use of streptomycin in treatment of bacterial endocarditis. *Am. J. Med.* 2:436-442, 1949.
43. Jawetz, E., Gunnison, J.B., and Coleman, V.R.: The combined action of penicillin with streptomycin or chloromycetin on enterococci *in vitro. Science* 111:254-256, 1950.
44. Simon, H.J.: Antimicrobial susceptibility of group D hemolytic streptococci (enterococci). *Am. J. Med. Sci.* 253:14-18, 1967.
45. Basker, M.J., and Sutherland, R.: Activity of amoxycillin, alone and in combination with aminoglycoside antibiotics against streptococci associated with bacterial endocarditis. *J. Antimicrob. Chemother.* 3:273–282, 1977.
46. Gutschik, C., Jepsen, O.B., and Mortensen, I.: Effect of combinations of penicillin and aminoglycosides on *Streptococcus faecalis:* A comparative study of seven aminoglycoside antibiotics. *J. Infect. Dis.* 135:832–836, 1977.
47. Hartwick, H.J., Kalmanson, G.M., and Guze, L.B.: In vitro activity of ampicillin or vancomycin combined with gentamicin or streptomycin against enterococci. *Antimicrob. Agents Chemother.* 4:383–387, 1973.
48. Westenfelder, G.O., Paterson, P.Y., Reisberg, B.E., and Carlson, G.M.: Vancomycin – streptomycin synergism in enterococcal endocarditis. *J. Am. Med. Assoc.* 223:37–40, 1973.
49. Sanders, C.C.: Synergy of penicillin-netilmicin combinations against enterococci, including strains highly resistant to streptomycin or kanamycin. *Antimicrob. Agents Chemother.* 12:195–200, 1977.
50. Jawetz, E., and Sonne, M.S.: Penicillin-streptomycin treatment of enterococcal endocarditis. A re-evaluation. *N. Engl. J. Med.* 274: 710–715, 1966.
51. Wilkowskie, C.J., Facklam, R.R., Washington, J.A., II, and Geraci, J.E.: Antibiotic synergism: Enhanced susceptibility of group D streptococci to certain antibiotic combinations. *Antimicrob. Agents Chemother.* 1970: 195–200, 1971.
52. Watanakunakorn, C.: Penicillin combined with gentamicin or streptomycin: synergism against enterococci. *J. Infect. Dis.* 124:581–586, 1971.
53. Moellering. R.C., Jr., Wennersten, C., and Weinberg, A.N.: Synergy of penicillin and gentamicin against enterococci. *J. Infect. Dis.* 124 (suppl.): S207–S209, 1971.

54. Moellering, R.C., Jr., Wennersten, C., and Weinstein, A.J.: Penicillin-tobramycin synergism against enterococci: A comparison with penicillin and gentamicin. *Antimicrob. Agents Chemother.* 3:526–5269, 1973.
55. Russell, E.J., and Sutherland, R.: Activity of amoxycillin against enterococci and synergism with aminoglycoside antibiotics. *J. Med. Microbiol.* 8:1–10, 1975.
56. McCracken, G.H., Nelson, J.D., and Thomas, M.L.: Discrepancy between carbenicillin- and ampicillin activity against enterococcocci and listeria. *Antimicrob. Agents Chemother.* 3:343–349, 1973.
57. Moellering, R.C., Jr.: Antimicrobial synergism -- an elusive concept. *J. Infect. Dis.* 140:639–641, 1979.
58. Matsumoto, J.Y., Wilson, W.R., and Washington, J.A. Synergy of penicillin and decreasing concentrations of aminoglycosides against enterococci from patients with endocarditis. Abstracts 11th International Congress of Chemotherapy and 19th Interscience Conference on Antimicrobial Agents and Chemotherapy. Abstract #363, 1979.
59. Soriano, F., and Greenwood, D.: Action and interaction of penicillin and gentamicin on enterococci. *J. Clin. Pathol.* 32:1174–1179, 1979.
60. Glew, R.H., and Moellering, R.C., Jr.: Effect of protein binding on the activity of penicillin in combination with gentamicin against enterococci. *Antimicrob. Agents Chemother.* 15:87–92, 1979.
61. Miles, C.P., Coleman, V.R., Gunnison, J.B., and Jawetz, E.: Antibiotic synergism requires simultaneous presence of both members of a synergistic drug pair. *Proc. Soc. Exp. Biol. Med.* 78:738–741, 1951.
62. Hewitt, W.L., Seligman, S.J., and Deigh, R.A.: Kinetics of the synergism of penicillin-streptomycin and penicillin-kanamycin for enterococci and its relationship to L-phase variants. *J. Lab. Clin. Med.* 67:792–807, 1966.
63. Standiford, H.C., deMaine, J.B., and Kirby, W.M.M.: Antibiotic synergism of enterococci: relation to inhibitory concentrations. *Arch. Intern. Med.* 126:255–259, 1970.
64. Moellering, R.C., Jr., Wennersten, C., Medrek, T., and Weinberg, A.N.: Prevalence of high-level resistance to aminoglycosides in clinical isolates of enterococci. *Antimicrob. Agents Chemother.* 1970: 335–340, 1971.
65. Ruhen, R.W., and Darrell, J.H.: Antibiotic synergism against group D streptococci in the treatment of endocarditis. *Med. J. Austral.* 2:114–116, 1973.
66. Zimmermann, R.A., Moellering, R.C., Jr., and Weinberg, A.N.: Mechanism of resistance to antibiotic synergism in enterococci. *J. Bacteriol.* 105: 873–879, 1971.

67. Krogstad, D.J., Korfhagen, T.R., Moellering, R.C., Jr., Wennersten, C., Swartz, M.N., Perzynski, S., and Davies, J.: Aminoglycoside-inactivating enzymes in clinical isolates of *Streptococcus faecalis:* an explanation for resistance to antibiotic synergism. *J. Clin. Invest.* 62:480–486, 1978.
68. Slocombe, B.: Transmissible aminoglycoside resistance in *Streptococcus faecalis. Current Chemotherapy 1978.* pp. 891–893.
69. Horodniceanu, T., Bouqueleret, L., El-Solh, N., Bieth, G., and Delbos, F.: High-level, plasmid-borne resistance to gentamicin in *Streptococcus faecalis* subsp. *zymogenes. Antimicrob. Agents Chemother.* 16:686–689, 1979.
70. Wennersten, C.B., and Moellering, R.C., Jr.: Mechanism of resistance to penicillin-aminoglycoside synergism in *Streptococcus faecium. Current Chemotherapy* (in press).

Donald Kaye, M.D.

7

TREATMENT OF ENTEROCOCCAL ENDOCARDITIS IN EXPERIMENTAL ANIMALS AND IN MAN

Infective endocarditis caused by enterococci deserves special attention. Enterococci are much more resistant to penicillin than are other streptococci, and the therapeutic approach to enterococcal endocarditis differs from the management of endocarditis caused by more penicillin-susceptible streptococci.

In recent years, experimental models of enterococcal endocarditis have been developed and used to evaluate certain therapeutic principles. In addition, significant changes have occurred in the susceptibility of enterococci to aminoglycosides which have raised questions about which antibiotic regimens constitute optimal therapy.

Animal Studies

The studies of therapy of enterococcal endocarditis in animals have mainly focused on the effectiveness of penicillins, vancomycin, and cephalosporins alone and in combination with aminoglycosides.

The first therapeutic animal study of enterococcal endocarditis was that of Sapico et al.[1] Using a dog model of *Streptococcus faecalis* endocarditis (with an enterococcus inhibited by 6.2 μg/ml penicillin and 400 μg/ml streptomycin), they demonstrated that single doses of streptomycin alone had no effect in reducing the level of bacteremia.

However, single doses of penicillin plus streptomycin produced a more rapid and more sustained drop in the bacteremia than penicillin alone.

Several investigators[2–4] have used a rabbit model of enterococcal endocarditis. They reported a clear advantage of penicillin plus an aminoglycoside over penicillin alone in reducing the number of enterococci in vegetations. Furthermore, they demonstrated that when the enterococci were susceptible to streptomycin (inhibited by 125 μg/ml) the advantage of adding streptomycin was present. However, when the strains were resistant to streptomycin (not inhibited by 7500 μg/ml) there was no consistent advantage in adding streptomycin (although in some experiments there was an advantage). The rate of killing of both the streptomycin-sensitive and streptomycin-resistant strains was more rapid with penicillin plus gentamicin, sisomicin or netilmicin than penicillin alone. There were no differences between streptomycin, gentamicin, sisomicin or netilmicin when added to penicillin in treatment of endocarditis caused by streptomycin-sensitive *S. faecalis.* Similarly, there were no differences between gentamicin, sisomicin or netilmicin when added to penicillin in treatment of streptomycin-resistant *S. faecalis* endocarditis. Table I is abstracted from one of these experiments[3] and shows the added effect of streptomycin against a streptomycin-susceptible strain and its lack of effect against a streptomycin-resistant strain. Gentamicin was effective against both strains.

Table 1. Colony Forming Units (CFU) of Enterococci in Vegetation (mean $\log_{10}$ CFU/g)*+

	Streptomycin-sensitive (MIC - 125 μg/ml)	Streptomycin-resistant (MIC —>7500 μ g/ml)
Penicillin	4.9	4.5
Penicillin plus streptomycin	2.3	4.1
Penicillin plus gentamicin	2.3	1.5

*Adapted from Carrizosa and Kaye[3]

+Therapy started 24 hours after infection and continued for 9 days.

In these studies[2] streptomycin added to vancomycin increased the rate of killing of streptomycin-sensitive enterococci in vegetations as compared with vancomycin alone. No differences were found between penicillin alone and vancomycin alone or between penicillin plus streptomycin and vancomycin plus streptomycin. In all of these reports[2–4] there was an excellent correlation between results of *in vitro* and *in vivo* experiments. When addition of an aminoglycoside to penicillin increased the rate of killing of enterococci *in vitro,* the same effect was reproducibly noted *in vivo.* When there was no *in vitro* effect, the *in vivo* effect was absent or inconsistent.

The more therapy was delayed after induction of endocarditis (6 hours, 24 hours or 3 days), the longer therapy had to be prolonged to sterilize vegetations.[3] With a delay of six hours, many vegetations were sterile after three days of penicillin plus aminoglycoside therapy. With a delay of 24 hours few vegetations were sterile even after nine days of penicillin plus aminoglycoside therapy. Furthermore, a shorter period of time before initiation of therapy seemed to increase the effect of addition of streptomycin to penicillin in treatment of streptomycin-resistant enterococcal endocarditis.

The peak blood levels of penicillin and aminoglycosides achieved in these studies were comparable to those achieved in humans with therapeutic doses (penicillin 15–32 μg/ml, streptomycin 12–43 μg/ml and gentamicin 9–12 μg/ml).

It has been demonstrated that *S. faecium* is much more resistant to kanamycin, netilmicin and tobramycin than *S. faecalis.*[5] Penicillin in combination with these aminoglycosides does not show a more rapid bactericidal effect against any *S. faecium* strains than penicillin alone. However, all of the strains are killed more rapidly with the addition of gentamicin to penicillin. These same effects were noted in the rabbit model of endocarditis.[5] A *S. faecium* strain that was inhibited by 31 μg/ml gentamicin, 125 μg/ml streptomycin and 250 μg/ml netilmicin was used to produce endocarditis. Penicillin plus streptomycin and penicillin plus gentamicin were equally effective in reducing titers of bacteria in vegetations more rapidly than penicillin alone or penicillin plus netilmicin, which were equivalent in efficacy.

Weinstein and Lentnek[6] and Abrutyn et al. [7] studied the effect of cephalosporins plus gentamicin on enterococcal endocarditis in rabbits. The enterococcus was inhibited by 26 μg/ml cephalothin and 24 μg/ml cefazolin. *In vitro* synergistic killing was demonstrated with these concentrations plus gentamicin. When the rabbits were treated, enterococcal vegetations could be sterilized with cephalothin or cefazolin plus gentamicin. However, in order to achieve 100% sterilization, peak serum levels were required that were 10-fold higher than the minimal inhibitory concentration for the enterococcus. These levels were achieved with doses of 500 mg/kg of cephalothin intramuscularly four times a day but not with 200 mg/kg four times a day. Doses of 40 mg/kg of cefazolin gave peak levels in serum that were 4.5 times the minimal inhibitory concentration. These doses of cefazolin plus gentamicin four times a day were incapable of sterilizing all vegetations. Extrapolating from these data, doses of cephalothin or cefazolin that give peak serum levels of 250–500 μg/ml (10 times the minimal inhibitory concentration for most enterococci) might be effective in enterococcal endocarditis in man in combination with an aminoglycoside. However, these serum concentrations do not take the protein binding of these cephalosporins into account and much higher concentrations might actually be required.

In contrast to the results with cephalosporins, Weinstein and Lentnek sterilized all vegetations with doses of penicillin of 250,000 units/kg plus gentamicin three times a day. Serum levels of penicillin peaked at 62 units/ml, which was 15 times the minimal inhibitory concentration of the enterococcus.

Lincoln et al.[8] studied the effect of nafcillin, oxacillin and methicillin plus gentamicin in therapy of enterococcal endocarditis in rabbits. The minimal inhibitory concentrations for the enterococcus were 3.2, 12.5, and 25 μg/ml for nafcillin, oxacillin and methicillin, respectively. An *in vitro* synergistic bactericidal effect could be demonstrated with each of these penicillins combined with gentamicin. Doses of these penicillins of 42.5 mg/kg intramuscularly four times a day plus gentamicin were ineffective in treatment of endocarditis. Doses of 85 mg/kg four times a day plus gentamicin were more effective but failed to sterilize all vegetations. Peak serum concentrations at least ten times the minimal inhibitory concentration were achieved only with nafcillin at a dose of 85 mg/kg. However, these minimal inhibitory concentrations did not take protein binding into account, and the protein binding of nafcillin is about 90%.

Carrizosa et al.[9] studied the minimal concentration of gentamicin required for bactericidal synergism with penicillin using an enterococcus that was resistant to 2,000 μg/ml of streptomycin. Vegetations from rabbits with enterococcal endocarditis were incubated *in vitro* in broth with penicillin alone or penicillin plus gentamicin. At least 3 μg/ml of gentamicin was required along with penicillin to sterilize vegetations; 1.6 μg/ml of gentamicin was inadequate. In contrast, broth cultures of enterococci were sterilized with penicillin plus 0.75 μg/ml gentamicin. Thus 4-fold higher concentrations of gentamicin were required to sterilize vegetations than to sterilize broth cultures of enterococci.

These studies in animals indicate that adding an aminoglycoside to penicillin markedly increased the rate of sterilization of vegetations in experimental enterococcal endocarditis. If the enterococcus were resistant to 2,000 μg/ml of streptomycin, *in vivo* synergistic killing activity was generally not present with streptomycin but was with gentamicin. *S. faecium* tended to show *in vivo* synergistic killing with penicillin plus gentamicin but not penicillin plus kanamycin, netilmicin, sisomicin, or tobramycin.

Cephalosporins and penicillinase-resistant penicillins were far less effective than penicillin or vancomycin in treatment of experimental enterococcal endocarditis. It seems from all of the studies that, for sterilization of the vegetation, peak serum concentrations of a penicillin or cephalosporin are required that are at least 10-fold higher than the minimal inhibitory concentration.

It is likely that the true required ratio is a serum level of free antibiotic (not protein bound) that is 4 to 8-fold greater than the minimal inhibitory concentration in broth. The required serum concentration of aminoglycoside is also a multiple of the amount necessary to demonstrate a synergistic killing effect *in vitro.* In the case of gentamicin, the required serum concentration is at least 4-fold higher than the *in vitro* concentration needed for a synergistic killing effect. Protein binding is not a factor with aminoglycosides which have very low binding capacities but may be a very important factor with some penicillinase-resistant penicillins and cephalosporins which are very highly protein bound.

Clinical Experience

Penicillin alone and with streptomycin. Results with treatment of enterococcal endocarditis were poor with penicillin alone even with use of relatively large daily doses.[10–12] Although occasional cures were reported, most patients relapsed when the penicillin was discontinued. Hunter in 1947[13] first reported the successful use of concurrent penicillin and streptomycin in the treatment of enterococcal endocarditis. Robbins and Tompsett[11] and Cates et al[14] in 1951 reported 5 of 9 patients and 3 of 3 patients respectively with enterococcal endocarditis cured with combined penicillin and streptomycin therapy. Most of the successfully treated patients received at least 6 weeks of combination therapy. Additional series were subsequently reported by Geraci and Martin[15], Koenig and Kaye[16], Vogler et al[17], Jawetz and Sonne[18], and Mandell et al[12] clearly indicating the efficacy of penicillin plus streptomycin therapy in enterococcal endocarditis. Most of the patients cured were treated with about 20,000,000 units of penicillin daily plus 1–2 grams of streptomycin daily for 6 weeks. Cure rates with penicillin plus streptomycin in these later series approximated 85%. Geraci and Martin[15] cured 12 of the last 14 (86%) patients treated and Mandell et al[12] (incorporating the cases of Robbins and Tompsett[11] and Koenig and Kaye[16]) cured 83%.

Penicillin plus streptomycin versus penicillin plus gentamicin. It is unclear if penicillin plus streptomycin is inadequate therapy for cure of enterococcal endocarditis caused by enterococci that are resistant to 2000 μg/ml of streptomycin (i.e. enterococci not synergistically killed with penicillin plus streptomycin). Standiford et al[19] and Moellering et al[20] in 1970 reported that these isolates constituted 40% of all blood isolates of enterococci. However, despite the high prevalence of these strains, Tompsett and Berman[21] in 1977 could find only three clear-cut failures of penicillin and streptomycin therapy in the literature. They also reported one case of their own that failed on four weeks of vancomycin and streptomycin and was retreated with penicillin and streptomycin only to relapse again. It is of interest that their failure was with an enterococcus that did not have high level streptomycin resistance and in fact demonstrated *in vitro* synergistic killing with penicillin plus streptomycin. They also cited a cure with penicillin and streptomycin of a patient whose enterococcus grew in 100,000 μg/ml streptomycin.

Roberts[22] reported that all fourteen of his patients with enterococcal endocarditis seen from 1970–1977 were treated with penicillin plus streptomycin. Despite the fact that 30–40% were highly resistant to streptomycin, there was no difference in clinical course between the patients who were infected with streptomycin-sensitive strains and highly resistant strains.

It is very difficult to evaluate the efficacy of penicillin plus streptomycin in patients infected with highly streptomycin-resistant enterococci. The streptomycin might be adding nothing to the regimen. Some patients can be cured with penicillin alone [15] and the exact percent is unknown. The older studies, in which penicillin alone was often ineffective, used smaller doses of penicillin daily than are used now. It is possible that with current dosage (e.g. 20 million units daily), penicillin alone might cure an appreciable number of patients. Furthermore, it is likely that the highly streptomycin-resistant strains have been causing infection only in relatively recent years and that endocarditis caused by these organisms is a new problem.

Enterococci are clearly becoming more resistant to streptomycin. In a series of reports from the same institution: only 2 of 18 strains isolated prior to 1960 were resistant to 50 μg/ml of streptomycin[16]; 7 of 19 strains isolated from 1958–1968 were resistant to 50 μg/ml[12]; and 30–40% of strains isolated after 1970 were highly resistant to streptomycin (i.e. resistant to 2000 μg/ml).[22]

There have been few published reports of the use of penicillin or ampicillin plus gentamicin in therapy of enterococcal endocarditis. Weinstein and Moellering[23] reported 4 cases of enterococcal endocarditis treated successfully with penicillin and gentamicin given for 25 to 42 days. The dose of gentamicin was 60 mg every 8 hours in three patients and 100 mg every 8 hours in one patient. In a study by El-Khatib et al[24], 13 heroin addicts were treated with penicillin plus gentamicin 3 mg/kg/day. Nine were cured and 4 died. Serra et al[25] successfully treated 7 patients with enterococcal endocarditis with penicillin or ampicillin combined with gentamicin. The usual dose of gentamicin was 40 mg every 8 hours.

Recently Wilson et al[26] reported 17 patients with enterococcal endocarditis caused by highly streptomycin-resistant enterococci (over 2000 μg/ml streptomycin for inhibition). Seven patients received penicillin plus 3 mg/kg gentamicin or less each day and 2 relapsed. Ten patients received penicillin plus more than 3 mg/kg gentamicin each day and 1 relapsed. All 3 relapses were retreated with penicillin plus gentamicin and 2 relapsed again; one died while the other was cured with ampicillin plus streptomycin. A relapse rate of 3/17 patients (18%) or 5/20 treatment courses (25%) is much higher than has ever been reported with penicillin plus streptomycin and is very disturbing. These results suggest either that penicillin plus gentamicin would not be as effective therapy as penicillin plus streptomycin in streptomycin-susceptible enterococcal endocarditis or that streptomycin-resistant enterococcal endocarditis is much more refractory to therapy with penicillin plus an aminoglycoside than streptomycin-sensitive enterococcal endocarditis.

Animal data[9] suggest that serum gentamicin levels of at least 3 μg/ml would be required for synergistic bactericidal activity in the vegetation. In the study by Wilson et al, mean peak gentamicin concentrations were 3.3 μg/ml in those who received 3 mg/kg or less each day and 5 μg/ml in those who received more than 3 mg/kg each day. While the range of peaks was not given, it is likely that many of these patients had peaks of less than 3 μg/ml and therefore had inadequate gentamicin levels for synergistic activity.

Of special interest is the recent report of Moellering et al[27] of a patient with enterococcal endocarditis who relapsed twice after courses of ampicillin and gentamicin. She was cured by using tobramycin as the aminoglycoside. Although the enterococcus was not highly resistant to streptomycin or gentamicin, these aminoglycosides did not show a synergistic *in vitro* bactericidal effect. This lack of aminoglycoside effect was apparently due to a defect in intracellular transport of the aminoglycoside. In contrast tobramycin did demonstrate a synergistic bactericidal effect. Although this strain is to date unique, its existence suggests the need for tests of *in vitro* synergism for all isolates of enterococci from patients with endocarditis.

Ampicillin. When ampicillin became available, it was noted to be slightly more active *in vitro* against enterococci than penicillin G. (The minimal inhibitory concentrations of ampicillin for enterococci were usually about one-half of the minimal inhibitory concentrations of pencillin G). Therefore, ampicillin was evaluated alone in the treatment of enterococcal endocarditis. Cures of enterococcal endocarditis have been reported with ampicillin alone.[28–31] However, failures have also occurred.[12,32] At present, the evidence suggests that enterococcal endocarditis should not be routinely treated with ampicillin alone.

Vancomycin. Vancomycin is accepted as the substitute antibiotic of choice in treatment of enterococcal endocarditis if penicillin or ampicillin cannot be given. However, there have been very few published reports evaluating vancomycin in therapy of enterococcal endocarditis. Friedberg et al[33] in 1968 reported four cures in patients with enterococcal endocarditis treated with vancomycin without a companion aminoglycoside. Subsequently, there have been three reports of 3 patients with enterococcal endocarditis treated and cured with vancomycin plus streptomycin[34–36] and a report of 2 cured with vancomycin plus gentamicin.[37] The dose of vancomycin was usually 2 grams a day and therapy was continued for 4–6 weeks. The problem with these reports is that there are few patients studied and that some of these received penicillin for varying periods of time prior to onset of vancomycin therapy. Therefore, from the published reports, it is very difficult to develop firm conclusions about the relative usefulness of vancomycin alone or with an aminoglycoside in enterococcal endocarditis.

Oral therapy. Oral therapy of enterococcal endocarditis with penicillin (with or without an aminoglycoside) has been almost uniformly unsuccessful. However, cures have been reported with use of oral amoxicillin plus a parenteral aminoglycoside. Seligman[38] used amoxicillin in doses of 6 grams daily (together with intramuscular gentamicin) and cured one patient, but the valve was resected making it difficult to evaluate the efficacy of the antibiotic therapy. Lidji et al[39] cured one patient with 24 grams of amoxicillin daily plus intramuscular streptomycin. This approach should be reserved for extraordinary cases where parenteral therapy is impossible. Very large doses must be used and adequate serum levels should be demonstrated.

Duration of therapy. The duration of therapy of enterococcal endocarditis with penicillin plus an aminoglycoside has generally been six weeks. However, Tompsett and Berman[21] have argued that four weeks of therapy is sufficient. They cured nine patients with four weeks of therapy and had no relapses. Geraci and Martin[15] also cured two patients with only four weeks of therapy. There were also at least two relapses following a four week course of penicillin and dihydrostreptomycin. It must be noted, however, that Geraci and Martin used smaller doses of penicillin than would be currently accepted (i.e. 5–10 million units a day were used). It is possible that four weeks of therapy may be as effective as six weeks of treatment.

The penicillin-allergic patient. In the penicillin-allergic patient, several approaches have been used in treatment of enterococcal endocarditis. Substitution of a cephalosporin for penicillin is not an acceptable alternative because of the high concentrations of cephalosporins required to inhibit enterococci. Furthermore, cephalosporins in combination with streptomycin have been unsuccessful in treatment of enterococcal endocarditis.[40] The two successful methods of treating enterococcal endocarditis in the penicillin-allergic patient are: 1) "desensitization" with penicillin and 2) use of vancomycin.

The "desensitization" procedure may actually desensitize to penicillin. However, it is possible that it does little more than provide the safety measure of skin testing with increasing amounts of penicillin. Therefore, a minor reaction will be noted before a potentially fatal anaphylactic reaction occurs. At any rate, this approach has been successful in the vast majority of patients with a history of hypersensitivity to penicillin. A detailed protocol for densitization to penicillin may be found in Chapter 14.

The use of vancomycin with an aminoglycoside as already discussed is the only other antibiotic regimen of proven efficacy available for treatment of enterococcal endocarditis.

Serum bactericidal activity. The serum bactericidal test (Chapter 15) has been used as a parameter of adequacy of therapy of enterococcal endocarditis. However, the methods used to determine serum bactericidal activity and the time at which the activity is measured have varied from report to report. A bactericidal titer of 1:4 to 1:10 seems to be predictive of adequate therapy.[12,18,25,26,34] While most seem to measure peak serum bactericidal activity, some investigators have measured the serum bactericidal titers at the nadir of serum concentrations. High serum bactericidal activity at the point of lowest serum concentrations obviously indicates even higher bactericidal activity at the point of peak concentrations. However, poor serum bactericidal activity at the nadir does not necessarily indicate inadequate therapy. For example, 3 of the 8 cures reported by Moellering et al[37] had nadir serum bactericidal activity titers of 1:2 or less.

It would seem most reasonable to use a 99.9% kill after 24 hours of incubation or sterilization of $10^4 - 10^5$ enterococci/ml after 48 hours of incubation as a criterion for bactericidal activity and to measure this at the time of anticipated peak serum bactericidal activity. My preference is for complete sterilization after 48 hours because of the observation that some cultures not demonstrating a 99.9% kill after 24 hours will be sterile at 48 hours. A 1:8 serum bactericidal activity, as used by many investigators, seems to be a reasonable parameter of adequate therapy. Using this approach the penicillin or ampicillin should be given by continuous drip or in divided doses every four hours. Vancomycin should be administered every six hours, streptomycin every 12 hours, and gentamicin every eight hours.

Side effects of therapeutic agents. Skin rashes and other manifestations of hypersensitivity are common in patients treated for enterococcal endocarditis with penicillin or ampicillin. In general, about 10% of patients receiving penicillin G for a period of weeks develop hypersensitivity reactions. The series of Mandell et al[12] is typical; these investigators reported penicillin hypersensitivity in 13% of their 38 patients. Most investigators seem to continue penicillin in the face of drug fever and rash while attempting to control the rash with antihistamines or if necessary corticosteroids.

Vancomycin, which was at one time reported to commonly cause severe thrombophlebitis and fever, nephrotoxicity, and hearing loss [36], seems to be well tolerated in recently reported series. [33,36,37] The change is probably related to differences in manufacturing. [36] Only two of 25 patients treated with vancomycin in these series developed a rise in serum creatinine (which was reversible). Rash, phlebitis or fever related to vancomycin were noted in three patients each out of 25. Three of ten patients observed with serial audiograms developed high frequency hearing loss which was reversible in one. [36] The hearing loss was associated with renal insufficiency in all three patients (serum creatinines of 1.3 – 1.6 mg/100 ml). The development of renal insufficiency requires lowering the vancomycin dose to amounts that achieve peak serum bactericidal levels of 1:8.

Mandell et al[12] reported vestibular toxic side effects in eight of 36 patients (22%) who received streptomycin. All received at least two grams of streptomycin daily for at least 14 days before onset of symptoms. In contrast, Tompsett[41] using 20 mg/kg per day of streptomycin (and never more than one gram) for four weeks reported no vestibular toxicity; when renal insufficiency was present, he reduced the dose. This 20 mg/kg dose of streptomycin in patients with normal renal function is unlikely to result in vestibular toxicity. In the presence of renal insufficiency, adjustment of the dose to yield peak serum concentrations of about 15–30 μg/ml is likely to result in bactericidal activity in serum at a 1:8 dilution (together with penicillin) and unlikely to cause eighth nerve toxicity.

Gentamicin resulted in a rise in serum creatinine in only one of nine patients treated with this agent in one series[37] and none of seven patients in another series.[25] However, in a large series, Wilson et al[26] reported a rise in serum creatinine in most patients treated with gentamicin. The serum creatinine rose by at least 0.5 mg/100 ml (mean 0.85 mg/100 ml) in 2/9 patients receiving 3 mg/kg or less gentamicin daily and in all 11 patients (mean 1.35 mg/100 ml) receiving more than 3 mg/kg of gentamicin daily. The mean time to rise of creatinine was 13.5 days in the lower dose group and 10.4 days in the higher dose group.

Mortality Rate. The mortality rate in treated patients with enterococcal endocarditis has varied in different series. In 1970 Mandell et al[12] reported an 83% cure rate in 36 patients treated with penicillin or ampicillin plus streptomycin. None of these patients had cardiac surgery and in fact with valve replacement the mortality rate probably would have been lower than the 17% observed. In more recent series, Serra et al[25] cured all seven patients treated with penicillin or ampicillin from 1972–1976. The reported experience in two series of narcotic addicts with enterococcal endocarditis treated from 1970–1974 [24,31] revealed mortality rates of 2/11 (18%) and 4/13 (31%) for a combined rate of 25%. At least three of the patients who were cured required valve replacement. In contrast to these mortality rates is the experience of Moellering et al[37], who treated a series of patients from 1964–1973. In 14 whom the investigators felt were treated appropriately, the mortality rate was 43%, and three of the eight cures required valve replacement. However, the investigators stressed that most of the deaths occurred in patients with other serious underlying diseases, and in two, death was caused by *Candida* endocarditis secondary to super-infection from intravenous catheters. All of the series concluded that deaths from enterococcal endocarditis do not result from uncontrolled infection when therapy is with adequate doses of penicillin, ampicillin or vancomycin in combination with an aminoglycoside. Deaths occur mainly from heart failure, emboli, rupture of mycotic aneurysms, superinfection, or underlying disease. It is my feeling that the cure rate of enterococcal endocarditis should approach that of non-enterococcal streptococcal endocarditis (85–90% in my experience) with appropriate use of valve replacement.

Conclusions and Recommendations

With present information, it seems that either streptomycin or gentamicin can be used when enterococci are inhibited by 2000 μg/ml or less of streptomycin (Table 2). The decision can be made on the basis of whether vestibular toxicity (more likely with streptomycin) or nephrotoxicity (more likely with gentamicin) might be of greater consequence in the particular patient being treated. If the enterococcus is not inhibited by 2000 μg/ml streptomycin, gentamicin is probably preferable therapy. My own preference is streptomycin for strains that are inhibited by 2000 μg/ml streptomycin. Vestibular toxicity can be diminished by achieving peak streptomycin serum levels of 15–30 μg/ml and avoiding levels above 30 μg/ml. However, peak gentamicin serum levels of at least 3μg/ml seem to be necessary for adequate bactericidal activity[9] and nephrotoxicity is common with these levels.[26] The recent report of Moellering et al[27] serves as a *caveat* against the choice of an aminoglycoside based only on *in vitro* susceptibility testing and strongly suggests the need for *in vitro* tests of synergism in enterococcal endocarditis.

A duration of 4 weeks of therapy may be adequate for treatment of most patients with enterococcal endocarditis using the penicillin (or ampicillin)-aminoglycoside regimen. Six weeks of treatment might be considered in patients with complicated courses. While insufficient information is available concerning duration of therapy for prosthetic valve enterococcal endocarditis, six to eight weeks would seem to be reasonable.

The doses for treatment of enterococcal endocarditis should be at least 20 million units of penicillin, 12 grams of ampicillin, 1 gram of streptomycin and 3 mg/kg body weight of gentamicin each day. The ampicillin and penicillin are given intravenously by continuous drip or every 4 hours. The streptomycin is given intramuscularly every 12 hours and the gentamicin intramuscularly or intravenously in equal, divided doses every 8 hours. It is my preference to use penicillin G rather than ampicillin even though ampicillin is somewhat more active *in vitro* than penicillin. This is because of my impression that rash is more likely to occur with ampicillin than penicillin G.

In the penicillin-allergic patient (Table 3), desensitization with penicillin should be the first approach. If this is unsuccessful, therapy with vancomycin, 500 mg every 6 hours, plus streptomycin or gentamicin (if the enterococcus is resistant to 2000 μg/ml streptomycin) should be used.

The use of serum bactericidal activity as a parameter of adequacy of therapy has not been demonstrated to be completely reliable in any form of endocarditis. However, it is the only criterion available that seems to correlate with bacteriologic response both in the experimental model and in patients. Experimental data seem to indicate that peak serum activity should be bactericidal for the infecting enterococcus at a 1:8 or greater dilution.

Table 2. Therapy of Enterococcal Endocarditis in the Patient Who Is Not Hypersensitive to Penicillin

Antibiotic	Dosage	Route	Duration	Comments
Penicillin G*	20 million units daily	IV by continuous drip or every four hours in divided doses	4–6 weeks	
Plus				
Streptomycin +	0.5 gram every 12 hours	IM	4–6 weeks	Causes vestibular toxicity
Or				
Gentamicin +	1 mg/kg every 8 hours	IM or IV	4–6 weeks	Causes nephro-and ototoxicity

* Ampicillin 2 grams every 4 hours IM or IV may be substituted for penicillin G but may cause more rashes.

\+ Gentamicin is used when the susceptibility of the enterococcus to streptomycin is unknown or when the enterococcus is resistant to 2000 μg/ml streptomycin. Streptomycin or gentamicin can be used if the enterococcus is susceptible to 2000 μg/ml streptomycin.

Table 3. Therapy of Enterococcal Endocarditis in the Patient Who is Hypersensitive to Penicillin

Antibiotic	Dosage	Route	Duration	Comments
Attempt desensitization to Penicillin and use Table 2				Should not be attempted in patients who have had anaphylaxis or other immediate type hypersensitivity reactions to penicillin
Vancomycin	0.5 gram every six hours	IV	4—6 weeks	Causes thrombophlebitis, 8th nerve toxicity, and occasionally, nephrotoxicity
Plus				
Streptomycin*	0.5 gram every 12 hours	IM	4—6 weeks	Causes vestibular toxicity
Or				
Gentamicin*	1 mg/kg every 8 hours	IM or IV	4—6 weeks	Causes nephro-and ototoxicity

* Gentamicin is used when the susceptibility of the enterococcus to streptomycin is unknown or when the enterococcus is resistant to 2000 μg/ml streptomycin. Streptomycin or gentamicin can be used if the enterococcus is susceptible to 2000 μg/ml streptomycin.

REFERENCES

1. Sapico, F.L., Keys, T.F. and Hewitt, W.L.: Experimental Enterococcal Endocarditis. II. Study of in Vivo Synergism of Penicillin and Streptomycin. Amer. J. Med. Sci. 263:128, 1972.
2. Hook, E.W., Roberts, R.B. and Sande, M.A.: Antimicrobial Therapy of Experimental Enterococcal Endocarditis. Antimic. Ag. Chemother. 8:564, 1975.
3. Carrizosa, J. and Kaye, D.: Antibiotic Synergism in Enterococcal Endocarditis. J. Lab. Clin. Med. 88:132, 1976.
4. Carrizosa, J. and Kaye, D.: Penicillin and Netilmicin in Treatment of Experimental Enterococcal Endocarditis. Antimic. Ag. Chemother. 13:505, 1978.
5. Moellering, R.C., Korzeniowski, O.M., Sande, M.A. and Wennersten, C.B.: Species-Specific Resistance to Antimicrobial Synergism in *Streptococcus faecium* and *Streptococcus faecalis.* J. Inf. Dis. 140:203, 1979.
6. Weinstein, A.J. and Lentnek, A.L.: Cephalosporin—Aminoglycoside Synergism in Experimental Enterococcal Endocarditis. Antimic. Ag. Chemother. 9:983, 1976.
7. Abrutyn, E., Lincoln, L., Gallagher, M. and Weinstein, A.J.: Cephalothin-Gentamicin Synergism in Experimental Enterococcal Endocarditis. J. Antimicrobial Chemotherapy. 4:153, 1978.
8. Lincoln, L.J., Weinstein, A.J., Gallagher, M. and Abrutyn, E.: Penicillinase-Resistant Penicillins Plus Gentamicin in Experimental Enterococcal Endocarditis. Antimicrob. Ag. Chemother. 12:484, 1977.
9. Carrizosa, J., Trestman, I.J. and Levison, M.E.: Minimal Concentrations of Gentamicin for Synergy with Penicillin in Enterococcal Endocarditis. Clin. Res. 27:341A, 1979.
10. Loewe, L., Candel, S. and Eiber, H.B.: Therapy of Subacute Enterococcus *(Streptococcus fecalis)* Endocarditis. Ann. Int. Med. 34:717, 1951.
11. Robbins, W.C. and Tompsett, R.: Treatment of Enterococcal Endocarditis and Bacteremia. Results of Combined Therapy with Penicillin and Streptomycin. Am. J. Med. 10:278, 1951.
12. Mandell, G.L., Kaye, D., Levison, M.E. and Hook, E.W.: Enterococcal Endocarditis. An Analysis of 38 Patients Observed at the New York Hospital - Cornell Medical Center. Arch. Int. Med. 125:258, 1970.
13. Hunter, T.H.: Use of Streptomycin in Treatment of Bacterial Endocarditis Am. J. Med. 2:436, 1947.
14. Cates, J.E., Christie, R.V. and Garrod, L.P.: Penicillin - Resistant Subacute Bacterial Endocarditis Treated by a Combination of Penicillin and Streptomycin. Brit. Med. J. 1:653, 1951.

15. Geraci, J.E. and Martin, W.J.: Antibiotic Therapy of Bacterial Endocarditis. VI. Subacute Enterococcal Endocarditis: Clinical, Pathologic and Therapeutic Consideration of 33 Cases. Circulation 10:173, 1954.
16. Koenig, G.M. and Kaye, D.: Enterococcal Endocarditis. Report of Nineteen Cases With Long-term Follow-up Data. N. Eng. J. Med. 264:257, 1961.
17. Vogler, W.R., Dorney, E.R. and Bridges, H.A.: Bacterial Endocarditis. Am. J. Med. 32:910, 1962.
18. Jawetz, E., and Sonne, M.: Penicillin-Streptomycin Treatment of Enterococcal Endocarditis. A Reevaluation. N. Eng. J. Med. 274:710, 1966.
19. Standiford, H.D., deMaine, H.B., Kirby, W.M.M.: Antibiotic Synergism of Enterococci. Arch. Int. Med. 126:255, 1970.
20. Moellering, R.C., Jr., Wennensten, C., Medrek, T. et al.: Prevalence of High Level Resistance to Aminoglycosides in Clinical Isolates of Enterococci. Antimic. Ag. Chemother. 10:335, 1970.
21. Tompsett, R. and Berman, W.: Enterococcal Endocarditis: Duration and Mode of Treatment. Trans. Am. Clin. Clim. Assoc. 89:49, 1977.
22. Roberts, R.: Discussion of Enterococcal Endocarditis: Duration and Mode of Treatment. Trans. Am. Clin. Clim. Assoc. 89:56, 1977.
23. Weinstein, A.J. and Moellering, R.C.: Penicillin and Gentamicin Therapy for Enterococcal Infections. J.A.M.A. 223:1030, 1973.
24. El-Khatib, M.R., Wilson, F.M. and Lerner, A.M.: Characteristics of Bacterial Endocarditis in Heroin Addicts in Detroit. Am. J. Med. Sci. 271:197, 1976.
25. Serra, P., Brandimarte, C., Martino, P., Carlone, S. and Giunchi, G.S.: Synergistic Treatment of Enterococcal Endocarditis. In Vitro and in Vivo Studies Arch. Int. Med. 137:1562, 1977.
26. Wilson, W.R., Wilkowske, C.J., Thompson, R.L. and Geraci, J.E.: Treatment of Streptomycin-Resistant Enterococcal (SRE) Infective Endocarditis. (I.E.) 11th International Congress of Chemotherapy and 19th Interscience Conference on Antimicrobial Agents and Chemotherapy. Abstract 1063, October 1–5, 1979.
27. Moellering, R.C., Murray, B.E., Schoenbaum, S.C., Adler, J. and Wennersten, C.B. A novel mechanism of Resistance to Penicillin - Gentamicin Synergism in *Streptococcus faecalis*. J. Inf. Dis. 141:81, 1980.
28. Johnson, D.G., Barnes, J.A. and McLeod, E.: Subacute Bacterial Endocarditis Caused by *Streptococcus faecalis* and Successfully Treated with Ampicillin. Med. J. Australia 2:1026, 1965.
29. Beaty, H.N., Turck, M. and Petersdorf, R.G.: Ampicillin in the Treatment of Enterococcal Endocarditis. Ann. Intern. Med. 65:701, 1966.

30. Parker, R.H., and Hoeprich, P.D.: Parenteral Sodium Ampicillin Therapy of Endocarditis, Salmonellosis, and other Bacterial Infections. Antimicrob. Agents Chemother. 618, 1965.
31. Reiner, N.E., Gopalakrishna, K.V. and Lerner, P.I.: Enterococcal Endocarditis in Heroin Addicts. J.A.M.A. 235:1861, 1976.
32. Louria, D.: Discussion of Paper. Activity of Broad-Spectrum Antibiotics Against Enterococci and Their Efficacy in Enterococcal Endocarditis. Ann. N.Y. Acad. Sci. 145:471, 1967.
33. Friedberg, C.K., Rosen, K.M. and Bienstock, P.A.: Vancomycin Therapy for Enterococcal and *Streptococcus viridans* Endocarditis. Successful Treatment of Six Patients. Arch. Int. Med. 122:134, 1968.
34. Cook, F.V., Coddington, C.C., Wadland, W.C. and Farrar, W.E., Jr.: Treatment of Bacterial Endocarditis with Vancomycin. Am. J. Med. Sci. 276:153, 1978.
35. Westenfelder, G.O., Paterson, P.Y., Reisberg, B.E. and Carlson, G.M.: Vancomycin-Streptomycin Synergism in Enterococcal Endocarditis. J.A.M.A. 223:37, 1973.
36. Hook, E.W. III, and Johnson, W.D.: Vancomycin Therapy of Bacterial Endocarditis. Am. J. Med. 65:411, 1978.
37. Moellering, R.C., Jr., Watson, B.K. and Kunz, L.J.: Endocarditis Due to Group D Streptococci. Comparison of Disease Caused by *Streptococcus Bovis* with that Produced by the Enterococci. Am. J. Med. 57:239, 1974.
38. Seligman, S.J.: Treatment of Enterococcal Endocarditis with Oral Amoxicillin and Intramuscular Gentamicin. J. Inf. Dis. 129:S213, 1974.
39. Lidji, M., Rubinstein, E. and Samra, H.: Bacterial Endocarditis on a Prosthetic Valve. Oral Treatment with Amoxicillin. Chest. 74:224, 1978.
40. Rahal, J.J., Myers, P.R. and Weinstein, L.: Treatment of Bacterial Endocarditis with Cephalothin, New Eng. J. Med. 279:1305, 1968.
41. Tompsett, R.: Discussion of Enterococcal Endocarditis: Duration and Mode of Therapy. Trans. Am. Clin. Climatol. Assoc. 89:57, 1977.

Merle A. Sande, M.D.
Oksana M. Korzeniowski, M.D.

8

THE ANTIMICROBIAL THERAPY OF STAPHYLOCOCCAL ENDOCARDITIS

With the introduction of antibiotics in the 1940's and 1950's it became possible to cure patients with endocarditis caused by *Staphylococcus aureus.* Unfortunately while mortality rates initially dropped to 25 to 50% they have remained unchanged for the last 30 years.[1]

This lack of progress has prompted an extensive search for explanations of treatment failures and for new modes of therapy. Recent recommendations have included routine use of two drugs (a β-lactam antibiotic and an aminoglycoside) for all cases[2] and a more radical suggestion that all patients with staphylococcal endocarditis undergo surgery.[3]

This chapter will review the *in vitro, in vivo,* and clinical studies dealing with attempts to improve the antimicrobial therapy of this disease and present initial results on some aspects of a multicenter study designed to evaluate the potential value of combination (β-lactam plus aminoglycoside) therapy.

In Vitro Studies

The vast majority (80 to 90%) of strains of *S. aureus* causing endocarditis are resistant to penicillin G but nearly all remain sensitive to penicillinase-resistant semisynthetic penicillins and cephalosporins. The activity of nafcillin against 28 strains recently isolated from patients with endocarditis from various parts of the USA and Canada is summarized in Table 1.

Table 1. Susceptibility to Nafcillin of 28 *Staphylococcus aureus* strains causing Endocarditis

Cumulative % of strains	Nafcillin concentration (μgm/ml) 0.06	0.12	0.25	0.50	1.0
inhibited[x]	6.8	47.6	81.6	100	---
killed[o]	0	27.2	78.2	96.6	100

x minimal inhibitory concentration determined with microtiter technique in heart infusion broth using 10^4 to 10^5 initial inoculum and recorded as the lowest dilution producing no visable growth after 24 hours of incubation.

o minimal bactericidal concentration determined by subculture after 24 hours of incubation onto blood agar plates and recorded as the lowest dilution producing <5 colonies of growth.

Sabath and others have reported a variable number of clinical isolates (1% to 40%) of *S. aureus* that are inhibited but not killed by easily achievable serum levels of β-lactam and other cell wall active agents (e.g., vancomycin).[4] The mechanism for this defect in bactericidal activity, so called "tolerance", seems to be a reduction in autolytic enzyme activity by the organism and was found in less than 7% of cells in a single population of organisms. This characteristic has been linked to clinical theraputic failures with single drug therapy.[5,6,7] In other cases, however, tolerant strains have apparently responded well to therapy with β-lactam drugs alone.[8] "Tolerance" was not demonstrated in any of the 28 endocarditis isolates of *S. aureus* identified above by the microtiter technique. It is possible that tolerance in those strains was missed because of the low initial inoculum used, the small volume of media subcultured, or the fact that these isolates had been subcultured several times prior to testing. When these 28 strains were incubated with concentrations of nafcillin (5 μgm/ml) which exceeded their minimum bactericidal concentrations (MBC) and a large inoculum [$>10^7$ colony forming units (CFU)] similar to that found in cardiac vegetations *in vivo*[9] and bactericidal rates determined over time, two distinct populations were identified. Nafcillin produced a pronounced drop in viable bacteria in 48 hours in 22 strains (mean reduction was 4.5 logs with a range of 3.8 to 7.3 logs). With 6 strains, nafcillin exhibited a reduced bactericidal effect (mean reduction 2.5 logs with a range of 1.23 to 2.7 logs). Thus 21% of strains exhibited a relative resistance to the bactericidal action of nafcillin, an incidence similar to that reported by Sabath.[4] Watanakunakorn however found no difference in the bactericidal rates of various β-lactam drugs between so called tolerant and nontolerant strains of *S. aureus.*[8] All of the strains were also susceptible to low concentrations of gentamicin (Table 2).

Table 2. Susceptibility to gentamicin of 28 *Staphylococcus aureus* strains causing endocarditis.

Cumulative % of strains	Gentamicin concentration (μgm/ml) 0.06	0.12	0.25	0.50
inhibited	3.4	20.4	71.4	100
killed	3.4	10.2	47.6	100

Gentamicin alone incubated with large populations of *S. aureus* (>10^7 CFU) at concentrations 4 to 5 times the minimal inhibitory concentration (MIC) failed to sterlize the culture after 48 hours. This failure was associated with the rapid emergence of the previously reported resistant dwarf colony forming strains.[10,11]

Previous studies have demonstrated that the combination of a penicillin and gentamicin have a more rapid and complete bactericidal action than either drug alone[12,9,10,11] against large numbers of *S. aureus.* The 28 isolates from patients with endocarditis described above were tested using time-kill curves *in vitro* (i.e. quantitive cultures of broth solutions containing an initial inoculum of 10^7 CFU incubated for 48 hours with either nafcillin (5 μgm/ml) alone, nafcillin (5 μgm/ml) plus gentamicin (0.5 μgm/ml) or nafcillin (5 μgm/ml) plus gentamicin (2 μgm/ml). Gentamicin combined with nafcillin produced a more rapid bactericidal action than nafcillin alone against all strains. One half of the strains demonstrated a greater than 2 log enhancement of bactericidal activity with the low concentration of gentamicin (0.5 μgm/ml) while all strains exhibited this response to nafcillin plus the higher concentration (2 μgm/ml) of gentamicin. This level of enhanced killing (>2 log difference) has been defined by Moellering as antibiotic synergism in his studies with *Streptococcus faecalis.*[13]

The following table summarizes the time of incubation when synergism (>2 log difference in viable counts) was demonstrated in these 28 strains.

Table 3. Percentage of strains exhibiting synergistic response to nafcillin and gentamicin

Gentamicin concentration	Time of incubation 4hrs	24hrs	48hrs
0.5 μgm/ml	7 %	39 %	43 %
2.0 μgm/ml	46 %	78 %	82 %

Only one strain incubated for 48 hours with 0.5 μgm/ml of gentamicin and nafcillin contained more viable organisms (4.7×10^2 CFU/ml) than was found in the flask containing nafcillin alone (8.0×10^1 CFU/ml). In all other determinations (3 for each strain) the combinations produced a greater drop in viable bacteria (83/84 for the 0.5 μgm/ml gentamicin and 84/84 for 2 μgm/ml gentamicin) than the nafcillin alone. Thus the combination seems to enhance the bactericidal effect for essentially all strains of *S. aureus.*

In Vivo Studies

Attempts to examine the significance of the above *in vitro* observations in an experimental model of endocarditis have flourished in the last 10 years. This review will concentrate on those conducted in our laboratory at the Univeristy of Virginia using a modification of the well characterized Freedman model of staphylococcal endocarditis in rabbits.[14]

We initially demonstrated that in general the relative rate at which antibiotics alone or in combination kill the organism in broth is predictive of the relative rate at which the drugs will eradicate the staphylococcus from the cardiac vegetations *in vivo.*[9] Antibiotics were administered in dosages and intervals to approximate serum levels considered therapeutic in man. To date four different strains have been examined.

A penicillin sensitive strain of *S. aureus* was initially studied, and animals were treated with antibiotics for 1 to 10 days. Vancomycin was the most rapidly bactericidal single drug against this strain both *in vitro* and in the rate of sterilization of cardiac vegetations in treated animals. Penicillin and cefazolin produced equivalent killing ratios *in vitro* and *in vivo.* Cefazolin has recently been found to be less effective in sterilizing vegetations in a similar rabbit model than other β-lactum antibiotics when disease was produced by β-lactamase producing strains of *S. aureus.*[15] This has been attributed to its increased susceptibility to destruction by the enzyme. Clindamycin was less rapidly bactericidal *in vitro* and proved less effective *in vivo.* A clindamycin resistant strain of *S. aureus* emerged during therapy in one animal and resulted in a therapeutic failure.

Rifampin alone was ineffective *in vitro* and *in vivo* in exhibiting a sustained bactericidal effect. Resistance develops rapidly (within 24 hours) when the drug is incubated with large numbers of bacteria ($>10^7$ CFU/ml) in broth. Highly resistant strains of *S. aureus* also emerged in 3 of 14 aniamls with endocarditis treated with rifampin alone, and all were associated with reappearance of bacteremia, fever, and eventual death of the animal. The combination of penicillin plus rifampin was less rapidly bactericidal than penicillin alone *in vitro,* a phenomena that was expressed *in vivo* by a reduced rate of sterilization of vegetations. Rifampin resistant strains did not emerge in the 11 animals treated with both drugs. Rifampin may, however, have a potentially valuable role to play in the treatment of acute *S. aureus* endocarditis. The drug seems to possess two unique properties: 1) it penetrates into phagocytic cells and kills intraleukocytic staphylococci[16], and 2) it reduces the bacterial titers and sterilizes abscesses *in vivo* more rapidly than other available antistaphylococcal drugs.[17] When renal tissue from the animals with endocarditis described above was cultured quantitatively, it was found that the combination of rifampin and penicillin was more effective than any other regimen tested in sterilizing the abscess-studded kidneys. Addition of rifampin has been effective in achieving cure in patients with *S. aureus* endocarditis caused by tolerant strains.[18] Since complications from staphylococcal endocarditis often result from intra-cardiac or metastatic abscesses, utilization of this drug in combination warrants further investigations.

The combination of gentamicin and penicillin was more rapidly bactericidal *in vivo* than penicillin alone. This enhanced *in vivo* action had been previously demonstrated in other experimental models.[19,20] This initial observation prompted expanded studies with nafcillin and gentamicin against 3 penicillinase producing strains of *S. aureus*[10], (unpublished observations,Korzeniowski, O and Sande, M). In all instances addition of gentamicin to nafcillin increased the rate at which the *S. aureus* was eradicated from the vegetations. Others have confirmed these results.[11] One of our strains (provided by Dr. L. Sabath) was "tolerant" to nafcillin *in vitro;* i.e. incubation of 10^7 bacteria with nafcillin (5 μgm/ml) only reduced titer to 10^6 in 24 hours and 10^5 in 48 hours. *In vivo,* however, nafcillin therapy was as effective in reducing the vegetation titers of tolerant staphylococci as the drug alone was in reducing titers of non-tolerant staphylococci. Others have also failed to show a lack of effectiveness of β-lactam antibiotics in the therapy of experimental endocarditis caused by "tolerant" strains of *S. aureus.*[21]

Clinical Studies

Treatment of *S. aureus* endocarditis with a single β-lactam antibiotic is usually successful in achieving a bacterologic cure. The occasional failure to eradicate the organism from the blood stream or cardiac vegetations has been attributed to "tolerance"[4,5], β-lactamase production by the large populations of organisms found in the cardiac vegetations[22], undrained staphylococcal abscesses, or so called "intrinsic methicillin resistance".[23] However, even though the bacteria may be effectively killed, the mortality rate remains high (25 – 50%) in the general patient population.

The majority of these deaths are due to the sequelae of the infection, i.e. congestive heart failure or cardiac arrhythmias secondary to valvular or myocardial tissue destruction or a vascular catastrophe (ruptured mycotic aneurysm or embolus).[3] Thus in an attempt to minimize valve destruction and vegetation propagation, rapid sterilization of the infected focus would seem to be a rational theraputic goal.

As noted above the addition of gentamicin to the β-lactam antibiotic increased the bactericidal rate in broth and increased the rate of sterilization of infected vegetations in experimental animals. In man the addition of the aminoglycoside to therapy with penicillinase-resistant penicillin markedly increased the serum bactericidal activity against strains of *S. aureus.*[24] Several published studies, however, suggest that the addition of gentamicin has no beneficial effect on the eventual outcome of the disease. Abrams and collegues treated 25 intravenous drug addicts (mean age 27.5 yrs) with staphylococcal endocarditis in a prospective randomized fashion with either a β-lactam drug alone or in combination with gentamicin.[25] Mortality was nil in both groups. This low mortality rate seems to be unique to the addict population (8 deaths in 216 reported cases - 4%) and has been attributed to the young age group and predominance of tricuspid valve involvement. Our recently completed multicenter study of 48 addicts with *S. aureus* endocarditis confirmed these results.[26] Patients were treated with nafcillin alone (mean duration 30 days) or in combination with gentamicin for the first two weeks. One patient (4%) in each group of 24 failed therapy, a single relapse in the combination therapy group and a death in the single drug group.

The Abrams study failed to show an accelerated clinical response with the combination therapy and reported no difference in toxicity. The multicenter study demonstrated an increase in the rate of sterilization of blood cultures, but only in patients with right-sided (tricuspid valve) infection. The mean number of days to negative blood cultures was 2.6 for patients treated with the combination and 3.6 for those treated with nafcillin alone. Clincial response was also more rapid in all patients treated with both drugs. The median duration of fever was three days in the combination group vs seven days in the single drug group, and leukocytosis was present for a median of three days in the combination group vs 11 days in the single drug group. Drug-related toxicity was similar in both groups.

In a retrospective study of staphylococcal endocarditis (primarily in non-addicts), Watanakunakorn and Baird reported a mortality rate of 40% in 15 patients treated with a penicillin plus gentamicin and 40% in 25 patients treated with the penicillin alone.[27] Death rates correlated with the age of the patient (11% mortality in patients $<$50 yrs of age and 63.6% in patients over 50 yrs) and with the presence of an underlying medical disease (diabetes mellitis, cardiac disease, alcoholism and/or cirrhosis). The majority of the 16 deaths occured early in therapy: 6 in the first week, 5 in the second week, and 4 in the third week. Extensive metastatic abscess formation was present in fatal cases.

The initial analysis of our prospective multicenter study in nonaddicts also demonstrates no significant difference in outcome of disease. Mortality rates ranged from 22 to 30%. Bacteremia was cleared more rapidly in patients receiving aminoglycoside but renal toxicity was increased.

These studies all suffer from the inherent difficulties in randomizing patients with similar ages, similar underlying diseases, and a similar stage of disease (equal organ involvement and degree of valve destruction). For example in our multicenter study patients expired from complications of the destructive effects of the organism. None could be attributed to a failure of antimicrobial therapy *per se.* The multicenter study supports the *in vitro* and *in vivo* observations of a more rapid eradication of the staphylococci from the blood stream when patients received the combination therapy. Whether this increased efficiency of antimicrobial action will have an impact on reducing valvular destruction and eventual mortality has not been answered.

While initial use of combination therapy can perhaps be justified by the accelerated response rate demonstrated in the multicenter study, it must be emphasized that these findings were in conflict with results in the other two published series (although the rate of clearance of bacteremia was not examined in those studies).[25,27] In addition, the increased renal toxicity found in the older patient population must be considered. We would therefore only use the gentamicin, β-lactam combination for the first several days to week of therapy while aminoglycoside serum levels are closely monitored. Therapy with the β-lactam alone is then continued for a total of at least 4 weeks. While such manipulations in antimicrobial chemotherapy may be beneficial, any major improvements in survival rates in staphylococcal endocarditis will probably result from earlier diagnosis of the disease coupled with rapid detection and aggressive treatment of complications. On the basis of the above studies, our recommendations for antibiotic therapy of endocarditis due to *S. aureus* are set forth below.

Table 4. Therapy of Endocarditis due to *Staphylococcus aureus* in Adults

Primary drug of choice	Dose (gms/day)	Duration
β-lactamase resistant penicillin:		
Nafcillin[(a)]	8–12	4–6 weeks
Oxacillin	8–12	4–6 weeks
Methicillin	12–16	4–6 weeks
Allergy to Penicillins:		
Rash (maculopapular)		
Cephalosporin		
Cephalothin	8–12	4–6 weeks
Cefazolin	4–8	4–6 weeks
Cefamandole or other	4–8	4–6 weeks
Anaphylaxis or hives		
Vancomycin	2	4–6 weeks

Special Considerations:

1) Addition of aminoglycoside to penicillin may speed sterilization of blood.		
Gentamicin[(b)]	1 mg/kg three times per day	5 days
Tobramycin	1 mg/kg three times per day	5 days
2) Myocardial abscess -- addition of rifampin may be of benefit.	300 mg twice daily	several weeks
3) Tolerance to cell wall active drugs. (β-lactam or vancomycin) add gentamicin/tobramycin and/or rifampin	check serum bactericidal titer	
4) Prosthetic valve infection -- err on the longside of therapy		6 weeks to 2 months

(a.) All of these drugs have potential side effects, for example:

Nafcillin: Neutropenia may occur after 2 to 3 weeks, and in 5% may reach levels of < 1000 mm^3.

Oxacillin: Hepatitis has been observed.

Methicillin: Probably has greatest incidence of interstitial nephritis.

(b.) Nephrotoxicity (doubling of serum creatinine) was observed in over 50% of patients with left-sided endocarditis who were treated for two weeks.

REFERENCES

1. Watanakunakorn, C., Tan J.S., Phair J.P. Some salient features of *Staphylococcus aureus* endocarditis. Amer. J. Med. 54: 473, 1973.
2. Hoeprich P.D. Infective endocarditis. In Hoeprich P.D. (ed) Infectious Diseases. Hagerstown, Harper and Row, 1972, p. 1045.
3. Richardson, T.J., Karp, R.B., Kirklin, J.W., Dismukes, W.E. Treatment of Infective Endocarditis: a 10-year Comparative Analysis. Circulation 58: 589, 1978.
4. Sabath, L.D., Wheeler, N., Laverdier, M., Blazevic D., Wilkinson, B.T. A New type of Penicillin resistance of *Staphylococcus aureus.* Lancet 1: 443, 1977.
5. Gopal, Bisno, A.L., Silverblatt, F.J., Failure of vancomycin treatment in *Staphylococcus aureus* endocarditis. J.A.M.A. 236: 1604, 1926.
6. Rozenberg-Arska, M., Fabius, G., Beens-Dekkers, M., Duursma, S. Sabath, L.D., Verhoef, T., Antibiotic Sensitivity and Synergism of "Penicillin-Tolerant" *Staphylococcus aureus.* Chemoth. 25: 352, 1979.
7. Mayhall, C.G., Medoff, G., Marr, T.T., Variation in the Susceptibility of strains of *Staphylococcus aureus* to oxacillin, Cephalothin, and gentamicin. Antimicrob. Agents Chemoth. 10: 707, 1976.
8. Watanakunakorn, C., Antibiotic-tolerant *Staphylococcus aureus.* Antimicrob. Chemoth. 4: 561, 1978.
9. Sande, M., Johnson, M., Antimicrobial therapy of experimental endocarditis caused by Staphylococcus aureus. J. Infect. Dis. 131: 367, 1975.
10. Sande, M., Courtney, K., Naficillin-gentamicin Synergism in experimental Staphylococcus endocarditis. J. Lab. Clin. Med. 88: 118, 1976.
11. Miller, M., Wexler, M., Steigbigel N., Single and combination antibiotic therapy of *Staphylococcus aureus* experimental endocarditis: emergence of gentamicin-resistance mutants. Antimicrob. Agents and Chemoth. 14: 336, 1978.
12. Watanakunakorn, C., Glotzbecker, C.: Enhancement of the effects of Anti-Staphyloccal Antibiotics by Aminoglycosides. Antimicrol. Agents Chemoth. 6: 802, 1974.
13. Moellering, R.C. Jr., Wennersten, C., and Weinberg, A.N. Studies on Antibiotic synergism against Enterococci. 1. Bacteriologic studies. J. Lab. Clin. Med. 77: 821, 1971.
14. Perlman, B.B., and Freedman, L.R., Experimental Endocarditis III. Natural history of catheter induced Staphylococcal Endocarditis following catheter removal. Yale J. Bio. Med. 44: 212, 1971.
15. Goodman, P., Petersdorf, R.G., Importance of β-lactamase Inactivation in treatment of experimental endocarditis caused by *Staphylococcus aureus.* Infect. Dis. 141: 331, 1980.

16. Mandell, G.L., Vest, T.K., Killing of intraleukocytic *Staphylococcus aureus* by rifampin: in vitro and in vivo studies. J. Infect. Dis. 125: 486, 1972.
17. Lobo, M.C., Mandell, G.L., Treatment of experimental Staphylococcal infection with rifampin. Antimicrob. Agents Chemother. 2: 195, 1972.
18. Faville, R.J.. Zaske, D.E., Kaplan, E.N., Crossley, K., Sabath, L.D., Quie, P.G., *Staphylococcus aureus* endocarditis; combined therapy with Vancomyicn and rifampin. J.A.M.A. 240: 1963, 1978.
19. Campos, M.E., Rabinorich, S., Smith, I.M., Therapy of Experimental Staphylococcal infection with antibiotic combination. J. Lab. Clin. Med. 83: 241, 1974.
20. Steigbigel, R.T., Greenman, R.C., Remington, J.S., Antibiotic combinations in the treatment of experimental *Staphylococcus aureus* infections. J. Infect. Dis. 131: 245, 1975.
21. Goldman, P.C., and Petersdorf, R.G., The significance of methicillin tolerance in experimental *Staphylococcal* endocarditis. Antimicrob. Agents Chemother. 15: 802, 1979.
22. Reymann, M.T., Holley, H.P., Cobbs, C.G., Persistent Bacteremia in Staphylococcal endocarditis. Am. J. Med. 65: 729, 1978.
23. Lacey, R., A new type of penicillin resistance of *Staphylococcus aureus?* J. of Antimicro. Chemoth. 3: 380, 1977.
24. Licht, J.H., Penicillinese-Resistant Penicillin/Gentamicin Synergism. Arch. Intern Med. 139: 1094, 1979.
25. Abrams, B., Sklaver, A., Hoffman, T., Greenman, R., Single or combination therapy of Staphylococcal endocarditis in intravenous drug abusers. Ann. Intern. Med. 90: 789, 1979.
26. Sande, M.A., Korzeniowski, O.M., Endocarditis Collaborative Group, 11th International Congress Chemotherapy 1980. Interscience Conference on Antimicrobial Agents and Chemotherapy 1979, abstract 362.
27. Watanakunakorn, C., Baird, I.M., Prognostic factors in *Staphylococcus aureus* endocarditis and results of therapy with a penicillin and gentamicin. Am. J. of Med. Sci. 273: 133, 1977.

Chatrchai Watanakunakorn, M.D.

ANTIMICROBIAL THERAPY OF ENDOCARDITIS DUE TO LESS COMMON BACTERIA

It is obvious that because the clinical experience in treating bacterial endocarditis caused by less common organisms is very limited, it is not possible to formulate a standard regimen. However, this chapter outlines the treatment regimens of bacterial endocarditis caused by selected organisms where meaningful information can be obtained from the literature.

Haemophilus Species Endocarditis

Among the various species in the genus *Hemophilus, H. aphrophilus, H. parainfluenzae* and *H. paraphrophilus* are much more common than *H. influenzae* in causing endocarditis.[1] Of the 37 patients with *H. aphrophilus* endocarditis who received known antibiotics and survived, 15 were treated with penicillin and streptomycin plus either tetracycline or chloramphenicol, 9 received penicillin and streptomycin.[1–5] Of the 14 patients with *H. aphrophilus* endocarditis who were treated with known antibiotics and died, 3 received penicillin and streptomycin and none received tetracycline or chloramphenicol in addition.[1–4]

Of the 35 patients with *H. parainfluenzae* endocarditis who received known antibiotics and survived, 5 were treated with ampicillin alone, 8 received ampicillin and an aminoglycoside (gentamicin, streptomycin or kanamycin), 4 received ampicillin, an aminoglycoside and either tetracycline or chloramphenicol.[1,4,6–13] In all, 25 of the 35 patients received ampicillin as part of their therapy. Of the 7 patients with *H. parainfluenzae* endocarditis who died despite treatment, only 3 received ampicillin as part of their therapy.[4,6–8] A single case of ampicillin-resistant *H. parainfluenzae* endocarditis has been reported; the patient was cured with chloramphenicol.[12]

There have been only 9 reported cases of *H. paraphrophilus* endocarditis.[1,9,14,15] It is possible that some cases reported as *H. parainfluenzae* endocarditis were actually caused by *H. paraphrophilus* because of the difficulties in correct identification.[14,15] All the 9 patients survived; 5 were treated with ampicillin alone, 2 with ampicillin and gentamicin, one with ampicillin and streptomycin and one with penicillin alone.

Among the different species of *Haemophilus, H. influenzae* is the least likely to cause endocarditis. Only 9 cases of *H. influenzae* endocarditis treated with antibiotics have been reported. The 5 survivors were treated with penicillin and streptomycin (3),[8,9] streptomycin alone (1)[8] and ampicillin alone (1).[16] The 4 patients who died were treated with sulfonamide (1), penicillin plus streptomycin (1), and ampicillin alone (2).[4,17]

From the available information in the literature, it appears that for *H. aphrophilus* endocarditis, penicillin plus streptomycin with or without tetracycline is the treatment of choice. As for *H. parainfluenzae* and *H. paraphrophilus* endocarditis, ampicillin with or without an aminoglycoside is the preferred treatment regimen. There is not enough experience with *H. influenzae* endocarditis, but it probably can be treated the same way as *H. parainfluenzae*.

Actinobacillus actinomycetemcomitans Endocarditis

Of the 38 patients with *A. actinomycetemcomitans* endocarditis who were treated with antibiotics, 26 patients survived and 12 died.[1,2,18,19] The majority of patients (19 of 26 survivors and 10 of 12 deaths) were treated with a penicillin and an aminoglycoside as part of their antibiotic therapy. Penicillin plus streptomycin with or without other antibiotics were used most often, namely in 14 of 26 survivors and 9 of 12 deaths. It appears that penicillin and streptomycin should be used to treat *A. actinomycetemcomitans* endocarditis unless laboratory studies indicate otherwise.

Cardiobacterium hominis Endocarditis

There have been 23 reported cases of endocarditis caused by the fastidious gram-negative bacillus, *C. hominis.*[1,20–24] Twenty of the 23 patients survived. Six patients were treated with penicillin alone and survived. Of the 12 patients treated with penicillin and streptomycin with or without other antibiotics, 9 survived. Gentamicin was the aminoglycoside used in conjunction with penicillin in 3 other patients; all of whom survived. These data suggest that penicillin with or without streptomycin can be used to treat *C. hominis* endocarditis, if adequate serum bactericidal concentration can be achieved.

Diphtheroid Endocarditis

Diphtheroids are a group of organisms that cause endocarditis usually in patients with a prosthetic valve. Thirty-three of the 50 cases of endocarditis due to diphtheroids treated with antibiotics were in patients with a prosthetic valve.[25–31] Various antibiotics and different combinations have been used with unpredictable results. Evaluation of the efficacy of antibiotic therapy is impossible. Fourteen of the 17 patients (82%) without a prosthetic valve survived, while only 19 of 33 patients (57%) with diphtheroid prosthetic valve endocarditis survived. Most of these latter patients required removal of the infected prosthesis.

The *in vitro* antimicrobial susceptibility of diphtheroids to different antibiotics is not uniform. Although many strains are susceptible to penicillin, minimal inhibitory concentrations (MIC) as high as > 100 μg/ml have been reported (Table 1)[25,30–33] However, all diphtheroids

Table 1. Susceptibility of Diphtheroids to Penicillin G

Author (Ref.)		Year	No. of Strains	MIC* (μg/ml)	
				Range	Median
Johnson	(25)	1970	13	0.2 –>50	1.6
Gerry	(30)	1976	9	0.02 – 50	2.5
Hande	(32)	1976	4	>6.0	
Van Scoy	(31)	1977	3	>5.0	
Heczko	(33)	1977	118	<0.04 –>100	<0.04

* Minimal inhibitory concentrations

that have been tested are susceptible to vancomycin (Table 2).[25,30–34] Vancomycin should be used to treat endocarditis due to diphtheroids, pending the results of *in vitro* susceptibility tests to penicillin, vancomycin and other antibiotics.[31]

Pseudomonas aeruginosa Endocarditis

There have been over one hundred cases of endocarditis caused by *Pseudomonas aeurginosa* reported in the literature, the majority of which

Table 2. Susceptibility of Diphtheroids to Vancomycin

Author (Ref.)		Year	No. of Strains	MIC* (µg/ml) Range	Median
Johnson	(25)	1970	5	0.4–1.56	0.8
Hande	(32)	1976	4	<0.5 –0.8	<0.4
Gerry	(30)	1976	1	1.2	
Van Scoy	(31)	1977	3	1.0	
Pearson	(34)	1977	7	1.0	
Heczko	(33)	1977	118	<0.04–3.1	<0.04

* Minimal inhibitory concentration

occurred in intravenous drug abusers.[35] The most extensive experience in treating this infection was recorded by Lerner's group in Detroit where most of their patients were intravenous drug abusers.[36] The current recommended treatment is the combination of carbenicillin (at 30 gm/d) and tobramycin or gentamicin (at 8 mg/kg/d) for at least 6 weeks. In their experience in treating 14 patients, 12 patients (85.7%) were cured and only 4 of 14 patients required surgery; this stands in contrast to previous less favorable results using lower doses of aminoglycosides (Table 3).[36] Obviously, vestibular, auditory and renal functions should be monitored closely in these patients. Further clinical studies using some of the newer beta-lactam compounds effective against *Pseudomonas aeruginosa* such as cefotaxime, cefoperazone and moxalactam are indicated.

Table 3. Treatment of *Pseudomonas aeruginosa* endocarditis*

Antibiotic Regimen	Recovery: Medical Therapy Alone	Medical & Surgical Therapy	Total (%)	
Carbenicillin 30 gm/d, plus Gentamicin 2.5–5 mg/kg/d	5/9	6/11	11/20	(55.0)
Carbenicillin 30 gm/d, plus Gentamicin or tobramycin 8 mg/kg/d	9/10	3/4	12/14	(85.7)

*Modified from Reyes *et al.*[36]

Pseudomonas cepacia Endocarditis

Endocarditis due to *Pseudomonas cepacia* occurs mainly in intravenous drug abusers and patients with cardiac valvular prostheses. Strains of *P. cepacia* are usually resistant to multiple antibiotics but all are susceptible to trimethoprim-sulfamethoxazole (TMP–SMZ).[37] Of the 11 reported patients with *P. cepacia* endocarditis in whom details of antibiotic therapy were known, 8 survived.[38–42] One of 3 patients treated with TMP-SMZ survived. Two patients who were treated with TMP-SMZ and kanamycin survived. Five of the 6 patients who were treated with TMP-SMZ in combination with polymyxin B survived.

Thus, TMP-SMZ in combination with either polymyxin B or kanamycin according to *in vitro* susceptibility and synergism studies has been used successfully in the treatment of endocarditis caused by *P. cepacia.* The dosage of TMP-SMZ varies from 240 mg to 960 mg of TMP and 1,200 mg to 4,800 mg of SMZ per day.

Pseudomonas maltophilia Endocarditis

P. maltophilia endocarditis occurs in patients with a cardiac valvular prosthesis and to a lesser degree in intravenous drug abusers. As in the case of *P. cepacia, P. maltophilia* strains are resistant to multiple antibiotics, but almost all are susceptible to TMP-SMZ.[37] Of the 7 patients with *P. maltophilia* endocarditis, 6 survived.[43] Four of the 6 received TMP-SMZ with or without polymyxin, kanamycin, amikacin or carbenicillin. Two patients were treated with chloramphenicol and one died.

Serratia marcescens Endocarditis

Serratia marcescens also causes endocarditis mainly in patients with a cardiac valvular prosthesis and in intravenous drug abusers. Of the 49 patients with *S. marcescens* endocarditis who were treated with antibiotics, 30 died (61%).[44–50] The majority of these patients had aortic and/or mitral valve involvement. Many different antibiotic regimens have been used,but Mills and his associates in San Francisco have had the most experience in treating this disease.[49,50] Only 2 of 13 patients treated with an aminoglycoside alone were cured, while 18 of 29 patients treated with an aminoglycoside in combination with another antibiotic (carbenicillin, cefoxitin, chloramphenicol, or TMP-SMZ) were cured.[50] The prognosis of patients with right-sided involvement was much better than ones with left-sided involvement.[50] Most patients with *Serratia* endocarditis of the aortic and/or mitral valve require cardiac surgery.[50] As with other types of gram-negative endocarditis, *in vitro* antimicrobial susceptibility and synergism studies are important in selecting the most appropriate antibiotic combination.

Endocarditis Due to Anaerobes

Almost 60 cases of endocarditis caused by anaerobes have been reported.[51–58] The infecting organisms included various species of the genera *Bacteroides, Fusobacterium, Clostridium, Propionibacterium* and *Peptostreptococcus, Eubacterium aerofaciens* and *Megasphaera elsdenii.* Different antibiotic regimens have been used including various combinations of sulfadiazine, penicillin, ampicillin, hetacillin, methicillin, cephalothin, tetracycline, choloramphenicol, kanamycin, streptomycin, carbenicillin, clindamycin and metronidazole. Due to the insufficient number of cases being treated with each regimen, the clinical efficacy of antibiotic therapy cannot be assessed. It seems that high doses of penicillin G should be used if the infecting anaerobe is not *Bacteroides fragilis*. Metronidazole is a promising agent in treating endocarditis caused by *Bacteroides fragilis* and other species resistant to penicillin G.[57] *In vitro*, metronidazole is active against the majority of anaerobes, especially *Fusobacterium, Clostridium* and *B. fragilis,*[59–62] and its action is reported to be bactericidal against susceptible anaerobes.[63–64]

Comment

It is clear from this review that clinical experience in treating endocarditis due to less common bacteria is limited. Table 4 lists the

Table 4. Mortality of Endocarditis Due to Less Common Bacteria

Bacteria	Death/Total	(%)
Haemophilus aphrophilus	14/51	(27.5)
Haemophilus parainfluenzae	7/42	(16.7)
Haemophilus paraphrophilus	0/9	(0)
Haemophilus influenzae	4/9	(44.4)
Actinobacillus actinomycetemcomitans	12/38	(31.6)
Cardiobacterium hominis	3/23	(13.0)
Diphtheroids	17/50	(34.0)
Pseudomonas aeruginosa	11/34	(32.4)*
Pseudomonas cepacia	3/11	(27.3)
Pseudomonas maltophilia	1/7	(14.3)
Serratia marcescens	22/42	(52.4)*

* Experience at a single institution

mortality of endocarditis caused by different organisms. Based on the information available in the literature, certain antibiotics or antibiotic combinations seem to be effective therapy. The duration of therapy is generally 4 to 6 weeks. Obviously *in vitro* quantitative antimicrobial susceptibility testing and synergism studies are useful in selecting appropriate antimicrobial agents. In general an antibiotic which inhibits cell wall synthesis in combination with an aminoglycoside should be used pending the results of *in vitro* studies. For endocarditis due to *P. aeruginosa*, it has been shown that treatment failure occurred when there was no *in vitro* synergism between carbenicillin and gentamicin or tobramycin against the infecting organism, whereas synergism between these antibiotics did not assure medical cure.[65] The peak serum bactericidal titer of >1:8 has been reported to be correlated well with successful therapy.[48] On the other hand a peak serum bactericidal titer of >1:8 is often unobtainable in the treatment of endocarditis due to gram-negative bacilli.[36–49] Furthermore, bacteriologic cure has been achieved in patients with peak serum bactericidal titer of <1:8.[36,50] The clinical relevance of serum bactericidal titer in the therapy of gram-negative bacillary endocarditis needs further study. Surgery is indicated when there is persistent infection in spite of the best available antimicrobial therapy.

REFERENCES

1. Ellner, J.J., Rosenthal, M.S., Lerner, P.I., and McHenry, M.C.: Infective endocarditis caused by slow-growing, fastidious, gram-negative bacteria. Medicine 58:145, 1979.
2. Page, M.I., and King, E.O.: Infection due to *Actinobacillus actinomycetemcomitans* and *Haemophilus aprophilus*. New Engl. J. Med. 175:181, 1966.
3. Bieger, R.C., Brewer, N.S., and Washington, J.A., II.: *Haemophilus aphrophilus*: A microbiologic and clinical review and report of 42 cases. Medicine 57:345, 1978.
4. Johnson, R.H., Kennedy, R.P., Marton, K.I., and Thornsberry, C.: *Haemophilus endocarditis*: New cases, literature review, and recommendations for management. South Med. J. 70:1098, 1977.
5. Varghese, R., Melo, J.C., Barnwell, P., Chun, C.H., and Raff, M.J.: Endocarditis due to *Haemophilus aphrophilus*. Report of a case with possible transmission from dog to man. Chest 72:680, 1977.
6. Blair, D.C., Walker, W., Sodeman, T., and Pagano, T.: Bacterial endocarditis due to *Haemophilus parainfluenzae*. Chest 71:146, 1977.
7. Chunn, C.J., Jones, S.R., McCutchan, J.A., Young, E.J., and Gilbert, D.N.: *Haemophilus parainfluenzae* infective endocarditis. Medicine 56:99, 1977.
8. Lynn, D.J., Kane, J.G., and Parker, R.H.: *Haemophilus parainfluenzae* and *influenzae* endocarditis: A review of forty cases. Medicine 56:115, 1977.
9. Geraci, J.E., Wilkowske, C.J., Wilson, W.R., and Washington, J.A., II.: *Haemophilus* endocarditis. Mayo Clin. Proc. 52:209, 1977.

10. Jemsek, J.G., Greenberg, S.B., Gentry, L.O., Welton, D.E., and Mattox, K.L.: *Haemophilus parainfluenzae* endocarditis. Two cases and review of the literature in the past decade. Am. J. Med. 66:51, 1979.
11. Cole, R.A., Winickoff, R.N.: *Haemophilus parainfluenzae* endocarditis. South. Med. J. 72:516, 1979.
12. Smith, P.W., Chambers, W.A., and Walker, C.A.: Ampicillin resistant *Haemophilus parainfluenzae* endocarditis. Am. J. Med. Sci. 278:173, 1979.
13. Blair, D.C., and Weiner, L.B.: Prosthetic valve endocarditis due to *Haemophilus parainfluenzae* biotype II. Am. J. Dis. Child 133:617, 1979.
14. DeSilva, M., Rubin, M.J., Lyons, R.W., Liss, J.P., and Rotatori, E.S.: *Hamophilus paraphrophilus* endocarditis in a prolapsed mitral valve. Am. J. Clin. Pathol. 66:922, 1976.
15. Hammond, G.W., Richardson, H., Lian, C.J., and Ronald, A.R.: Two cases of *Haemophilus paraphrophilus* endocarditis of prolapsed mitral valves - *Haemophilus paraphrophilus* or *parainfluenzae*. Am. J. Med. 65:537, 1978.
16. Watanakunakorn, C.: Unpublished data.
17. Laird, W.P., Nelson, J.D., Weinberg, A.G., and Huffines, F.D.: Fatal *Haemophilus influenzae* endocarditis diagnosed by echocardiography in an infant. Pediatrics 64:292, 1979.
18. Vandepitte, J., DeGeest, H., and Jousten, P.: Subacute bacterial endocarditis due to *Actinobacillus actinomycetemcomitans*. Report of a case with a review of the literature. Am. J. Clin. Pathol. 30:842, 1977.
19. Affias, S., West, A., Stewart, J.W., and Haldane, E.V.: *Actinobacillus actinomycetemcomitans* endocarditis. Canad. Med. J. 118:1256, 1978.
20. Rahal, J., and Simberkoff, M.S.: Bactericidal activity of chloramphenicol in endocarditis and meningitis. Prog. Abs. Intersci. Conf. Antimicrob. Ag. Chemother. 17th, NY, Abstr. No. 5, 1977.
21. Geraci, J.E., Greipp, P.R., Wilkowske, C.J., Wilson, W.R., and Washington, J.A., II: *Cardiobacterium hominis* endocarditis. Four cases with clinical and laboratory observations. Mayo Clin. Proc. 53:49, 1978.
22. Jabanputra, R.S., and Moysey, J.: Endocarditis due to *Cardiobacterium hominis*. J. Clin. Pathol. 30:1033, 1977.
23. Wormser, G.P., Bottone, E.J., Tudy, J., and Hirschman, S.Z.: *Cardiobacterium hominis*: Review of prior infections and report of endocarditis on a fascia lata prosthetic heart valve. Am. J. Med. Sci. 276:117, 1978.
24. Prior, R.B., Spagna, V.A., and Perkins, R.L.: Endocarditis due to strain of *Cardiobacterium hominis* resistant to erythromycin and vancomycin. Chest 75:85, 1979.

25. Johnson, W.D., and Kaye, D.: Serious infections caused by diphtheroids. Ann. N.Y. Aca. Sci. 174 (Art 2):568, 1970.
26. Thomas, T.V., and Heilbraunn, A.: Prosthetic aortic valve replacement complicated by diphtheroid endocarditis and aortopulmonary fistula. Chest 59:679, 1971.
27. Jackson, G., and Saunders, K.: Prosthetic valve diphtheroid endocarditis treated with sodium fusidate and erythromycin. Brit. Heart J. 35:931, 1973.
28. Boyce, J.M.H.: A case of prosthetic valve endocarditis caused by *Corynebacterium hofmanni* and *Candida albicans*. Brit. Heart J. 37:1195, 1975.
29. Wanat, F.E., and Wychulis, A.R.: Diphtheroid endocarditis after aortic valve replacement. Chest 68:379, 1975.
30. Gerry, J.L. and Greenough, W.B., III: Diphtheroid endocarditis. Report of nine cases and review of the literature. Johns Hopkins Med. J. 139:61, 1976.
31. Van Scoy, R.E., Cohen, S.N., Geraci, J.E., and Washington, J.A., II: Coryneform bacterial endocarditis. Mayo Clin. Proc. 52:216, 1977.
32. Hande, K.R., Witebsky, F.G., Brown, M.S., Schulman, C.B., Anderson, S.E., Levine, A.S., MacLowry, J.D., and Chabner, B.A.: Sepsis with a new species of *Corynebacterium*. Ann. Intern. Med. 85:423, 1976.
33. Heczko, P.B., Kasprowicz, A., and Pulverer, G.: Susceptibility of human skin aerobic diphtheroids to antimicrobial agents in vitro. J. Antimicrob. Chemother. 3:141, 1977.
34. Pearson, T.A., Braine, H.G., Rathbun, H.K.: *Corynebacterium* sepsis in oncology patients. Predisposing factors, diagnosis, and treatment. J.A.M.A. 238:1737, 1977.
35. Cohen, P.S., Maguire, J.H., and Weinstein, L.: Infective Endocarditis caused by gram-negative bacteria: a review of the literature, 1945–1977. Prog. Cardiovasc. Dis. 22:205, 1980.
36. Reyes, M.P., Brown, W.J., and Lerner, A.M.: Treatment of patients with pseudomonas endocarditis with high dose aminoglycoside and carbenicillin therapy. Medicine 57:57, 1978.
37. Moody, M.R., and Young, V.M.: *In vitro* susceptibility of *Pseudomonas cepacia* and *Pseudomonas maltophilia* to trimethoprim-sulfamethoxazole. Antimicrob. Ag. Chemother. 7:836, 1975.
38. Seligman, S.J., Madhavan, T., and Alcid, D.: Trimethoprim-sulfamethoxazole in the treatment of bacterial endocarditis. J. Infect. Dis. 128 (Suppl):S754, 1973.
39. Neu, H.C., Garvey, G.J., and Beach, M.P.: Successful treatment of *Pseudomonas cepacia* endocarditis in a heroin addict with Trimethoprim-sulfamethoxazole. J. Infect. Dis. 128 (Suppl):S768, 1973.
40. Speller, D.C.E.: *Pseudomonas cepacia* endocarditis treated with cotrimoxazole and kanamycin. Brit. Heart J. 35:47, 1973.

41. Noriega, E.R., Rubinstein, E., Simberkoff, M.S., and Rahal, J.J.: Subacute and acute endocarditis due to *Pseudomonas cepacia* in heroin addicts. Am. J. Med. 58:29, 1975.
42. Hamilton, J., Burch, W., Grimmett, G., Orme, K., Brewer, D., Frost, R., and Fulkerson, C.: Successful treatment of *Pseudomonas cepacia* endocarditis with trimethoprim-sulfamethoxazole. Antimicrob. Ag. Chemother. 4:551, 1973.
43. Yu, V.L., Rumans, L.W., Wing, E.J., McLeod, R., Sattler, F.N., Harvey, R.M., and Derensinski, S.C.: *Pseudomonas maltophilia* causing heroin-associated infective endocarditis. Arch. Intern. Med. 138:1667, 1978.
44. Quintiliani, R., and Gifford, R.H.: Endocarditis from *Serratia marcescens.* J.A.M.A.: 208:2055, 1969.
45. Williams, J.C., Jr., Johnson, J.E., III: *Serratia marcescens* endocarditis. Arch. Intern. Med. 125:1038, 1970.
46. Khan, F.A. and Khan, A.R.: *Serratia marcescens* endocarditis. Ann. Intern. Med. 79:454, 1973.
47. Harris, J.A., and Cobbs, C.G.: *Serratia* endocarditis in patients with a Starr-Edwards valve: report of a case of bacteriologic cure with antimicrobial therapy. South. Med. J. 66:1117, 1973.
48. Bryan, C.S., Marney, S.R., Alfrod, R.H., and Bryant, R.E.: Gram-negative bacillary endocarditis. Intrepretation of the serum bactericidal test. Am. J. Med. 58:208, 1975.
49. Mills, J., and Drew, D.: *Serratia marcescens* endocarditis: a regional illness associated with intravenous drug abuse. Ann. Intern. Med. 84–28, 1976.
50. Cooper, R., and Mills, J.: *Serratia* endocarditis. Arch. Intern. Med. 140:199, 1980.
51. Fellner, J.M., and Dowell, V.R., Jr.: Anaerobic bacterial endocarditis. New Engl. J. Med. 283:1188, 1970.
52. Case, D.B., Goforth, J.M., and Silva, J., Jr.: A case of *Clostridium perfringens* endocarditis. Johns Hopkins Med. J. 130:54, 1972.
53. Masri, A.F., and Grieco, M.H.: Bacteroides endocarditis. Am. J. Med. Sci. 263:357, 1972.
54. Nastro, L.J., and Finegold, S.M.: Endocarditis due to anaerobic gram-negative bacilli. Am. J. Med. 54:482, 1973.
55. Sans, M.D., and Crowder, J.G.: Subacute bacterial endocarditis caused by *Eubacterium aerofaciens*. Am. J. Clin. Pathol. 59:576, 1973.
56. Al-Ibrahim, M.S., and Holzman, R.S.: Treatment of *Bacteriodes* endocarditis with carbenicillin. Am. J. Med. Sci. 273:105, 1977.
57. Galgiani, J.N., Busch, D.F., Brass, C., Rumans, L.W., Mangels, J.I., and Stevens, D.A.: *Bacteroides fragilis* endocarditis, bacteremia and other infections treated with oral or intravenous metronidazole. Am. J. Med. 65:284, 1978.

58. Brancaccio, M., and Legendre, G.C.: *Megasphaera elsdenii* endocarditis. J. Clin. Microbiol. 10:72, 1979.
59. Chow, A.W., Patten, V., and Guze, L.B.: Susceptibility of anaerobic bacteria to metronidazole: relative resistance of non-spore-forming gram-negative bacilli. J. Infect. Dis. 131:182, 1975.
60. Sutter, V.L., and Finegold, S.M.: Susceptibility of anaerobic bacteria to 23 antimicrobial agents. Antimicrob. Ag. Chemother. 10:736, 1976.
61. Dubois, J., and Pechere, J.C.: Activity of ten antimicrobial agents against anaerobic bacteria. J. Antimicrob. Chemother. 4:329, 1978.
62. Appelbaum, P.C. and Chatterton, S.A.: Susceptibility of anaerobic bacteria to ten antimicrobial agents. Antimicrob. Ag. Chemother. 14:371, 1978.
63. Ralph, E.D., and Kirby, W.M.M.: Unique bactericidal action of metronidazole against *Bacteroides fragilis* and *Clostridium perfringens*. Antimicrob. Ag. Chemother. 8:409, 1975.
64. Tally, F.P., Goldin, B.R., Sullivan, N., Johnston, J., and Gorbach, S.L.: Antimicrobial activity of metronidazole in anaerobic bacteria. Antimicrob. Ag. Chemother. 13:460, 1978.
65. Reyes, M.P., El-Khatib, M.R., Brown, W.J., Smith, F., and Lerner, A.M.: Synergy between Carbenicillin and an Aminoglycoside (Gentamicin or Tobramycin) against *Pseudomonas aeruginosa* Isolated from Patients with Endocarditis and Sensitivity of Isolates to Normal Human Serum. J. Infect. Dis. 140:192, 1979.

James J. Rahal, Jr., M.D.
Michael S. Simberkoff, M.D.

10

TREATMENT OF FUNGAL ENDOCARDITIS

Fungal endocarditis is among the most difficult of the infections of the heart to recognize and treat. Symptoms of infection are frequently minimal or nonspecific. Consequently, there may be long delays before the diagnosis is considered and this may result in formation of bulky vegetations, local abscesses and metastatic emboli. In addition, blood cultures are frequently sterile or only intermittently yield the pathogen. This further delays definitive diagnosis and intiation of therapy. Evaluation of therapeutic regimens has been hampered by the relatively small incidence of these infections at individual institutions. Further, a lack of criteria for initial classification of these infections and definitions for follow-up has made it difficult to compare results at differing centers.

The majority of fungal endocardial infections is caused by *Candida* species with a distinctly lesser number due to *Aspergillus.* This review will deal primarily with these two categories plus a third group of miscellaneous fungal endocarditides. Three clinical situations predominate in which such infections occur. These are: (1) prolonged intravenous antibiotic administration, usually for the treatment of bacterial endocarditis; (2) intravenous narcotic abuse; and (3) cardiac surgery for prosthetic or homograft valve replacement, insertion of a Teflon graft, valvuloplasty, or other procedures involving endocardial trauma. Each of these situations presents somewhat different problems in therapy which will be considered in the following discussions.

Candida Endocarditis

Evaluation of past experience with the therapy of *Candida* endocarditis is obfuscated by two major factors. The first is that relapse has been documented as long as 20 months after completion of therapy.[1,2] Therefore, cure should be defined as absence of infection (a) for at least two years after all antifungal therapy has been discontinued, or (b) at surgery or autopsy at least six months after termination of treatment. The majority of cures reported to date have not described the results of clinical follow-up for more than 6–12 months. Thus, reports of survival after combined medical and surgical therapy of 50–73% in natural valve infection must be viewed with reservation.[3,4] The second major complicating factor in evaluating outcome is the lack of adequate clinical criteria for the diagnosis of endocarditis in patients with established candidemia. Medical "cures" of patients with candidemia occurring after antibiotic therapy for bacterial endocarditis or after cardiac valve replacement may be due to eradication of an endophlebitic or wound infection. For these reasons we propose that patients with candidemia in the presence of natural heart valves be classified into one of three major groups for purposes of future reporting (Table 1). The first group, *Possible Endocarditis* includes patients whose candidemia is associated with a removable focus of infection such as an indwelling vascular catheter. The absence of a heart murmur or the presence of a known, unchanging murmur, endopthalmitis, chorioretinitis and/or infected skin lesions (as seen in disseminated candidiasis without endocarditis) make the diagnosis of endocarditis possible but less than probable. Thus, patients with any combination of these findings would be categorized in Group I. In the second group, *Probable Endocarditis,* heroin addiction in the absence of vegetations by echocardiography would make the diagnosis of endocarditis probable but not definite. Patients in this group may or may not have a stable murmur, splenomegaly, Osler nodes, Janeway lesions, petechiae or a rising anticandida antibody titer. *Definite Endocarditis* would then be defined as candidemia in the presence of either a new heart murmur, arterial emboli or aneurysms, vegetations detectable by echocardiography, or isolation of *Candida* from arterial emboli.

Patients whom we would include in Group I on the basis of clinical criteria have been treated and cured by medical and surgical therapy. In these latter instances surgery obviously proved the presence of endocarditis. However, this does not mean that all such patients require operation. Cures have been reported with medical therapy alone among heroin addicts who would be included in Group II.[3,5] In the absence of echocardiographic evidence of vegetations in such patients, it is possible that successful medical therapy might be explained by adequate penetration of amphotericin into early or small vegetations, in contrast to

Table 1. Candidemia in the Presence of Natural Heart Valves

Group I Possible Endocarditis - Medical Therapy
any one or more of the followinq
- A. Removable focus
- B. No murmur or stable murmur
- C. Endophthalmitis or chorioretinits
- D. Infected skin lesions

Group II Probable Endocarditis - Medical Therapy + Surgery (Conditional)
Presence of A. and B., with or without any of C.-F.:
- A. Heroin addiction
- B. Echocardiogram without vegetations
- C. Stable murmur
- D. Splenomegaly
- E. Osler nodes, Janeway lesions, petechiae
- F. Rising antibody

Group III Definite Endocarditis - Medical Therapy + Early Surgery (Mandatory)
Any one or more of the following:
- A. New or changing murmur
- B. Arterial emboli or aneurysms
- C. Vegetations by echocardiography
- D. Isolation of Candida from arterial emboli or aneurysms in the absence of documented candidemia.

its inadequate penetration into large, established vegetations.[1] Experimental studies in rabbits support this hypothesis since amphotericin therapy, initiated shortly after establishment of *Candida* endocarditis, reduced the number of organisms from $10^{8.8}$ to $10^{3.1}$ per gram of vegetation after six days.[6]

Replacement of heart valves for bacterial or fungal endocarditis carries a definite risk of late morbidity and mortality, particularly among heroin addicts. These patients rarely discontinue heroin use after valve replacement and frequently develop subsequent prosthetic valve endocarditis. Reinfection of a prosthetic valve from an occult metastatic focus may also occur. Thus, among eight patients treated by Utley, et al with antifungal agents and valve replacement, six died of later bleeding, pneumonia, cardiac arrest, valve dehiscence, persistent infection or recurrent endocarditis.[7]

In our own previously reported and more recent experience[8], six heroin addicts with criteria for definite *Candida* endocarditis on natural valves have been treated with amphotericin B, 5-fluorocytosine and valve replacement with one survivor for five years. In addition, two heroin addicts and one non-addict with prosthetic valve *Candida* endocarditis have survived for 2–5 years after medical therapy and valve replacement. We have also cured two patients with infections on natural valves with amphotericin B therapy and no surgery. In one of these, 5-fluorocytosine was given also. These patients had fungemia due to *Candida tropicalis* and *Torulopsis glabrata* occuring after prolonged intravenous antibiotic therapy. Both patients would have fulfilled our present criteria for definite endocarditis and valve resection because of arterial embolization. However, one is alive and well five years after medical therapy and the other died seven years following treatment, and there was no evidence of endocarditis at autopsy. Thus, of eleven patients with either prosthetic or natural valve endocarditis, six have survived for two or more years (Table 2).

Our current approach to *Candida* fungemia in patients with natural valves is to give medical therapy alone for those in Groups I and II, using amphotericin B and 5-fluorocytosine. Treatment is discontinued after two weeks in Group I patients with catheter-associated candidemia (at least two positive blood cultures) if the course remains uncomplicated. In the remainder of Group I and II patients, a full therapeutic course of 2–3 grams of amphotericin B plus 5-fluorocytosince is planned. Blood cultures in hyperosmolar media may yield *Candida* during therapy at the time that routine cultures are negative.[9,10] Positive blood cultures by this or other means during treatment, prolonged fever, development of a new murmur, heart failure, pericarditis, conduction disturbance, emboli or vegetations demonstrable by echocardiography are considered to be strong indications for surgery. In the absence of demonstrable vegetations the risk of major embolization during medical therapy may be less than that in patients with a positive echocardiogram. Though this appears to be true for bacterial endocarditis[11], it has not been defined in fungal endocarditis. Obviously, relapse of candidemia after a completed course of therapy would require early valve replacement and retreatment. In reality, relatively few patients should fall into Group II since the majority with candidemia and associated systemic signs might be expected to have demonstrable vegetations by echocardiographic results. In one of our patients a false positive result led to surgery in a patient with candidemia in whom mitral valve prolapse was found rather than endocarditis.

It is widely agreed that patients with criteria for *Definite Endocarditis* (Group III) should be treated with amphotericin B and 5-fluorocytosine, and that valve replacement should be carried out within 48–72 hours to reduce the danger of major emboli.[4] Prolonged preoperative therapy does not aid in survival and surgery should not be delayed for this purpose. Surgical debridement of an infected valve, in association with medical therapy, has resulted in cures documented by eight year follow-up in one instance[12] and by autopsy in another.[13] This procedure cannot be recommended unless anatomic considerations make valve replacement impossible.

Table 2. Fungal Endocarditis: Treatment and Follow-up of Survivors

PATIENT #	AGE	SITE OF INFECTION	ORGANISM	TREATMENT	STATUS-DURATION OF FOLLOW-UP
1.	17	Mitral Valve	*Candida tropicalis*	Amphotericin B	Alive - 5 years
2.	57	Aortis Valve	*Torulopsis glabrata*	Amphotericin B 5-Fluorocytosine	Died - 7 years after infection autopsy-no active endocarditis
3.	59	Mitral Valve Prosthesis	*Candida albicans*	Surgery plus Amphotericin B	Alive - 2 years
4.	23	Aortic Valve	*Candida parapsilosis*	Surgery plus Amphotericin B	Alive - 5 years
5.	27	Mitral Valve Prosthesis	*Candida parasilosis*	Surgery plus Amphotericin B 5-Fluorocytosine	Alive - 5 years
6.	38	Mitral Valve Prosthesis	*Candida parapsilosis*	Surgery plus Amphotericin B	Alive - 3 years

In patients with a prosthetic heart valve the clinician's dilemma in distinguishing between candidemia secondary to a non-cardiac focus and *Candida* endocarditis is increased by the fact that most candidemia in such patients occurs in the early post-operative period when multiple potential extra-caridac sources exist.[4] Because *Candida* infection of a prosthetic valve appears to have a still poorer prognosis than that on natural valves, the indications for surgery must be more liberal. Thus, in patients with a prosthetic valve, candidemia occurring after discharge from the hospital and without an obvious peripheral focus must be considered an indication for valve replacement in addition to medical therapy. Only in the immediate post-operative period would fever and candidemia alone allow antifungal therapy without surgery. Since petechiae occur frequently in the absence of infection following cardiac surgery this sign alone is not an indication of valve infection. Measurement of *Candida* precipitins is a sensitive method for detection of serious infections, but its specificity varies widely with different techniques. A 4-fold rise in antibody may increase specificity. Since *Candida* precipitins have been found by some investigators in almost half of patients following prosthetic valve insertion and in bacterial endocarditis, this test must be used with caution in defining early post-operative *Candida* endocarditis.[14] Detection of *Candida* antigenemia appears to be a highly sensitive and more specific test for systemic *Candida* infection than is measurement of antibody.[15,16] However, its role in defining the presence of endocarditis has not been established. Following initiation of medical therapy for early post-operative candidemia, the presence of persistent fever, candidemia, congestive heart failure, valve dysfunction, a new heart murmur, emboli, splenomegaly, nephritis or evidence of vegetations by echocardiography would provide strong indications for replacement of the prosthetic valve. Each of these must be weighed separately in deciding upon valve replacement and definite criteria cannot be stated for all patients.

Aspergillus Endocarditis

In contrast to *Candida* endocarditis, the prognosis of *Aspergillus* endocarditis appears to be equally grim whether it occurs on a natural or prosthetic valve. There are no known cures after medical therapy alone and few after medical treatment plus valve resection. At least 80% of cases of *Aspergillus* endocarditis occur on prosthetic valves.[17] Many of the remainder are associated with disseminated aspergillosis in immuno-compromised patients in whom both endocarditis and myocardial abscesses develop.[18] Thus, *Aspergillus* endocarditis rarely occurs in heroin addicts with natural heart valves or as a result of prolonged intravenous therapy in immunocompetent hosts. Positive blood cultures are extremely rare in *Aspergillus* endocarditis (10–15%) accounting for the small proportion of pre-mortem diagnoses (25%).[17,19]

The diagnosis is usually made by culture and histologic examination of excised arterial emboli, or at cardiac surgery. Arterial blood cultures have been suggested to aid in diagnosis but their superior yield as compared to venous cultures has not been demonstrated.[17] The number of patients treated with antifungal therapy and valve replacement remains small and sporadic recoveries documented for more than a year have been reported.[17,19,20] Experience to date has clearly demonstrated that survival cannot be expected with medical therapy alone. Early valve replacement, in conjunction with medical therapy, is mandatory when *Aspergillus* is isolated from peripheral emboli, or demonstrated by histologic examination of embolic material. Positive blood cultures occur rarely in disseminated aspergillosis without endocarditis. However, in the presence of a prosthetic valve, *Aspergillus* fungemia must be considered diagnostic of endocarditis. There is insufficient evidence at present to evaluate serologic methods in the diagnosis of *Aspergillus* endocarditis.[21,2] A proportion of *Aspergillus* strains is sensitive to 5-fluorocytosine, and the combination of this drug plus amphotericin B may be both synergistic and fungicidal.[23,24] Combined treatment is therefore preferred although proof of its superiority over amphotericin B alone does not exist. The combination of rifampin and amphotericin B is also synergistic against *Aspergillus*[24,25] but there is no recorded clinical experience with such therapy for endocarditis.

Miscellaneous Fungal Endocarditis

Histoplasma endocarditis is usually a complication of disseminated histoplasmosis but may rarely present as an isolated endocardial infection. Like endocarditis due to *Aspergillus,* blood cultures are usually negative and premortem diagnoses are most often made by culture and histologic examination of peripheral emboli. Large emboli are common in *Histoplasma* endocarditis as in other fungal endocarditides. In a recent review of nine cases treated with amphotericin B alone, three long term (5–18 years) survivors were recorded and two had received a total dose of four grams or more.[26] Thus, it would seem that a trial of medical therapy alone may be justified despite the risk of major embolization. *Histoplasma* infection of prosthetic valves has been reported.[27] Although experience is too limited to form any firm conclusion, the principle of early valve resection for any definite fungal prosthetic valve infection appears appropriate for that due to *Histoplasma.*

Torulopsis glabrata fungemia occurred in 53 patients at the Massachusetts General Hospital during a five year period.[28] Twenty seven were considered to have clinically significant fungemia, seven had disseminated disease and two had fungemia after insertion of prosthetic aortic valves. The setting of fungemia was usually that of prolonged antibiotic administration, intravenous catheters, and gastrointestinal or cardiac surgery. In one patient with a prosthetic valve, fungemia disappeared after six weeks of amphotericin B and 5-fluorocytosine therapy. The results of prolonged follow-up are not known. In another reported case of *Torulopsis* fungemia with a prosthetic valve, amphotericin B therapy failed to eradicate the organism from blood cultures, but 5-fluorocytosine treatment did so.[26] Subsequent cardiac surgery revealed yeasts by histologic examination but cultures were not taken. In one of our patients, *Torulopsis* endocarditis developed on a natural valve 14 months after catheter-related fungemia. Fungemia persisted despite amphotericin B therapy for six months with a total dose of 2.2 grams. Surgery could not be carried out and the patient was subsequently cured by combined amphotericin B - 5-fluorocytosine therapy with a seven year follow-up. Thus, *Torulopsis glabrata* fungemia has many of the characteristics of that due to *Candida albicans.* It may be less virulent and for this reason may be more susceptible to antifungal therapy, particularly 5-fluorocytosine in combination with amphotericin B. As with *Candida albicans,* we favor a two week course of antifungal therapy for patients with two or more positive blood cultures containing *Torulopsis* in the presence of an intravenous catheter without other signs of infection. If a prosthetic heart valve is present, treatment for 4-6 weeks is probably indicated. The indications for prosthetic valve replacement would be the same as for patients with *Candida* fungemia in this setting.

A large variety of miscellaneous fungi have been described as causes of both natural and prosthetic valve endocarditis. These include *Saccharomyces, Phialophora, Paecilomyces, Mucor, Penicillium,* and others.[30–33]. Most have been diagnosed at post-mortem examination and there is insufficient experience with each to draw therapeutic conclusions. Factors such as the duration and severity of illness, presence of vegetations by echocardiography, underlying disease, and occurrence of emboli or other metastatic foci of infection should be used to decide whether valve replacement is indicated in addition to medical therapy. When a prosthetic valve is present, its early replacement would seem to be the most conservative approach.

Antifungal Agents

The optimal dose and duration of amphotericin B is not known and the value of 5-fluorcytosine as an additional agent has not been demonstrated by clinical trials. The two drugs are synergistic against approximately 25% of yeast-like pathogens.[34] In lethal *Candida* infection of mice the survival rate in animals treated with either drug alone is increased from 15% to 80% by combined therapy.[35] However, in experimental *Candida*[6] and *Aspergillus*[36] endocarditis, no enhanced killing of fungi on infected valves occurs when both drugs are combined. *In vivo* results may vary depending upon the presence of *in vitro* synergy and whether such synergy is fungistatic or fungicidal.

Because of the unfavorable overall prognosis of fungal endocarditis, combined therapy is reasonable despite the potential bone marrow and hepatic toxicity of 5-fluorocytosine. Blood isolates should be tested for *in vitro* susceptibility to amphotericin B, 5-fluorocytosine and the combination. Organisms resistant to 5-fluorocytosine (minimal inhibitory concentration $> 25\ \mu g/ml$) may still be susceptible to a synergistic effect of both drugs.[34,37] If both resistance to 5-fluorocytosine and absence of synergy with amphotericin B are demonstrated *in vitro*, then treatment with 5-fluorocytosine is not indicated.

Most reports have described the use of 1.5–3.0 grams of amphotericin B as a full therapeutic course. The previously recommended daily dose of 1 mg per kilogram is larger than necessary to achieve therapeutic blood levels against the majority of fungi.[38] Nephrotoxicity can be reduced by using a maximum daily dose of 0.5–0.6 mg/kg/day or 25–50 mg per day. A test dose of 1 mg is given in 100 ml 5% dextrose in water over 20–30 minutes. If fever, chills or hypotension occur, subsequent doses should be preceded by 25–50 mg of hydrocortisone, or the latter can be added to the amphotericin infusion. For patients with serious, progressive disease such as endocarditis, the test dose should be followed by 5 and 10 mg infusions during the first 24 hours and a 25 mg dose within 48 hours. Subsequent increments are given on a daily or every other day schedule at a rate of 25–50 mg per day with adjustments to maintain the serum creatinine below 3.0 mg%. Serum potassium concentrations should be followed carefully since significant hypokalemia secondary to renal tubular dysfunction may require potassium replacement.

Fluorocytosine is given in a daily dose of 150mg/kg when renal function is normal. Diminished renal function due to amphotericin eventually occurs in all patients and should lead to an appropriate reduction in the dose of 5-fluorocytosine. One fourth of the daily dose is given every six hours when creatinine clearance is greater than 40 ml per minute, every 12 hours for clearance of 20–40 ml per minute and every 24 hours for clearance of 10–20 mg per minute. Fluorocytosine can be hemodialyzed, the rate varying with dialysis flow rates. Following valve replacement treatment should be continued for at least six weeks unless the patient has received a total dose of 3.0 grams of amphotericin B before the sixth postoperative week. A newer antifungal agent, miconozole, is active against a wide variety of fungal pathogens. Published clinical trials to date have not included patients with fungal endocarditis.[39]

REFERENCES

1. Rubinstein, E., Noriega, E.R., Simberkoff, M.S., and Rahal, J.J., Jr.: Tissue penetration of amphotericin B in Candida endocarditis. *Chest 66:* 376, 1974.
2. Galgiani, J.N. and Stevens, D.A.: Fungal endocarditis: Need for guidelines in evaluating therapy. *J. Thorac. Cardiovasc. Surg. 73:*293, 1977.
3. Premsingh, N., Kapilla, R., Tecson, F., Smith, L.G., and Louria, D.B.: Candida endocarditis in two patients. *Arch. Intern. Med. 136:* 208, 1976.
4. McLeod, R., and Remington, J.S.: Postoperative fungal endocarditis in Duma, R.J. (ed.): Infections of prosthetic heart valves and vascular grafts. (Baltimore: University Park Press, 1977), Chapter 9, p. 163.
5. Mayrer, A.R., Brown, A., Weintraub, R.A., Ragni, M. and Postic, B: Successful medical therapy for endocarditis due to *Candida parasilosis. Chest 73:*546, 1978.
6. Sande, M.A., Bowman, C.R., and Calderone, R.A.: Experimental *Candida albicans* endocarditis: Characterization of the disease and response to therapy. *Antimicrob. Agents Chemother.. 17:* 140, 1977.
7. Utley, J.R., Millsa, J. and Roe, B.B.: The role of valve replacement in the treatment of fungal endocarditis. *J. Thorac. Cardiovasc. Surg. 69:* 255, 1975.
8. Rubinstein, E., Noriega, E.R., Simberkoff, M.S., Holzman, R., and Rahal, J.J.. Jr.: Fungal endocarditis: Analysis of 24 cases and review of the literature. *Medicine 54:* 331, 1975.
9. Rosner, R.: Isolation of Candida protoplasts from a case of Candida endocarditis. *J. Bacterial. 91*: 1320, 1966.
10. Watanakunakorn, C., Carleton, J., Goldberg, L.M. and Hamburger, M. Candida endocarditis surrounding a Starr-Edwards prosthetic valve. *Arch. Intern. Med. 121:* 243, 1968.
11. Mintz, G.S., Kotler, M.N., Segal, B.L. and Parry, W.R.: Survival of patients with aortic valve endocarditis. The prognostic implications of the echocardiogram. *Arch. Intern Med. 139:* 862, 1979.
12. Turnier, E., Kay, J.H., Bernstein, S. Mendez, A.M. and Zubiate, P.: Surgical treatment of Candida endocarditis. *Chest 67:* 262, 1975.
13. Gladstone, J.L., Friedman, S.A., Cerruti, M.M. and Jomain, S.L. Treatment of Candida endocarditis and arteritis. *J. Thorac. Cardiovasc. Surg. 71:* 835, 1976.
14. Dee, T.H.: Mycoserology: its status as a diagnostic adjunct, in Rytel, M.W. (es.): Rapid Diagnosis in Infectious Disease (Boca Ration: CRC Press, Inc., 1979) Ch. 12 p. 157.
15. Kerkering, T.M., Espinel-Ingeroff, A., and Shadomy, S. Detection of Candida antigenemia by counter immunoelectrophoresis in patients with invasive candidiasis. *J. Infect. Dis. 140:* 659, 1979.

16. Weiner, M.H. and Coats-Stephen, M. Immunodiagnosis of systemic candidiasis: mannan antigenemia detected by radioimmunoassay in experimental and human infections. *J. Infect. Dis. 140:* 989, 1979.
17. Kammer, R.B. and Utż, J.P.: Aspergillus species endocarditis. *Amer. J. Med. 56:* 506, 1974.
18. Walsh, T.J., and Hutchins, G.M.: Aspergillus mural endocarditis. *Amer. J. Clin. Pathol. 71:* 640, 1979.
19. Carrizosa, J., Levison, M.E., Lawrence, T. and Kaye, D.: Cure of *Aspergillus ustus* endocarditis on prosthetic valve. *Arch. Intern. Med. 133:* 486, 1974.
20. Lawrence, T., Shockman, A.T. and MacVaugh, H.: Aspergillus infection of prosthetic aortic valves. *Chest 60:* 406, 1971.
21. Shaffer, P.J., Medoff, G., and Kobayashi, G.S. Demonstration of antigenemia by radioimmunoassay in rabbits experimentally infected with Aspergillus. *J. Infect. Dis. 139:* 313, 1979.
22. Weiner, M.H. and Coats-Stephen, M: Immunodiagnosis of systemic aspergillosis. I. Antigenemia detected by radioimmunoassay in experimental infection. *J. Lab. Clin. Med. 93:* 111, 1979.
23. Lauer, B.A., Reller, L.B. and Schroter, P.J.: Susceptibility of Aspergillus to 5-fluorocytosine and amphotericin B alone and in combination. *J. Antimicrob. Chemother. 4:* 375–380, 1978.
24. Kitahara, M., Seth, V.K., Medoff, G. and Kobayashi, G.S.: Activity of amphotericin B, 5-fluorocytosine, and rifampin against six clinical isolates of Aspergillus. *Antimicrob Agents Chemother. 9:* 915, 1976.
25. Ribner, B., Keusch, G.T. Hanna, B.A. and Perloff, M.: Combination amphortericin B-rifampin therapy for pulmonary Aspergillus in a leukemic patient. *Chest. 70:* 681. 1976.
26. Goodwin, R.A, Jr., Shapiro, J.L., Thuman, G.H., Thusman, S.S. and Des Prez, R.M. Disseminated histoplasmosis: Clinical and pathologic correlations. *Medicine 59:* 1, 1980.
27. Alexander, W.J., Mowry, R.W., Cobbs, C.G., and Dismukes, W.E. Prosthetic valve endocarditis caused by Histoplasma. *J. Amer. Med. Assoc. 242:* 1399, 1979.
28. Berkowitz, I.D., Robboy, S.J., Karchmer, A.W. and Kunz, L.J.: *Torulopsis glabrata* fungemia - A clinical pathological study. *Medicine 58:* 430, 1979.
29. Sharpe, D.N., Singh, B.N., Cornere, B.M. and Allwood, G.K.: *Torulosis glabrata* endocarditis complicating aortic homograft valve treated with 5-fluorocytosine: Case report with discussion of antifungal chemotherapy. New Zealand Medical Journal 81:294, 1975.
30. Stein, P.D., Folkens, A.T. and Hruska, K.A.: Saccharomyces fungemia. *Chest 58:* 173, 1970.
31. Khicha, G.J., Berroya, R.B., Escano, F.B., and Lee, C.S.: Mucormycosis in a mitral prothesis. *J. Thorac. Cardiovasc. Surg. 63:* 903–905, 1972.

32. Upshaw, C.B. Jr.: Penicillium endocarditis of aortic valve prosthesis. *J. Thorac. Cardiovasc. Surg. 68:* 428, 1974.
33. Slifkin, M., and Bowers, H.M., Jr.: *Philophora mutabilis* endocarditis. *Amer. J. Clin. Pathol. 63:* 120, 1975.
34. Shadomy, S., Wagner, G., Espinel-Ingroff, A., and Davis, B.A.: *In vitro* studies with combinations of 5-fluorocytosine and amphotericin B. *Antimicrob. Agents Chemother. 8:* 117, 1975.
35. Rabinovich, S., Shaw, B.D., Bryant, T., and Donta, S.T.: Effect of 5-fluorocytosine and amphotericin B on *Candida albicans* infection in mice. *J. Infect. Dis. 130:* 28, 1974.
36. Carrizosa, J., Kohn, C., and Levison, M.E.: Experimental Aspergillus endocarditis in rabbits. *J. Lab. Clin. Med. 86:* 746, 1975.
37. Medoff, G., Comfort, M. and Kobayashi, G.S.: Synergistic action of amphotericin B and 5-fluorocytosine against yeast-like organisms. *Proc. Soc. Exp. Biol. Med. 138:* 571, 1971.
38. Bennett, J.E.: Medical intelligence: drug therapy chemotherapy of systemic mycoses. *N. Engl. J. Med. 290:* 30, 320, 1974.
39. Wade, T.R., Jones, H.E. and Chanda, J.J.: Intravenous miconzaole therapy of mycotic infections. *Arch. Intern. Med. 139:* 784, 1979.

C. Glenn Cobbs, M.D.
Wiley K. Livingston, M.D.

11

SPECIAL PROBLEMS IN THE MANAGEMENT OF INFECTIVE ENDOCARDITIS

Patients with infective endocarditis may present a wide variety of clinical manifestations and provide the clinician with a number of diagnostic and therapeutic challenges. While many of the symptoms and signs are due directly to multiplication of microorganisms at the endocardial site, others are the result of complications of the disorder. Operationally the complications of infective endocarditis may reflect cardiac disorders or lesions in other organs.[1] The purpose of this chapter is to consider primarily the diagnosis and treatment of non-cardiac complications.

Mycotic Aneurysms

Mycotic aneurysm describes a lesion caused by microbial infection in or near a vessel with subsequent aneurysmal dilatation. It may result from infected embolus or suppuration in adjacent tissue. Mycotic aneurysms may complicate vascular surgery or arise *de novo* in damaged vessels such as the abdominal aorta in patients with atherosclerosis. Mycotic aneurysms are an especially important complication of infective endocarditis and are discovered in 2–10% of patients; in about one quarter of cases in which they occur the aneurysms are multiple.[2,3] There has been a clinical impression that avirulent bacteria such as viridans streptococci are more likely to cause mycotic aneurysms than virulent ones such as *Staphylococcus aureus*[4,5] and it has been suggested that this is probably related to the duration of the disease prior to initiation of therapy. Recent work in animal models may provide new insights into the pathogenesis of this lesion and the influence of the particular variety of bacteria. Using dogs, Molinari and workers injected elastic silicone rubber emboli coated with different bacteria into the carotid artery.[6,7] They found that dogs embolized into the carotid circulation with virulent organisms such as *Staphylococcus aureus* developed mycotic aneurysms, often within 24 h of the embolic event, whereas animals inoculated with particles coated with viridans streptococci were more likely to develop brain abscess after several days. Although bacteria were obviously delivered to the intimal surface by this process, the subsequent inflammatory changes began in the adventitia and spread inwardly. Other authors have documented this same direction of spread in clinical specimens.[8] It has been postulated that stasis in the lumen following embolization permits bacterial spread to the *vasa vasorum* with resulting inflammatory response and weakening of the arterial wall.[7,9] The dog models described give only a rough approximation of events which may occur in human disease and the precise role of bacterial virulence and host mechanisms in this disorder remains uncertain.

The sites of mycotic aneurysms which become apparent clinically will be a function of circulatory factors which are poorly defined and the ease with which a lesion can be recognized. Mycotic aneurysms are detected most commonly in the central nervous system, particularly when they are symptomatic.[10] We are aware of no *post mortem* studies in patients with infective endocarditis in which mycotic aneurysms have been carefully searched for in the entire vascular tree. Clearly, asymptomatic aneurysms occur in the central nervous system (as well as other sites) but whether there is a special susceptibility of vessels in the cerebral circulation for this lesion or whether their frequency in this site reflects the high incidence of arteriography of cerebral vessels is unclear.

Symptomatic mycotic aneurysms of vessels supplying extremities generally produce pain, tenderness and a palpable mass[11], in contrast to abdominal visceral aneurysms which are more difficult to diagnose clinically.[12] Mycotic aneurysms found in extremities should be repaired, and ligation of the vessel with complete resection of the aneurysm is the best procedure. If collateral circulation is not sufficient to allow resection, any graft introduced should bypass the infected area as widely as possible in order to prevent recurrent infection.[12,13] In addition prosthetic devices must not be utilized to restore circulation at the site of active infection; if grafting is necessary vein grafts should be used. Mycotic aneurysms discovered in abdominal viscera should be handled similarly. If the lesion cannot be resected, embolization of the involved artery may suffice.[14] Obviously careful cultures must be obtained of any material available at the time of surgical exploration. Management of cerebral mycotic aneurysms is discussed below (see section on "central nervous system complications").

Embolization

Approximately half of patients with endocarditis manifest evidence of systemic embolization, and up to 20% of patients with endocarditis will have admission prompted by an embolic event.[15,16] Emboli appear to be more common when endocarditis involves a prosthetic heart valve.[16] The presence of a bulky foreign body, paravalvular leak, and/or ring abscess probably predisposes to the formation of larger vegetations than when infection involves a native valve.

In patients with right-sided endocarditis, particularly complicating intravenous drug abuse, pulmonary embolism maybe seen in as many as 64% of patients.[17] *S. aureus* endocarditis involving the tricuspid valve is often associated with septic pulmonary emboli. Such patients complain of fever, chest pain, and pleurisy, and chest roentgenograms often reveal metastatic pulmonary abscess and/or empyema. In this circumstance the pulmonary symptoms and signs often dominate the clinical picture.

Although systemic embolism may complicate infective endocarditis caused by any variety of bacteria, some authors have stated that embolic phenomena occurring within the first two weeks of illness are more likely to reflect *Staphylococcus aureus* disease, whereas emboli occurring after two weeks are usually due to endocarditis caused by less virulent bacteria such as viridans streptococci.[2] Patients with infective endocarditis due to anaerobic bacteria also appear to experience a high rate of embolization.[18] Systemic emboli are most commonly appreciated in the central nervous system, coronary vessels, kidney and spleen.[19] It is likely that emboli lodge in vessels supplying muscles and other organs as well but that their presence is not appreciated as easily in these sites.

Fungal endocarditis, whether occurring on a native or prosthetic heart valve, is associated with bulky vegetations and large emboli. These emboli may be the only source of diagnostic material, especially in the case of fungi which are not easily recovered from blood such as *Histoplasma capsulatum* or aspergillus.[20]

Emboli frequently cause ischemic damage to organs involved. In the central nervous system the middle cerebral artery is the most common site of lodgement and sudden onset of focal neurologic deficits occurs following embolization. If the particular area of brain is supplied by collaterals the neurologic disorder may be transient. One author has reported transient ischemic attacks in association with major embolic events in as many as 25% of patients.[21] As noted above embolization associated with endocarditis caused by virulent microorganisms may result in formation of mycotic aneurysms at the site of the lodgement.

It is difficult to predict which patients are at risk for major emboli. Echocardiograms may be useful; if large vegetations are detected, there appears to be an approximate 30% incidence of subsequent embolization.[22] In addition, these authors found the chances of a clinically significant embolic event are increased in patients with certain echocardiographic findings: (1) vegetations associated with flail leaflets of the aortic or mitral valve, (2) the presence of significant aortic regurgitation and mitral preclosure, (3) vegetations present on both mitral and aortic valves, and (4) involvement of the mitral chordae or left ventricular endocardium with vegetation. Vegetations were rarely appreciated by echocardiogram during the first 2 weeks of clinically apparent endocarditis. Clearly vegetations may persist well beyond bacteriologic cure and emboli may occur after otherwise successful antimicrobial therapy. As the resolution power of most echocardiograms is 2 mm, smaller vegetations will be missed by this technique, and major embolic events may occur in patients whose echocardiogram revealed no vegetations.

Management of Embolization

When an embolus is suspected, emergency arteriography is indicated, and if vital organ function is impaired, surgical removal is necessary. This is often impractical in the central nervous system, myocardium, lung, kidney and spleen, but is feasible when vessels supplying the extremities are involved. Anticoagulants do not prevent emboli in infective endocarditis and because of potentially severe bleeding complications experienced by patients with infective endocarditis, anticoagulants are contraindicated in most patients.[19] Exceptions may include patients with prosthetic valves and patients with venous thrombophlebitis unrelated to their endocarditis. Theoretically, antiplatelet agents may help prevent emboli in infective endocarditis, but at present their role remains undefined.[2] In the patient with more than one major embolic event valve replacement is indicated and this procedure should also be considered in the patient with one embolus plus vegetations demonstrable by echocardiogram. Patients who experience a major cerebral embolic event have a mortality of 50–80%.[2,21] Clearly future emphasis should be placed on prevention of this disorder.

Central Nervous System Complications

Perhaps one third of patients with infective endocarditis develop neurologic complications, and according to one study these patients have a higher mortality rate, 58% compared to 20% for those patients without such complications.[2] The incidence of central nervous system involvement is greater when the infectious agent is more virulent - e.g. *Staphylococcus aureus, Streptococcus pneumoniae,* gram-negative bacilli, and anaerobes - than when viridans streptococci are implicated.[2,18,23] In addition, for reasons which are unclear, older patients appear to be at increased risk for these disorders.[4]

Potential neurologic complications of infective endocarditis are listed in Table 1. In addition to the previously mentioned mycotic aneurysms and emboli, they include brainstem syndromes, cranial nerve palsies,

Table 1. Neurologic Complications of Infective Endocarditis.

DISORDER	COMMENT
Brainstem syndrome	Usually secondary to emboli, and may present as dyskinesias, nausea, vomiting, or hiccuping.
Cranial nerve palsies	Uncommon complication. When they occur, usually secondary to emboli. Most commonly manifested as disorder of extra-ocular movement.
Decreased level of consciousness	Multiple causes, including metabolic (acid-base, electrolyte imbalance, hypoxia, severe hyperthermia), cardiac dysrrhythmias, drug toxicity, meningitis, intracranial mass lesion, subarachnoid hemorrhage, massive cerebral infarction, septic shock.
Meningitis	May be culture (+) or (-). May be a manifestation of leaking mycotic aneurysm, brain abscess, cerebral infarction due to embolus, thrombosis, vasculitis, or bacteremic infection.
Peripheral neuropathy	Acute mononeuropathy probably results from immune injury. Uncommon.
Psychiatric	Behavioral disorders may result from anatomic lesions, diffuse vasculitis, or may reflect chronic illness, depression, or drug toxicity. More common in older patients, and denotes a poorer prognosis.
Seizures	Focal seizures usually reflect infarction. Generalized seizures can be associated with mycotic aneurysm, brain abscess, meningitis, cerebral hypoxia, uremia, and drug toxicity. High dose penicillin therapy in renal failure particularly likely to result in neurotoxicity.
Stroke syndrome	Emboli are the major cause, but may be seen with intracerebral hemorrhage. The patient may develop signs of hemiplegia, aphasia, sensory loss, or ataxia.
Subarachnoid hemorrhage	Usually secondary to leaking mycotic aneurysm. However, cutaneous petechiae and purpura, presumably as a result of immunologic injury to vessels, may have a counterpart in the CNS, and gross bleeding can result from these lesions.
Visual disorders	May result from cranial nerve dysfunction, iridocyclitis, endopthalmitis, or involvement of optical tracts and cortex. Embolus to the central retinal artery is an ophthalmologic emergency.

(continued)

Miscellaneous	Symptoms of lightning-like pains in the extremities, diffuse myopathy, and even findings suggestive of a demyelinating disease may be present. Infective endocarditis may masquerade as hepatic, collagen-vascular, or uremic encephalopathy. Patients may present with more than one of the categories listed above.

meningo-encephalitis, peripheral nerve disorders, psychiatric abnormalities, seizures, and visual disturbances.[1,24] There seems to be little correlation between the type of neurologic disorder and any particular cardiac lesion.[25] Brainstem emboli may present as hiccuping or nausea and vomiting. Meningitis may be associated with multiplication of the etiologic microorganism in the subarachnoid space or complicate a parameningeal lesion such as brain abscess, leaking mycotic aneurysm, cerebral infarction, thrombosis, or immune-mediated arteritis. Decreased level of consciousness, behavioral disturbances or seizures may be seen in inflammatory disorders due to infective endocarditis but careful evaluation should also be undertaken for unsuspected hypoxia, uremia, or toxicity due to penicillin or lidocaine. Visual disturbances may be produced by several pathogenetic mechanisms, including cranial nerve palsies caused by cortical or brain stem lesions, involvement of visual tracts or cortex with resulting hemianopsia, or direct injury to the eye. Emboli may occlude the central artery of the retina, producing unilateral blindness. Finally, immunologically mediated lesions such as Roth spots, which probably share a common pathogenetic mechanism with cutaneous petechiae, and iridocyclitis may cause visual disturbances.

Intracranial mycotic aneurysms are most commonly found along the branches of the middle cerebral artery, often at the bifurcations, tend to be peripheral, and may develop during otherwise successful antimicrobial therapy.[4,8,19] They may elicit injury through pressure effects, or by secondary thrombosis leading to infarction. Most commonly they become clinically apparant when they bleed. When this occurs the bleeding is usually vigorous and not preceeded by a warning leak.[8] Frequently there are focal neurologic signs, and meningismus if the bleeding is into the subarachnoid space; often there are also manifestations of ischemia due to the intense vasospasm which accompanies the bleed.

When a patient with infective endocarditis demonstrates any neurologic impairment, an aggressive evaluation is necessary. Figure 1 illustrates an approach to the management of patients with infective endocarditis and a neurologic disorder. Physical examination and appropriate laboratory tests should be performed for possible hypoxia, uremia, dysrhythmias, acid-base disorders, or drug toxicity, in addition to evaluation for possible focal neurologic signs. Should focal abnormalities or evidence of increased intracranial pressure be present, computed tomography (CT) scanning should be performed without delay. If a large abscess is detected, then neurosurgical evaluation should be obtained. Multiple small (less than 1

Figure 1.

Infective endocarditis and neurologic deterioration:
decreased level of consciousness; focal signs; seizure; visual, psychiatric, cranial nerve dysfunction*

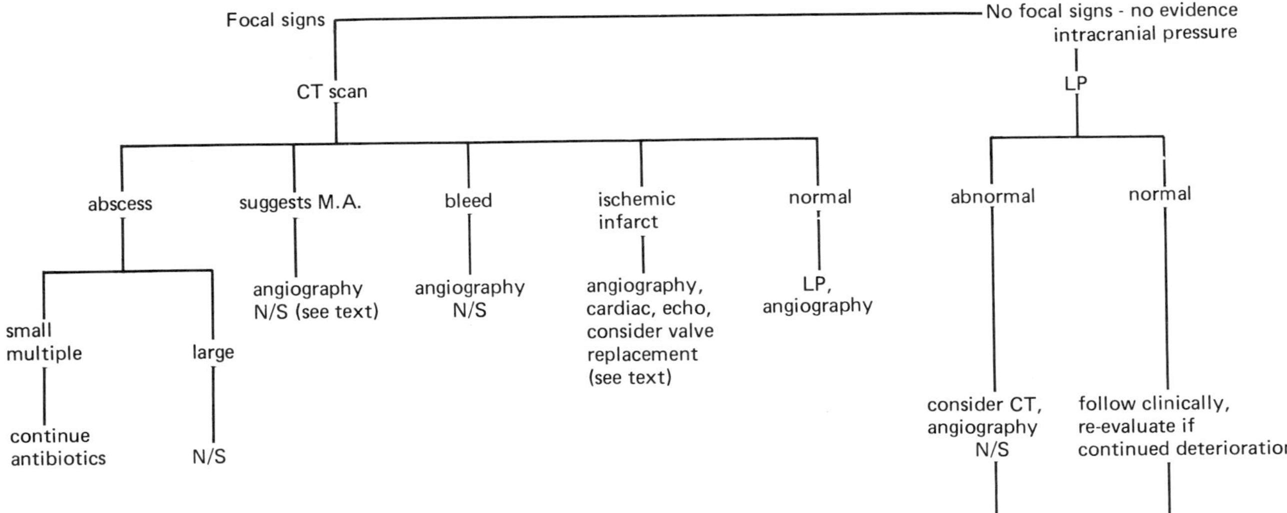

*Evaluate for hypoxia, uremia, acid-base disturbance, dysrhythmia, drug effects.

Figure 1. Proposed flow chart in the patient presenting with infective endocarditis and unexplained neurologic deterioration. Obviously every patient will not precisely fit the categories outlined and individualization of diagnostic and therapeutic management will be required. Abbreviations: CT-computed tomography, L.P. - lumbar puncture, M.A. - mycotic aneurysms, N/S - Neurosurgery

cm) abscesses should resolve with antimicrobial therapy alone.[4], and it is essential in this or any other neurological disorder in patients with infective endocarditis that the patient receive antimicrobial agents which cross the blood-brain barrier in high concentrations.

If a cerebral infarction is demonstrated, angiography should be performed. If no other abnormalities are found, conservative medical therapy is indicated, and an echocardiogram should be performed if not recently done. If vegetations are noted, valve replacement should be considered.

If the CT scan demonstrates a hemorrhage, four vessel cerebral angiography should be scheduled and neurosurgical assistance requested. The precise role of the CT scan remains to be defined in the evaluation of mycotic aneurysms which have not bled.

If no mass lesions are located, then lumbar puncture should be performed. There may be increased intracranial pressure and/or examination of cerebral spinal fluid may reveal cells. The glucose may be normal or depressed. If there are abnormalities of the cerebral spinal fluid, or if the patient continues to have unexplained neurologic deterioration, four vessel cerebral angiography should be performed. Neurosurgical intervention is recommended if a peripheral cerebral mycotic aneurysm is discovered and has bled.

Because there is an overall 65% chance of rupture of mycotic aneurysms and 28–80% mortality in those which bleed[8,26], it has previously been recommended that all aneurysms, whether they have bled or not, be repaired without delay once they are identified.[27] However, it has been shown with angiography that up to 30% of mycotic aneurysms may disappear on medical therapy alone.[2,26] We recommend that single peripheral cerebral aneurysms which have bled be clipped; if asymptomatic peripheral aneurysms are easily accesible to neurosurgery, they too should be clipped because of the low risk of such an operation.[28] Asymptomatic aneurysms, which in the opinion of the neurosurgeon may be more difficult to repair, should be followed by angiography at intervals of 1–2 weeks. Multiple aneurysms should also be radiographically followed. Enlargement of an aneurysm while on therapy has been considered by some authors an indication for immediate surgical repair. However, if angiograms are obtained early in the course of infective endocarditis, many aneurysms will appear to enlarge. Since these aneurysms may nevertheless resolved with appropriate medical treatment alone, at our institution surgical intervention is reserved for those aneurysms which bleed; an aneurysm which enlarges following *completion* of antimicrobial therapy should also be surgically repaired.[28]

Opinions vary on the course to be taken if the aneurysm remains the same size on subsequent studies, but it is probably best to wait until after completion of antimicrobial therapy to operate. Follow-up angiograms obtained in patients after completion of antimicrobial therapy have demonstrated eventual resolution in some cases.[28] The patient with a mycotic aneurysm should be kept at bed rest with sedation if necessary. The roles of hypotensive therapy and of antifibrinolytic agents remain controversial. Angiography should also be performed approximately 2 weeks after any surgery to evaluate the results of that surgery and to ascertain whether new mycotic aneurysms have developed.

Mycotic aneurysms in the circle of Willis pose a special problem, because of the chance that the friable aneurysm may fragment, requiring ligation of the parent artery producing severe neurological deficit. These patients should probably be monitored with angiography, and after antimicrobial therapy has been completed, the aneurysms may be fibrotic enough to allow surgery. There is no good solution for treating the enlarging proximal cerebral mycotic aneurysm. Newer neurosurgical techniques, such as extra-to-intracranial anastomosis of major vessels may prove valuable in these patients.

Any patient with a cerebral mycotic aneurysm should be closely followed by a neurosurgeon. For more detailed descriptions of approaches to patients with intracranial mycotic aneurysms, the reader is referred to several recent reviews.[2,8,26,28] Occasionally patients with infective endocarditis are found to have mycotic aneurysms and heart failure, and valve replacement is necessary. If possible, the mycotic aneurysm must be repaired before open heart surgery since that operation necessitates anticoagulation with attendent risk of aneurysmal bleeding. When emergency cardiac surgery is required, the use of a xenograft is recommended to avoid the risk of prolonged anticoagulation.

The patient with infective endocarditis and neurologic deterioration, who has no evidence of increased intracranial pressure or focal findings, should have lumbar puncture performed. If the cerebrospinal fluid is normal, subsequent re-evaluation with repeat lumbar puncture or CT scan is probably indicated while continuing evaluation for possible metabolic disorders. Except in the event of a major hemorrhage, an abnormal cerebrospinal fluid formula is not specific for any lesion and may indicate any one of the disorders previously discussed.[2] Further evaluation with CT scan and angiography may be necessary. Antimicrobial coverage should be modified if necessary to insure adequate levels in the cerebrospinal fluid. If unusual gram-negative bacilli or exceptionally resistant microorganisms are involved, intrathecal or intraventricular administration through an Omaya reservior may be required.

The approach to each patient with infective endocarditis and neurologic deterioration must be individualized in order to take into consideration special circumstances and provide optimum care. In an emergent situation prompt neurosurgical evaluation is essential.

Culture Negative Endocarditis

Recently there have appeared several reviews of culture negative endocarditis.[29,30,31,32] Since the first descriptions of infective endocarditis in the 19th century, patients have been observed with clinical signs and symptoms of the disorder and blood cultures which were persistently negative utilizing methods available at the time. In 1913 Dr. Libman popularized the concept of "culture negative endocarditis", describing it as a particularly virulent form of the disorder.[33] Presently most authorities report 10–15% of patients with infective endocarditis have negative blood cultures.[34]

The frequency of positive blood culture in patients with infective endocarditis depends on several factors: (1) the volume of blood cultured, (2) the facility with which a particular microorganism can be grown from the culture medium employed, (3) the duration cultures are held and the care with which they are observed, (4) presence of prior antimicrobial agents or inhibitory factors in serum, (5) the frequency with which pathologic tissue can be examined in order to make the diagnosis (development of techniques for open heart surgery have provided us the ability to look at valves in living patients to determine if in fact they are infected), (6) the frequency with which the physician is misled by diseases mimicking infective endocarditis. The reader is referred to chapter 15 for a detailed consideration of the microbiologic issues relating to blood culture negative endocarditis.

There have been a number of reports of infective endocarditis caused by fastidious bacteria (Chapter 15) and these have been summarized in two recent reviews.[35,36] In addition recent reports have described some patients with infective endocarditis caused by streptococci requiring thiol or pyridoxal supplemented media for growth.[37,38,39] Anaerobic bacteria may also be difficult to culture and will be missed if appropriate media are not utilized. Mycobacterial endocarditis is rare, but cases caused by *M. chelonei* have been reported in the past few years, and recently contamination of xenograft valves with these microorganisms prior to surgery has been reported.[40,41] This latter should be considered in patients with xenograft valves who present with the clinical syndrome of infective endocarditis and negative blood cultures.

While candida is usually cultured easily from blood, some other fungi are more difficult to grow. Patients with aspergillus endocarditis almost always have negative blood cultures, and when *H. capsulatum* causes endocarditis cultures are also usually sterile. *Coxiella burnetti* (Q fever) and *Chlamydia psittaci* (psittacosis) may cause endocarditis and will not grow in usual media. While a few cases of endocarditis due to viral infection have been reported, most authors doubt the existence of such an entity.[31]

Cell wall defective bacterial variants have received some attention as possible causes of culture negative endocarditis, but there is presently insufficient evidence to justify elaborate culture proceedures aimed at their isolation and identification.[5,42] Hypertonic medium is probably worthwhile for use in patients who have previously received cell wall active antimicrobial agents.

There are a number of non-infectious disorders which may mimic infective endocarditis: they include atrial myxoma, pulmonary embolism, collagen vascular disease, and marantic endocarditis. Systemic lupus erythematosis and acute rheumatic fever with congestive heart failure may be particularly difficult to distinguish clinically from endocarditis. Immune complexes and autoantibodies have been described in patients with infective endocarditis who were not subsequently found to have collagen vascular disease. As many as 50% of patients may have rheumatoid factor in serum[43], and anti-nuclear antibodies in high titer have been described in a few patients.[44] Therefore special care must be taken in making a diagnosis of collagen vascular disorder based on a limited number of serologic tests alone.

Marantic or non-bacterial thrombotic endocarditis (NBTE) may be especially common in patients with mucin-secreting adenocarcinomas. Patients with NBTE may have fever, leukocytosis, petechiae, and emboli sufficiently large to occlude even major vessels. Histologic examination of emboli or heart valves reveals platelets and fibrin, but virtually no cellular reaction.[45]

Approach to Patients with Suspected Infective Endocarditis and Negative Cultures

A detailed history may be useful in defining the causative agent in culture negative endocarditis. Infections with Brucella and Q fever, for example, are commonly associated with contact with domestic animals and their secretions. Psittacosis usually follows close contact with psittacine birds, especially imported varieties. Residence or travel in certain locations may provide clues to the possibility of fungal infections, e.g. coccidiodomycosis. The immunocompromised patient may be at risk for infection by Candida or Aspergillus.

Table 2 illustrates an approach to the patient with suspected blood culture negative endocaridits. Once appropriate blood cultures (including hypertonic and anaerobic media) have been obtained, they should be held for 4 weeks with periodic blind subculturing. Some of the more recently developed blood culture media contain L-cysteine and pyridoxal, which may improve recovery of fastidious streptococci. Commerical preparations contain different additives ,and it is necessary to inspect each type of medium used in any particular laboratory to determine if the substances required for growth by fastidious microorganisms are included. If available, the Bactec[R] automated system appears to be capable of adequately detecting bacteremia. If non-automated systems are utilized, we recommend the use of Tryptic Soy Broth as the basic blood culture medium.

Table 2. Diagnostic Approach to the Patient with Culture Negative Endocarditis

General

1. History: epidemiology (attention to animal exposure, travel history, immune status)

2. Physical exam: particular attention to optic fundus for chorioretinitis.

3. Culture techniques: aerobic, anaerobic, hypertonic bottles; optimal blood/-medium ratio; hold 4—6 weeks; close inspection of culture bottles; blind subculture at least once each week; +/- add penicillinase if patient has taken beta lactam antibiotics prior to cultures.

4. Consider culturing other sites: bone marrow, +/- petechiae

5. Examine peripheral smear for intraleukocytic microorganisms.

6. Serial echocardiograms

7. Acute and convalescent serologic testing for: Chlamydia *psittaci*, Brucella - including *B. canis*, Q fever, *Aspergillus* sp., *Histoplasma capsulatum*, *Candida albicans*, Teichoic acid antibodies.

8. Consider non-bacterial causes: Check anti-nuclear antibodies, anti-DNA antibodies, LE prep, rheumatoid factor, anti-streptolysin O, skin or muscle biopsy. (Remember some of these will be abnormal in patients with infective endocarditis.)

Special Circumstances

1. Recoverable embolus: culture for pyogenic bacteria, fungi, mycobacteria, stain sections with Gram's stain, and special stains for fungi, acid-fast microorganisms.

2. Valvular material from surgery or autopsy: culture and stain as above.

3. Patient has Xenograft valve: consider *Mycobacterium chelonei*

Examination of peripheral blood smears for intraleukocytic bacteria may be useful.[46] Some authors have reported increased cultural yield from bone marrow aspirates but others have not confirmed this observation.[47,48] Large occlusive emboli may be particularly common in fungal endocarditis, and if such an embolus is surgically approachable, it must be appropriately cultured and stained. Valvular material obtained from surgery should similarly be carefully cultured and examined microscopically; electron microscopy may be useful in this circumstance.

Serologic testing for Q fever, *Chlamydia psittaci, Aspergillus* sp., *Histoplasma capsulatum,* Brucella (including *B. canis*) and teichoic acid antibodies may help identify the presence of antibody to microorganisms responsible for the disorder. Some authors have found serial echocardiograms to be helpful in delineating involvement of the heart valves and identifying vegetations.[49,50] The role of newer techniques such as Gallium 67 myocardial imaging, gas-liquid chromatography, and CT scanning remains to be determined.

Antimicrobial therapy appears to have improved the prognosis of patients with culture negative endocarditis, although without a precise etiologic diagnosis one can never be sure therapy played a significant role in the patients' recovery. In a recent series Pesanti suggested culture negative endocarditis patients may be divided into 2 groups on the basis of their response to empiric antimicrobial therapy.[29] In one group, patients defervesced within one week following initiation of antimicrobial treatment and the overall survival was 92%. In the group who did not defervesce within one week only 50% lived, and death was related to emboli and congestive heart failure.

If used, empiric therapy might include penicillin, 20 million units per day, plus an aminoglycoside (e.g. gentamicin). If there is a prosthetic heart valve involved, therapy should also include agents active against *Staphylococcus epidermidis*, e.g. vancomycin. In the immunocompromised host Amphotericin B should be included in initial coverage. The penicillin allergic patient should be treated with vancomycin 30 mgm/kg/day in 4 divided doses (maximum daily dose of 2.0 grams) plus an aminoglycoside. Dosages of antibiotics should be reduced in the patient with renal insufficiency. Therapy should be continued for a total of 6 weeks. These antibiotics will not treat most non-bacterial causes of culture negative endocarditis. However, valve tissue which has been examined in patients with negative blood cultures has usually revealed gram-positive cocci, suggesting that culture negative endocarditis is generally caused by common bacteria which for some reason are rendered inculturable.[29,31]

Renal Complications of Infective Endocarditis

Infective endocarditis may cause renal injury in three ways: vegetations disrupted from the endocardial site may embolize renal vessels, the kidney may be damaged as a result of immune mechanisms, and the toxic or side effects of chemotherapeutic agents administered for treatment of the disease may affect the kidney.

Post mortem examinations of patients dying with infective endocarditis reveal an incidence of detectable embolization to the kidney in 38–69% of cases depending on the series.[51] Frequency of renal embolization will obviously be a function of duration of infection, type of microorgansim (fungal endocarditis associated with larger emboli), and perhaps peculiarities of renal circulation. Emboli will be detected *ante mortem* when clinical suspicion is sufficiently high to warrant specific tests. The clinical manifestations of renal emboli include flank pain, fever, gross or microscopic hematuria, and proteinuria. Frank renal failure is quite unusual as a result of renal emboli since these emboli rarely occlude sufficient vascular supply to impair renal function.[44,51,52] Arteriograms of the renal vascular bed remain the most precise test for delineation of renal emboli. Sonar and CT scans play as yet an undefined role in the evaluation of this disorder.

Most patients with proven renal embolization have few clinical manifestations and usually only painless hematuria is noted. Avirulent microorganisms such as viridans streptococci are not detected in the urine of patients with renal emboli. In contrast, when *Staphylococcus aureus* is the etiologic agent, it may be recovered from a urine culture due either to inoculation from a cortical abscess or from the *Staphylococcus aureus* bacteremia itself.[53] Since most patients with renal embolization have little functional impairment, therapy is generally unnecessary.

Glomerulonephritis is associated with infective endocarditis caused by a wide variety of bacterial agents, and the incidence varies widely in different series depending upon the degree with which it is sought.[54] For many years glomerulonephritis occurring in patients with infective endocarditis was divided into two varieties: diffuse glomerulonephritis mimicking that which occurs following streptococcal infections, and focal "embolic" glomerulonephritis thought due to emboli. Most authors believe that diffuse glomerulonephritis is immunologically mediated, but only recently has focal "embolic" glomerulonephritis been recognized as possibly resulting from the same type injury. Ninety percent of patients with infective endocarditis have detectable circulating immune complexes[21], and the continuous bacteremia may also be associated with elevated titers of IgG, IgM, rheumatoid factor, cryoglobulins, macroglobulins, and/or anti-nuclear antibodies.[19,55] The role of these molecules in producing the changes associated with infective endocarditis remains to be defined. Many of the pathologic changes seen in both varieties of glomerulonephritis appear to be due to the deposition of immune complexes in the microcirculatory bed of the kidneys. Electron microscopic and immunofluorescent examination of kidney biopsy specimens or tissue obtained at autopsy have shown similar findings in both diffuse and focal nephritides.[51] There may be diffuse, granular staining of C3 along capillary walls, and some specimens demonstrate mesangial, subendothelial or subepithelial deposits of antigen-antibody complexes, the location perhaps depending on the size of the complexes and whether they were formed during antibody or antigen excess.[51,56,57,58] Whether diffuse glomerulonephritis represents one end of the spectrum and the focal embolic variety the other is unclear. It is conceivable that there are two varieties of immune injury occurring; however at the present time there is no method with which one can separate these disorders.

As one might anticipate, renal failure is most common in patients with diffuse glomerulonephritis and in patients with infective endocarditis of long duration.[44] It is presently recognized in less than 10% of patients with infective endocarditis[59] and is generally completely reversible following initiation of effective antimicrobial therapy. In contrast, in the pre-antibiotic era renal failure occurred in 25–35% of patients and contributed significantly to morbidity and mortality.[59] Renal failure secondary to glomerulonephritis may be confused with that resulting from acute tubular necrosis, but the former is most likely to be associated with hematuria, hypertension, and to manifest a more gradual onset. The prognosis of renal failure caused by glomerulonephritis is generally not related to the histologic nature of the lesions but to the initiation of adequate antimicrobial therapy for the infectious process.[54] In a few patients renal failure has been noted to continue after completion of therapy. A detailed discussion of the management of patients with acute renal failure is beyond the scope of this chapter; however attention to fluid and electrolyte management, acid-base balance, and circulatory status is obviously important in the treatment of these problems. Some patients require dialysis.

Recent collaborative studies of management of infective endocarditis, particularly that caused by *Staphylococcus aureus*, have re-emphasized the frequency of renal toxicity associated with high dose antimicrobial therapy.[60] Penicillin type drugs, particularly nafcillin, methicillin, and penicillin G, may cause interstitial nephritis with hematuria, eosinophiliuria and fever. When these drug reactions are suspected in patients with potential or actual immunologic renal injury, a distinction may be very difficult. The presence of eosinophilia and eosinophiliuria may be of some help in the distinction, but often the antimicrobial agent must be discontinued to determine if renal function improves. In addition, renal tubular damage may result from use of aminoglycosides particularly when combined with cephalosporins. Nephrotoxicity also has been described with vancomycin, and rifampin may cause renal failure, particularly when given intermittently.[61]

Metastatic Abscesses

In spite of persistent bacteremia, infective endocarditis caused by viridans streptococci rarely results in metastatic abscess formation. Meningitis may be noted, but this is uncommon. In contrast, staphylococcal bacteremia with or without endocarditis may be associated with metastatic localization more commonly. The organs classically involved include the central nervous system, heart, lung, and kidneys. Despite the frequency of metastatic abscess caused by *Staphylococcus aureus*, it is noteworthy that in the central nervous system these are generally small and require no surgical intervention.[2] However, when staphylococcal abscess involves the myocardium, the results may be devastating. Myocardial rupture, purulent pericarditis, and other sequelae of heart muscle involvement may occur. Heart block, intractable dysrhythmias, and pericarditis all suggest myocardial abscess and are associated with a poor prognosis.[62] Renal cortical abscesses are commonly silent, although they may be associated with flank pain, fever, and an active urinary sediment. Splenic abscesses are characterized by abdominal pain, fever, and occasionally left pleural effusion; a rub may be heard. They are surgically remediable. Enterococcal bacteremia is more likely to result in metastatic infection and meningitis than disease caused by viridans streptococci. Fungal endocarditis is sometimes associated with CNS lesions, particularly endophthalmitis and osteomyelitis. Newer techniques such as gallium scanning and computerized scanning of the body are proving valuable in diagnosing these metastatic lesions.

Persistence of Infection

Therapeutic failure in the face of presumably appropriate therapy for infective endocarditis may be suggested by symptoms and signs of ongoing disease, by persistence of microbial organisms in the circulation or by other abnormal laboratory studies. Most commonly treatment failure is manifested by fever and bacteremia. The duration of bacteremia after the initiation of presumably appropriate therapy of infective endocarditis is variable and depends upon the etiologic microorganism. Usually, after therapy for viridans streptococcal endocarditis has begun, blood cultures will become sterile in 24–48 hours. In contrast, patients with *Staphylococcus aureus* endocarditis may have persistently positive blood cultures for several days. When bacteremia persists, it is important for the physician to carefully repeat the physicial examination with special attention to possible sites of occult abscess such as in liver, spleen, kidney, brain, and heart. Mycotic aneurysms, recurrent embolization and evidence of immunologically mediated vasculitis may also be responsible for lack of clinical improvement. The CT scan may be especially useful for delineation of abscesses or other lesions in the central nervous system or abdomen. One must also look for evidence of associated disorders which might mimic persistent endocarditis: specifically, toxic or hypersensitivity reactions to antimicrobial agents being administered, concomitant collagen vascular disease such as acute rheumatic fever or disseminated lupus erythematosis, and septic phlebitis at the site of administration of antimicrobial therapy.

When patients with infective endocarditis appear to have persistent infection while receiving presumably appropriate therapy, blood cultures should be repeated and, if the patient is receiving a beta lactamase susceptible agent, penicillinase should be added to the culture media. Assay of serum for teichoic acid antibodies is sometimes useful in assessing the response to therapy in patients with *Staphylococcus aureus* disease. Persistently elevated levels of anti-teichoic antibody suggest poor response.[63] If the infecting microorganism is recovered from blood after presumably appropriate therapy, special testing should be carried out.

Serum antimicrobial activity against the microorganism should be assayed with the Schlicter test (Chapter 15). The minimum concentrations of the antibotics which are being administered necessary for inhibition and killing of the microorgansim should also be redetermined. In the case of gram-positive microorganisms the laboratory should look for evidence of tolerance (Chapter 15) and inoculum effect.

When bacteremia persists in spite of what appears to be appropriate antimicrobial therapy, localized suppuration is usually responsible. Probably most common is abscess in or near the infected valve itself, but abscesses in viscera or adjacent to mycotic aneurysms may be present. In patients with *Staphylococcus aureus* endocarditis and persistent bacteremia valve debridement or replacement is often necessary for control of infection[64] (Chapter 13).

In general the approach to persistent infection in patients with infectious endocarditis is dependent upon careful assessment of antimicrobial therapy and the role of surgical intervention.

ACKNOWLEDGEMENTS

The authors wish to acknowledge the assistance of Dr. Richard B. Morawetz of the Department of Neurosurgery, University of Alabama in Birmingham, and Dr. Holt A. McDowell of the Department of Surgery, University of Alabama in Birmingham in the preparation of this manuscript.

REFERENCES

1. Snow, R.M., Cobbs, C.G.: Treatment of complications of infective endocarditis, in Kaye D. (ed): Infective Endocarditis, Baltimore, University Press, 1976, 213–227.
2. Pruitt, A.A., Rubin R.H., Karchmer, A.W., Duncan,G.W.: Neurologic complications of bacterial endocarditis. Medicine (Baltimore) 57:329, 1978.
3. Stengel, A., Wolferth, C.C.: Mycotic aneurisms of intravascular origin. Arch. Intern. Med. 31:527, 1923.
4. Ziment, I.: Nervous system complications in bacterial endocarditis. Am. J. Med. 47:593, 1969.
5. Weinstein, L., Rubin, R.H.: Infective endocarditis - 1973. Prog. in Cardiovasc. Dis. 16:239, 1973.
6. Molinari, G.F.: Septic cerebral embolism. Stroke 3:117, 1972.
7. Molinari, G.F., Smith, L., Golstein, M.N., Satran, R.: Pathogenesis of cerebral mycotic aneurisms. Neurology (Minneap) 23:325, 1973.

8. Bohmfalk, G.L., Story, J.L., Wissinger, J.P., Brown, W.E.: Bacterial intracranial aneurism. J. Neurosurg. 48:369, 1978.
9. Nakata, Y., Shionoya, S., Kamiya, K.: Pathogenesis of mycotic aneurism. Angiology 19:593, 1968.
10. Cates, J.E., Christie, R.V.: Subacute bacterial endocarditis. Q J Med. New Series 20:93, 1951.
11. Yellin, A.E.: Ruptured mycotic aneurysm, a complication of parenteral drug abuse. Arch. Surg. 112:981, 1977.
12. Patel, S., Johnston, K.W.: Classification and management of mycotic aneurisms. Surg. Gynecol. Obstet. 144:691, 1977.
13. Anderson, B.C., Butcher, H.R. Jr., Ballinger, W.F.: Mycotic aneurysms. Arch. Surg. 109:712, 1974.
14. Porter, L., Houston, M., Kadir, S.: Mycotic aneurisms of the hepatic artery: Treatment with arterial embolization. Am. J. Med. 67:697, 1979.
15. Anderson, D., Bulkley, B.H., Hutchins, G.M.: A clinicopathologic study of prosthetic valve endocarditis in 22 patients: Morphologic basis for diagnosis and therapy. Am. Heart J. 94:325, 1977.
16. Garvey, G.J., Neu, H.C.: Infective endocarditis - an evolving disease. Medicine (Baltimore) 57:105, 1978.
17. Banks, T., Fletcher, R., Ali, N.: Infective endocarditis in heroin addicts. Am. J. Med 55:444, 1973.
18. Nastro, L.J., Finegold, S.M.: Endocarditis due to anaerobic gram-negative bacilli. Am. J. Med. 54:482, 1973.
19. Weinstein, L., Schlesinger, J.J.: Pathoanatomic, pathophysiologic and clinical correlations in endocarditis. N. Engl. J. Med. 291:832, 1122, 1974.
20. Kammer, R.B., Utz, J.P.: Aspergillus species endocarditis: The new face of a not so rare disease. Am. J. Med. 56:506, 1974.
21. Freedman, L.R.: Endocarditis updated. D M 26:6, 1979.
22. Stewart, J.A., Silimper, D, Harris, P., Wise, N.K., Fraker, T.D., Kisslo, J.A.: Echocardiographic documentation of vegetative lesions in infective endocarditis: Clinical implications. Circulation 61:374, 1980.
23. Watanakunakorn, C., Tan, J.S., Phair, J.P.: Some salient features of staphylococcus aureus endocarditis. Am. J. Med. 54:473, 1973.
24. Editorial. Neurologic complications of infective endocarditis. Br. Med. J. 2:619, 1970.
25. Jones, R., Siekert, R.G., Geraci, J.E.: Neurologic manifestations of bacterial endocarditis. Ann. Intern. Med. 71:21, 1969.
26. Bingham, W.F.: Treatment of mycotic intracranial aneurysms. J. Neurosurg. 46:428, 1977.
27. Ziment, I., Johnson, B.L. Jr.: Angiography in the management of intracranial mycotic aneurysms. Arch. Intern. Med. 122:349, 1968.
28. Morawetz, R.B., Acker, J.D.: Management of mycotic (bacterial) intracranial aneurysms. Contemp. Neurosurg. In press.

29. Pesanti, E.L., Smith, I.M.: Infective endocarditis with negative blood cultures: An analysis of 52 cases. Am. J. Med. 66:43, 1979.
30. Cannady, P.B. Jr., Sanford, J.P.: Negative blood cultures in infective endocarditis: A review. South Med. J. 69:1420, 1976.
31. Editorial. Infective endocarditis with negative blood cultures. Br. Med. J. 2:4, 1979.
32. Editorial. Culture-negative endocarditis. Lancet 2:1164, 1977.
33. Libman, E.: The clinical feature of cases of subacute bacterial endocarditis that have spontaneously become bacteria-free. Am.J. Med. Sci. 146:625, 1913.
34. Hall, B., Dowling, H.F.: Negative blood cultures in bacterial endocarditis: A decades experience. Med. Clin. North Am. 50:159, 1966.
35. Ellner, J.J., Rosenthal, M.S., Lerner, P.I., McHenry, M.C.: Infective endocarditis caused by slow-growing, fastidious, gram-negative bacteria. Medicine (Baltimore) 58:145, 1979.
36. Cohen, P.S., Maguire, J.H., Winstein, L.: Infective endocarditis caused by gram-negative bacteria: A review of the literature, 1945-1977. Progr. Cardiovasc. Dis. 22:205, 1980.
37. Roberts, R.B., Knieger, A.G., Schiller, N.L., Gross, K.C.: Viridans streptococcal endocarditis: The role of various species including pyridoxal-dependent streptococci. Rev. Inf. Dis. 1:955, 1979.
38. Carey, R.B., Brause, B.D., Roberts, R.B.: Antimicrobial therapy of vitamin B_6-dependent streptococcal endocarditis. Ann. Intern. Med. 87:150, 1977.
39. McCarthy, L.R., Bottone, E.J.: Bacteremia and endocarditis caused by satelliting streptococci. Am. J. Clin. Pathol. 61:585, 1974.
40. Tyras, D.H., Kaiser, G.C., Barner, H.B., Laskowski, L.F., Marr, J.J.: Atypical mycobacteria and the xenograft valve. J. Thorac. and Cardiovasc. Surg. 75:331, 1978.
41. Repath, F., Seaburg, J.H., Sanders, C.V., Domer, J.: Prostheic valve endocarditis due to Mycobacterium chelonei. South Med. J. 69:1244, 1976.
42. Feingold, D.S.: Biology and pathogenicity of microbial spheroplasts and L-forms. N. Engl. J. Med. 281:1159, 1969.
43. Williams, R.C., Kunkel, H.G.: Rheumatoid factors and their disappearance following therapy in patients with SBE. Arth. Rheum. 5:126, 1962.
44. Gutman, R.A., Striker, G.E., Gilliland, B.C., Cutler, R.E.: The immune complex glomerulonephritis of bacterial endocarditis. Medicine (Baltimore) 51:1, 1972.
45. Editorial. Non-bacterial thrombotic endocarditis. Br. Med. J. 1:197, 1978.
46. Gleckman, R.: Culture negative bacterial endocarditis: Confirming the diagnosis. Am. Heart J. 94:125, 1977.
47. Johnston, C.L., Dalton, H.P.: Bone-marrow culture in infectious diseases (letter). Lancet 1:420, 1968.

48. Jacobs, P., et al: Bone marrow culture in vitro: Current status and some clinical applications. So. African Med. J. 55:701, 1979.
49. Peterson, K.L.: Infective endocarditis: Role of newer diagnostic techniques. Chest 72:553, 1977.
50. Dillon, T., Meyer, R.A., Korfhagen, J.C., Kaplan, S., Chung, K.J.: Management of infective endocarditis using echocardiography. J. Pediatr. 96:552, 1980.
51. Wilson, J.W., Houghton, D.C., Bennett, W.M., Proter, G.A.: The kidney and infective endocarditis, in Rahimtoola SH (ed): Infective Endocarditis, Grune & Stratton, 1978.
52. Levison, M.E., Response to therapy, in Kaye D (ed): Infective Endocarditis, Baltimore, University Press, 1976, p. 185.
53. Lee, B.K., Crossley, K., Gerding, D.N.: The association between Staphylococcus aureus bacteremia and bacteriuria. Am. J. Med. 65:303, 1978.
54. Beufils, M., Gilbert, C., Morel-Maroger, L., et al: Glomerulonephritis in severe bacterial infections with and without endocarditis. Adv. Nephrol. 7:217, 1978.
55. Phair, J.P., Clarke, J.: Immunology of infective endocarditis. Prog. Cardiovasc. Dis. 22:137, 1979.
56. Boulton-Jones, J.M., Sissons, J.G.P., Evans, D.J., Peters, D.K.: Renal lesions of subacute infective endocarditis. Br. Med. J. 2:11, 1974.
57. Keslin, M.H., Messner, R.P., Williams, R.C.: Glomerulonephritis with subacute bacterial endocarditis. Arch. Intern. Med. 132:578, 1973.
58. Morel-Maroger, L., Sraer, J., Herreman, G., Godeau, P.: Kidney in subacute endocarditis. Arch. Path. 94:205, 1972.
59. Lerner, P.I., Weinstein, L.: Infective endocarditis in the antibiotic era. New Engl. J. Med. 274:199, 259, 388; 1966.
60. Sande, M.A., Korzeniowski, O.M., Endocarditis Collaborative Group: Comparison of Nafcillin (N) with Nafcillin + Gentamicin (NG) in the treatment of addicts with *S. aureus* endocarditis. ICAAC, Abstract 362, 1979.
61. Calderwood, S.B., Moellering, R.C.: Common adverse effects of antimicrobial agents on major organ systems. Surg. Clin. North Am. 60:65, 1980.
62. Roberts, N.K., Somerville, J.: Pathologic significance of electrocardiographic change in aortic valve endocarditis. Br. Heart J. 31:395, 1969.
63. Tuazon, C.U., Sheagren, J.N.: Teichoic acid antibodies in the diagnosis of serious infections with Staphylococcus aureus. Ann. Intern. Med. 84:543, 1976.
64. Reyman, M.T., Holley, H.P., Cobbs, C.G.: Persistent bacteremia in staphylococcal endocarditis. Am. J. Med. 65:724, 1978.

William E. Dismukes, M.D.

12

PROSTHETIC VALVE ENDOCARDITIS: FACTORS INFLUENCING OUTCOME AND RECOMMENDATIONS FOR THERAPY

Prosthetic valve endocarditis (PVE) has been called "a clear cut example of endocarditis as a result of medical progress".[1] This complication of heart valve replacement plus other complications such as hemolytic anemia, systemic arterial embolization and obstruction of the prosthesis due to thrombi are potentially life-threating problems which must be detected promptly and treated vigorously.[2] PVE and hemolytic anemia appear to be the most common complications. Whereas reoperation for significant and refractory hemolysis due to paravalvular leak or dysfunction of the prosthesis is usually unnecessary, an aggressive surgical approach including replacement of the infected prosthesis has been increasingly utilized in the management of PVE with encouraging results. Not only does the prosthesis or foreign body increase the susceptibility of an individual patient to endocarditis but the infected prosthesis also makes eradication of the endocarditis difficult. Early reports suggested that PVE was nearly always fatal; however, recent experiences have shown that appropriate antimicrobial therapy together with prompt operative intervention have significantly improved survival.[3–6]

Incidence

PVE has generally been classified according to the time period in which the disorder occurs.[7] Early PVE is defined as endocarditis occurring within 60 days of the original prosthetic valve placement. In contrast, late PVE is defined as endocarditis occurring 60 days or more after the insertion of the valve prosthesis. Sixty days was originally arbitrarily chosen in an attempt to separate patients whose infection was probably related to operation from those whose infection probably arose from a source unrelated to the surgery and postoperative period. As shown in Table 1, Watanakunakorn, in a detailed analysis, has reported the incidence of early PVE to vary from 0 to 7.1% among different medical centers, with an average of 1.14%.[8] This analysis also showed that the incidence of early PVE was significantly higher in the period up to 1969 (2.53%), as compared to the period up to 1976 (0.75%). The incidence of

Table 1. Incidence of Prosthetic Valve Infective Endocarditis*

	STUDY PERIOD		
	UP TO 1969	UP TO 1976	TOTAL
No. of reports	10	11	21
No. of operations	2,572	9,301	11,873
No. of cases of early endocarditis	65	70	135
Incidence (per 100 patients)	2.53+	0.75+	1.14
No. of patients followed ($\geq$6 mo)	2,454	8,363	10,873
No. of cases of late endocarditis	35	95	130
Incidence (per 100 patients)	1.43	1.13	1.20
Overall incidence of endocarditis	3.96	1.88	2.34

+ $p < 0.001$ (X^2 test with Yates' correction)
* from Watanakunakorn [8]

late PVE for patients followed for at least six months after surgery varied from 0% to 3.2% among different medical centers, with an average of 1.20%. There was no significant difference in the incidence of late PVE in the period prior to 1969 and in the more recent period (1.43% vs. 1.13%). The overall incidence of PVE (early plus late) varied from 0 to 9.52% among different series with an average of 2.34%.

Using another approach in an attempt to define the risk of infection after palliative or reparative cardiovascular surgery, Kaplan and co-workers retrospectively analyzed 278 patients with infective endocarditis treated at 26 medical centers throughout the United States in 1972.[9] Two hundred and fifteen or 77% of the 278 endocarditis patients had not undergone any previous heart surgery. By contrast, only 23% (63 of 278) had previously undergone some type of cardiovascular surgery before developing endocarditis. Thirty-four of the 63 (54%) had undergone placement of a prosthetic heart valve before onset of infection.

A variety of heart valve substitutes have been employed: totally artificial plastic and metal valve prostheses as well as bioprosthetic valves that combine cloth covered supporting struts with homologous or heterologous tissue. Although suggestions have been made that tissue valves may be less susceptible to infection, until recently there have been no data regarding incidence of PVE by valve types. Rossiter and his colleagues reviewed 2,184 patients who underwent prosthetic valve replacement at Stanford University Medical Center from 1963 to 1977.[10] Eight hundred thirty-seven patients received Hancock porcine heterograft valves and 1,347 patients received mechanical Starr-Edwards (SE) valves. The average followup for SE aortic valve replacement (AVR) patients was 4.94 ± 2.81 years, compared with 1.67 ± 0.98 years for heterograft AVR patients. Similarly, the average followup for SE mitral valve replacement (MVR) patients was 6.02 ± 2.53 years, compared with 2.35 ± 1.54 years for heterograft MVR recipients. Average followup was longer in the patients who received mechanical valves since no heterograft valves were inserted prior to 1971. PVE occurred in 51 patients; early PVE in nine and late in 42. There was no significant difference between the total heterograft and Starr-Edwards valve groups in terms of linear rates of endocarditis per patient year. The incidence of PVE for the 14 year period was 1.9% (16/837) for heterograft recipients and 2.6% (35/1347) for mechanical valve recipients.

Magilligan et al, reported a similar incidence of heterograft PVE.[11] Eleven of 373 patients or 2.4% who received heterograft valves developed PVE. Interestingly, in the Magilligan series, all 11 heterograft PVE cases were late ones, whereas in the series reported by Rossiter, there was an increased incidence of early PVE in heterograft recipients.[10] Among a smaller group of porcine heterograft recipients followed over a 3 year period, Downham reported a 10% incidence of PVE: 7 episodes in 68 patients.[12] In the single largest series of endocarditis following homograft aortic valve replacement, Clarkson and Barratt-Boyes reported a 2.6% incidence of PVE (14 of 539 patients.).[13]

Earlier reports suggested that endocarditis of prosthetic aortic valves was more common than mitral valve PVE. However, subsequent analyses have provided varying results regarding this question. Watanakunakorn reported that in the period up to 1969, the incidence of aortic PVE was much higher than that of mitral PVE (4.17% vs. 1.50%,) $p < 0.01$).[8] But, in the period up to 1976, there was no difference in incidence of aortic valve PVE (1.94%) verses mitral valve PVE (1.25%). In the study by Rossiter et al, aortic valve PVE was signficantly more common than mitral valve PVE in both the Starr-Edwards valve recipients and the heterograft valve recipients.[10] In contrast, in the study by Magilligan et al, in which 11 cases of heterograft PVE were described, seven were mitral and four, aortic.[11]

Microbiology

Two important observations can be made about the microbiology of PVE. First, the microorgansims which cause PVE are somewhat different from those which cause native valve endocarditis (NVE). Secondly, the bacteriology of early PVE differs from the bacteriology of late PVE.

In NVE, streptococci, excluding enterococci, and *Staphylococcus aureus* are the most common causative agents. Among 139 cases of NVE seen at the Massachusetts General Hospital over the nine year period, 1964–1972, 45% were caused by nonenterococcal streptococci, and 22% by *S. aureus.*[14] Similarly, among 107 episodes of NVE observed at the Columbia–Presbyterian Medical Center from 1968–1973, streptococci, excluding enterococci, accounted for 52% and *S. aureus* for 13%.[15] At the University of Washington Hospitals over the 10 year period from 1963 to 1972, 91 patients were treated for NVE. Streptococci, excluding enterococci, were the infecting organisms in 33% of cases, and *S. aureus* in 28%.[16] In these three series, enterococci accounted for 11%, 7%, and 9%, of cases respectively, and *S. epidermidis,* diphtheroids, and aerobic gram-negative bacilli were uncommon causes of NVE.

In contrast, in both early and late cases of PVE, *S. epidermidis* is the most common causative organism, as depicted by data from two large reviews shown in Table 2. Delgado and Cobbs based their tabulation of causative microorganisms on data from 18 published studies, and Karchmer and Swartz based their review on 13 published studies. [17,14] Ten studies were common to both tabulations. In the review by Delagdo and Cobbs, *S. epidermidis* was the responsible agent in 96 of 340 episodes of PVE or 28%, and in the second review, *S. epidermidis* accounted for 77 of 305 cases or 25%. Nonenterococcal streptococci were the second most common organism, accounting for 16% of cases in each review. *S. aureus* caused 14–20% of cases, gram-negative bacilli, 12-22%, enterococci, 4–9%, diphtheroids, 4–8%, and fungi, 5–13%.

More recent data confirm these earlier observations about the microbiology of PVE. At the University of Alabama Medical Center and the Massachusetts General Hospital (MGH) over the four year period, 1976–1979, 105 episodes of PVE were recognized and studied (Table 3). Thirty-nine of these were early cases and 66 were late cases. Again, the most common causative microorganism was *S. epidermidis,* accounting for 42 of the 105 cases or 40%. Interestingly, there were fewer cases caused by *S. aureus* (7%) and gram-negative bacilli (9%), compared with the findings in the two reviews.

The microbiology of early PVE differs from that of late PVE. As illustrated in both Table 2 and Table 3, *S. epidermidis* is the most common cause of early PVE. In the combined Alabama-MGH series, 67% of early PVE cases were due to *S. epidermidis,* and in the two reviews 28% and 27% of the early cases were caused by *S. epidermidis.* Other important causes of early PVE include *S. aureus,* aerobic gram negative bacilli, diphtheroids, and fungi.

Table 2. Microbiology of PVE: Findings of Two Reviews

CAUSATIVE MICROORGANISM	Delgado & Cobbs[17]				Karchmer & Swartz[14]			
	EARLY		LATE		EARLY		LATE	
	178		162		151		154	
	No.	(%)	No.	(%)	No.	(%)	No.	(%)
S. epidermidis	53	(27)	43	(25)	41	(27)	36	(23)
S. aureus	36	(18)	23	(14)	30	(20)	22	(14)
Aerobic gram-negative bacilli	44	(22)	20	(12)	30	(20)	19	(12)
Streptococci (viridans and other nonenterococci)	7	(4)	46	(27)	9	(6)	41	(27)
Enterococci	9	(5)	16	(9)	6	(4)	14	(9)
S. pneumoniae	4	(2)	1	(1)	2	(1)	---	---
Diphtheroids	15	(8)	7	(4)	12	(8)	6	(4)
Miscellaneous	---	---	2	(1)	---	---	---	---
Fungi	26	(13)	8	(5)	18	(12)	9	(6)
Culture negative	---	---	---	---	3	(2)	7	(5)

Table 3. Microbiology of Combined Series of 105 Cases of PVE at University of Alabama Medical Center and Massachusetts General Hospital,* 1976–1979

MICROORGANISM	39 EARLY CASES		66 LATE CASES		ALL CASES	
S. epidermidis	26	(67)	16	(24)	42	(40)
S. aureus	1	(2.5)	6	(9.0)	7	(6.6)
Aerobic gram negative bacilli	1	(2.5)	8	(12)	9	(8.6)
Streptococci (viridans & other nonenterococci)	1	(2.5)	14	(21)	15	(14)
Enterococci	---	---	5	(7.5)	5	(4.8)
S. pneumoniae	---	---	1	(1.5)	1	(1.0)
Diphtheroids	7	(18)	7	(11)	14	(13)
Miscellaneous	1	(2.5)	3	(4.5)	4	(3.8)
Fungi	1	(2.5)	3	(4.5)	4	(3.8)
Culture negative	1	(2.5)	3	(4.5)	4	(3.8)

*Data on the Massachusetts General Hospital cases were kindly provided by A.W. Karchmer, M.D.

Similarly, virtually any organism can cause late PVE. The major difference in the microbiology of early and late PVE however, is that *S. epidermidis* and nonenterococcal streptococci are equally important causes of the latter. In the Alabama-MGH series, 24% of the late cases were caused by *S. epidermidis* and 21% by nonenterococcal streptococci. Very similar frequencies were reported in both reviews. Whereas nonenterococcal streptococci account for 21–27% of the late PVE cases, these organisms are far less common causes of early PVE, accounting for only 2.5%–6% of cases.

Source of Infection and/or Predisposing Factors

Early PVE. Endocarditis occuring early after valve replacement is almost always due to contamination during open heart surgery or to infectious complications in noncardiac areas during the immediate post-operative period.[18–20] Bacteremia, whether acquired intra-operatively or secondary to a contaminated IV line or to a noncardiac infection in the postoperative period, e.g., pneumonia and sternal wound infection, results in seeding of the newly implanted valve prosthesis with subsequent endocarditis. However, not every patient with postoperative bacteremia developes endocarditis. Sande et al, and Dismukes and Karchmer showed that gram-negative bacteremia in some patients with a prosthetic valve can be managed by elimination of extracardiac sources of the bacteremia plus short term antibiotic therapy.[21,22] More specifically, patients with bacteremia, extra cardiac sources of bacteremia and no signs of PVE and in whom the bacteremia is rapidly cleared by elimination of the extracardiac source can probably be satisfactory managed with two to three weeks of antibiotics. On the other hand, patients in whom gram-negative bacteremia persists after elimination of the extracardiac sources of infection or patients in whom there is sustained bacteremia but no identifiable cardiac source should be considered as having PVE, whether or not there are signs of endocarditis, and treated as such.

Late PVE. In contrast to early PVE, the pathogenesis of late PVE more nearly resembles that of classical subacute bacterial endocarditis. In both, the predisposing factor often appears to be an incidental septic event such as a urinary tract infection or a skin infection. In addition, in some patients the predisposing factor may be a minor surgical procedure such as dental manipulation or a genitourinary tract procedure. Finally, in a large group of patients, no significant predisposing event or factor can be identified. In patients with late PVE caused by *S. epidermidis,* diphtheroids, and Candida species, it is possible that the newly implanted prostheses are seeded by these organisms at the time of operation. Because of the low pathogenic potential of these organisms, the clinical expression of disease may not occur until several months following open heart surgery.

Clinical Features

The clinical manifestations of early and late PVE are generally very similar.[7,8,14,17,22,23] Fever is present in almost every patient. In fact, the absence of fever makes the diagnosis of endocarditis occurring on or around the prosthesis very unlikely. Conversely, the presence of unexplained fever in any patient with an artificial heart valve should raise a strong suspicion of PVE. A new or changing murmur is present in approximately one-half of the cases. The murmurs of mitral insufficiency and/or aortic insufficiency are especially important since these may signify paravalvular leak secondary to dehiscense of the seat of the prosthesis from the periannular tissue. However, absence of a regurgitant murmur does not preclude the presence of paravalvular leak. In patients in whom the infection primarily involves the central structures of a mechanical valve, e.g., the disc or ball, the endocarditis may cause an obstructing lesion with resulting absent to muffled prosthetic heart sounds and a new or an unusual murmur. Petechiae, especially in the conjunctivae, are the most common peripheral skin or mucous membrane manifestation of PVE and occur in 30 to 60 percent of patients. Roth spots, Osler nodes, and Janeway lesions, peripheral stigmata of subacute NVE, are less common findings than petechiae in PVE and appear to be more common in late PVE than early PVE. Systemic emboli, including emboli to the central nervous system, kidneys, spleen, and major peripheral vessels, have been reported in 7 to 28 percent of patients with PVE. Splenomegaly occurs in approximately one-third of patients and appears to be more common in late PVE.

Diagnostic and Monitoring Studies

Multiple positive blood cultures are the most definitive criterion on which to base a diagnosis of PVE. Among 79 cases of PVE observed at the Massachusetts General Hospital over the period 1964–1975, in only three cases were all blood cultures negative.[22] All three of these were late cases. In the other 76 cases there were at least two positive blood cultures and in the majority of patients there were five or more positive blood cultures. In the review by Karchmer and Swartz of 305 cases of PVE, only 10 or 3 percent were culture negative,[14] and in the recent series shown in Table 3, only 4% of cases were culture negative. Experience suggests, therefore, that most patients with PVE will have positive blood cultures.

Several studies or procedures are particularly helpful in assessing the overall cardiac and hemodynamic status of patients with suspected or established PVE. Daily auscultation of the heart is essential in order to detect new or changing murmurs (especially regurgitant murmurs), changes in valve sounds in patients with mechanical prostheses and the appearance of new sounds, e.g., gallops or friction rubs. In patients with aortic valve PVE, any change in pulse pressure which might signify development or progression of aortic insufficiency should be noted. Similarly, narrowing of the pulse pressure should suggest worsening heart failure or possible valve obstruction or thrombosis due to vegetations.[24] Serial electrocardiograms may detect varying degrees of heart block or other arrhythmias which may signifiy involvement of the conduction system by an intraseptal abscess, caused by extension of the paravalvular infection.[25,26]

Investigators have emphasized the potential importance of echocardiography in evaluating patients with NVE.[27,28] Although there are a few reports indicating that thrombosed prosthetic valves or vegetations which were suspected by echocardiography were confirmed at the time of operation or autopsy,[24,29–31] the precise role of echocardiography in assessing patients with PVE has yet to be established. In general, the echoes generated by the different mechanical prostheses are so intense that subtle changes which might indicate vegetation or abnormal valve motion may not be distinguishable. Both M-mode and two dimensional studies are probably required to optimally detect vegetations, and assess prosthesis and left ventricular function. Echocardiography may prove more useful in assessing patients with biosynthetic tissue valves[29] since in this group there is less hardware to cause interference.

In patients with PVE, cardiac cinefluoroscopy may demonstrate an abnormal rocking motion of the valve due to disruption of the suture line and consequent dehiscence of the valve with paravalvular leak. [32] In addition, demonstration of incomplete excursion of radiopaque elements of the prosthetic valve suggests invasion by clot or vegetation. Cinefluoroscopy should probably be performed early in the assessment of all patients in whom PVE is suspected or proven, in order that a baseline can be determined. When auscultatory or other clinical findings suggest an acute change in the function of the valve prosthesis, repeat cinefluoroscopy is indicated.

In patients in whom there is progressive or severe heart failure, cardiac catheterization and angiography may be necessary in order to assess the degree of prosthesis dysfunction, assess left ventricular performance, clarify whether there is dysfunction of a second valve, assess the coronary circulation in patients with known or suspected ischemic heart disease in whom a saphenous vein bypass graft may be included at operation, detect fistulae and aneurysms, and detect filling defects or lucencies adjacent to valves which may indicate vegetations.[33] Although concern exists about dislodging thrombi and vegetations at the time of catheterization and angiography in patients with endocarditis, experience indicates that the risk is extremely small and the potential for obtaining helpful management information appears to far outweigh any risk of the procedure.

Pathologic Features

Detailed evaluation and analysis of the autopsy and operative findings in PVE patients have provided significant insight into the nature of the pathologic process and have aided greatly in the formulation of approaches to management. Delgado and Cobbs[17] reviewed the pathologic findings from three published autopsy series[7,25,34] plus the combined surgical and autopsy experience at the University of Alabama Medical Center.[6] Their findings are summarized in Table 4. The most important and most common complication of PVE is valve ring abscess,

Table 4. Cardiac Pathology in PVE Described at Autopsy and Surgery*

STUDY REFERENCE	TOTAL NO. OF PATIENTS	RING ABSCESS	STENOSIS	MYOCARDIAL ABSCESS	PERICARDITIS
Arnett[25]	22	14	6	16	2
Anderson[34]	22	11	6	8	2
Dismukes[7]	16	8	2	3	2
Richardson[6]	32	28	1	9	0
Total	92	61	15	36	6

*from Delgado and Cobbs.[17]

i.e., infection of the tissue at the interface between the seat of the prosthesis and the endocardium of the patient. Valve ring abscess occurs in approximately two thirds of patients with PVE, and usually involves multiple sutures used to secure the valve to the surrounding periannular tissue. All autopsy and surgical studies of PVE indicate that the presence of a valve ring abscess is almost always accompanied by dehiscence of the prosthesis. Similarly, the clinical finding of a regurgitant murmur usually indicates paravalvular leak and more importantly, valve ring abscess. The recognition that antibiotics alone are inadequate to treat pus and necrotic tissue in the periannular area has been one of the major determinants in the formulation of a more aggressive surgical management of PVE in recent years.

Vegetations on the mechanical struts and in the opening between the valve ring and ball or disc may cause total or partial occlusion of the valve. This complication is far less common than either valve ring abscess or myocardial abscess. Thrombosis with obstruction, when it does occur, is more common in mitral PVE than in aortic PVE. Purulent pericarditis has been noted in approximately 10% of autopsy cases and appears to be more common in staphylococcal infection. Mycotic aneurysms and diffuse myocarditis are uncommon complications of PVE.

Mortality

Earlier reports have emphasized that the mortality of PVE is very high. Watanakunakorn analyzed mortality data from several published studies and divided the studies into two time periods, up to 1969, and up to 1974.[8] Early PVE was associated with a significantly higher mortality than late PVE, 72% vs 45% ($p < 0.001$.) There was no difference in the mortality of early PVE in the two time periods, 74% vs 70%. Similarly, there was no difference in the mortality of late PVE during the two periods, 48% vs 44%. Among 47 patients studied at the University of Alabama Medical Center over the ten year period ending June, 1977, the mortality rate of 71% in early PVE was significantly different from the 30% mortality in late PVE, $p < 0.025$.[6]

Our most recent experience provides more encouraging results regarding outcome. In the combined series of 105 PVE patients seen at the Massachusetts General Hosptial and at the University of Alabama Medical Center over the four year period 1976 through 1979, the mortality rate was only 29% (Table 5). The mortality rate of early PVE was 41% and that of late PVE, 21%, $p < 0.05$. More detailed analysis of these data will be presented under management, as well as comments about two other factors which appear to significantly influence outcome: the type of infecting microorganism and the degree of severity of congestive heart failure.

Table 5. Prosthetic Valve Endocarditis: Combined Alabama-MGH series
Outcome in 105 Cases by Mode of Therapy

MODE OF THERAPY	TOTAL NUMBER	SURVIVED				DIED			
		E*	L**	TOTAL	%	E	L	TOTAL	%
Medical	39	4	23	27	69	4	8	12	31
Medical-Surgical	66	19	29	48	73	12	6	18	27
Total	105	23	52	75	71	16	14	30	29

*E, early **L, late

Management

Antimicrobial therapy. The same principles which underlie the successful antimicrobial treatment of NVE apply to the therapy of PVE. These include: 1) use of bactericidal antibiotics, either singly or in combination, 2) parenteral administration of antibiotics, 3) adjustment of dosages of antibiotics in patients with renal dysfunction, 4) use of bacteriologic studies to determine the *in vitro* sensitivity of the infecting microorganism and to assay the *in vivo* effectiveness of the antibiotic regimen being used, 5) treatment for a prolonged duration, in the range of 6 to 8 weeks, and 6) acquisition of post treatment blood cultures. In general, there is unaminous agreement among investigators about these principles.

However, there are other considerations regarding therapy about which more controversy exists. The question often arises whether to withhold antimicrobial therapy pending identification of an etiologic agent. Although withholding therapy for 24–48 hours while awaiting a report of positive blood cultures may not unfavorably affect outcome, experience suggests that in the following situations therapy should be immediately begun after blood cultures are obtained:

1. when the signs and symptoms suggest acute PVE, especially in the early postoperative period;
2. when the patient is critically ill with congestive heart failure secondary to recent onset of valvular insufficiency (in patients with tissue prostheses) or paravalvular leak (in patients with mechanical prostheses and valve ring abscesses);
3. when the clinical diagnosis is likely and either cardiopulmonary bypass surgery for valve replacement is urgently needed or antimicrobial therapy is necessary for some other disorder.

In a patient who has received antibiotics prior to evaluation for PVE, it may be necessary to observe the patient off antibiotics several days while obtaining serial blood cultures. The clinical status of the patient dictates the degree of emergency regarding the initiation of therapy. Since any microorganism can be a pathogen in the presence of an intravascular foreign body and cause PVE, every effort should be made before therapy to identify the infecting organism in order to insure treatment with the appropriate antimicrobial agent(s). A report from the bacteriology laboratory of a positive blood culture for organisms often considered contaminants, such as *S. epidermidis,* micrococci, diphtheroids, or Candida species, etc., must not be categorically dismissed by the physician. Instead, it should raise the index of suspicion of PVE and should provide the impetus to obtain additional blood cultures. One other important consideration regarding blood cultures: studies have shown that PVE caused by diphtheroids or other fastidious bacteria may not result in high grade bacteremia.[22] As a consequence, the blood cultures in such patients may not all be positive, and there may be a several day interval from the time of obtaining the culture to the time of the culture becoming positive.

I will not comment further about the antimicrobial therapy of streptococcal PVE. The therapy for this entity is generally similar to that for streptococcal NVE, as discussed fully in chapters two through seven. Instead, emphasis will be placed on the controversies surrounding the antimicrobial treatment of staphylococcal and diphtheroid endocarditis. For more detailed discussions of specific antimicrobial regimens for various other organisms, the reader is referred to several reviews.[17,35–37]

Staphylococcus aureus. As indicated above, the mortality of PVE due to *S. aureus* is in the range of 50 to 90%. In all cases of suspected or proven endocarditis due to this organism, therapy should be initiated with a penicillinase-resistant penicillin providing the patient has no history of penicillin allergy. Since 80 to 85% of *S. aureus* isolates are resistant to penicillin G, this drug should not be used in initial treatment. High dose penicillin G in the range of 20 million units per day can be substituted if the MIC of the organism is less than 0.1 μg/ml.

Data obtained *in vitro* by time kill experiments and *in vivo* by animal models of experimental endocarditis have suggested that the combination of nafcillin and gentamicin affords more rapid killing of *S. aureus* than nafcillin alone.[38,39] However, the enhanced efficacy of this combination in patients has not been established (Chapter 8).[40–42]

At present, parenteral nafcillin for at least six weeks is generally considered the regimen of choice for the treatment of PVE due to *S. aureus.* In patients with a history of penicillin allergy, either a cephalosporin or vancomycin can be substituted.[43] In patients with endocarditis caused by methicillin-resistant strains of *S. aureus,* vancomycin is the antibiotic of choice. In addition, vancomycin or the combination of nafcillin plus gentamicin has been advocated for patients whose *S. aureus* isolate is considered to be "tolerant"[44] and for patients who do not respond to conventional therapy.[45]

Recent limited clinical experiences together with *in vitro* and *in vivo* laboratory studies suggest that rifampin may also be useful in treatment regimens for patients with persistent staphylococcal bacteremia. Massanari and Donta as well as Faville and his co-workers have ascribed striking clinical and laboratory evidence of improvement to the addition of rifampin in three patients with *S. aureus* endocarditis.[46,47] Supportive laboratory data show that many isolates of *S. aureus* are exquisitely sensitive to rifampin;[48] rifampin is synergistic with nafcillin and vancomycin against *S. aureus*,[49] rifampin has the capacity to kill intraleukocytic staphylococci,[50] and rifampin is effective in the treatment of experimental murine staphylococcal infections.[51] However, until the role of rifampin in the therapy of serious *S. aureus* disease has been more definitively established, rifampin probably should not be part of the initial treatment regimen but should be reserved for use in patients with persistent bacteremia while on "appropriate therapy".

Staphylococcus epidermidis. S. epidermidis PVE is often fatal; mortality rates vary from 56–75%.[6,52] *S. epidermidis* isolates recovered from patients with PVE are commonly methicillin-resistant. Among isolates from 87 *S. epidermidis* PVE patients in six different hospitals, 66% were reported to be methicillin-resistant.[52] The mortality rate for PVE due to methicillin-resistant strains of *S. epidermidis* was higher than that for PVE due to methicillin-sensitive strains, 59 versus 44%.

At the University of Alabama Medical Center during 1979, antibiotic sensitivity testing was performed on 2,915 isolates of *S. epidermidis;* 55% were found to be methicillin-resistant, 83%, penicillin resistant, and only 10%, cephalothin resistant. However, routine susceptibility testing of *S. epidermidis* isolates may fail to detect resistant organisms.[53,54] More sophisticated testing reveals heteroresistant isolates characterized by colony subpopulations which are resistant to a specific antibiotic to which the majority of the colonies are sensitive. This heteroresistance may explain in part the failure of patients with methicillin-resistant *S. epidermidis* infections to improve bacteriolgoically and clinically when treated with antibiotics to which the isolates have been shown to be sensitive by routine testing.

For example, the use of cephalosporins alone or in combination with other agents to treat *S. epidermidis* PVE in humans has given disappointing results.[52] Results of *in vitro* and animal *in vivo* studies also suggest problems with cephalosporins: 1) the existence of cephalosporin resistant subpopulations in methicillin-resistant strains of *S. epidermidis*,[53] 2) enhancement of heteroresistance to beta-lactam antibiotics when such agents are used in treatment,[55] 3) the poor bactericidal activity of cephalosporins against methicillin-resistant strains,[56] and 4) the failure of cephalothin alone to sterilize valvular vegetations in rabbits infected with these strains.[55]

If the *S. epidermidis* isolate is "methicillin-sensitive", the regimen of choice is probably a combination of nafcillin, gentamicin, and rifampin. On the other hand, if the *S. epidermidis* isolate is "methicillin-resistant", or the patient has a history of hypersensitivity to penicillin, vancomycin should probably be substituted for nafcillin. The rationale for the addition of rifampin and gentamicin to either nafcillin or vancomycin is based largely on the following observations. First, *S. epidermidis* clinical isolates including both methicillin-sensitive and methicillin-resistant ones, are almost always sensitive to rifampin and vancomycin, and often sensitive to gentamicin, tobramycin or amikacin. Archer et al, reported that all initial *S. epidermidis* isolates from 33 PVE patients were susceptible to 0.1 μg/ml of rifampin and $\leq$ 6.25 μg/ml of vancomycin.[53] Although subpopulations resistant to vancomycin were not found, rifampin alone was shown to induce the rapid emergence of rifampin-resistant strains. In addition, fifteen of 25 (56%) methicillin-resistant isolates were sensitive to gentamicin, tombramycin or amikacin; gentamicin resistant subpopulations were not noted among the susceptible strains.[53] Second, *in vitro* time kill experiments have shown enhanced killing of *S. epidermidis* by the addition of rifampin to either nafcillin, vancomycin, cephalothin or cefamandole, or gentamicin.[54,57] Third, the combinations of rifampin and vancomycin, rifampin and gentamicin, and vancomycin and gentamicin have been demonstrated to act synergistically against methicillin-resistant *S. epidermidis* in a rabbit experimental endocarditis model.[55] Fourth, rifampin is effective in preventing experimental *S. epidermidis* endocarditis.[58] Fifth, limited clinical experience with rifampin combined with other antimicrobials, especially vancomycin or a cephalosporin, in the treatment of *S. epidermidis* PVE has resulted in several bacteriological and clinical cures plus an enhancement of the serum bactericidal activity when compared with regimens not containing rifampin.[51,54]

Although many different treatment regimens have been utilized for the therapy of *S. epidermidis* endocarditis, it is safe to say that the optimum regimen has not been established. Out recent limited clinical experience plus the experimental data cited above strongly suggest that the combination of vancomycin and rifampin with or without gentamicin may be the most effective regimen for *S. epidermidis* PVE, especially that caused by methicillin-resistant strains. A multi-center prospective randomized clinical trial in PVE patients has been initiated to address this question.

Diphtheroids. Diphtheroids, which are important causative agents of PVE, are fastidious gram positive coccobacilli which are often difficult to isolate and maintain in cultures. As a result, the bacteriology laboratory may be unable to perform MIC's, MBC's, and serum bactericidal studies. When the isolate can be shown to be penicillin sensitive, the combination of penicillin and gentamicin has been commonly employed as the treatment regimen.[59,60] Murray and her co-workers demonstrated that 16 of 18 strains of diphtheroids from PVE patients were synergistically killed by penicillin plus gentamicin.[60] These investigators also showed that susceptibility of the diphtheroid isolate to gentamicin appears to predict synergy between penicillin and gentamicin. No synergism was shown for the two isolates which was highly gentamicin resistant. All 18 strains were sensitive to vancomycin, whereas only 38% were susceptible to cephalothin, and 66% to cefamandole. These data suggest that for diphtheroid PVE patients whose isolates are gentamicin sensitive, whether or not there is susceptibility to penicillin, the regimen of choice is probably penicillin and gentamicin. Vancomycin with or without an aminoglycoside appears to be an effective alternative.[43] Similarly, vancomycin is the drug of choice in patients who have a history of penicillin allergy.

The survival rate in the 18 patients with diphtheroid PVE was 55%.[60] Survival rates were similar for early and late cases, and for those treated medically and by a medical-surgical approach. There were no relapses.

Surgery. Surgery has been increasingly utilized over the past decade in the management of patients with PVE and the addition of surgery to the treatment regimen has significantly improved survival in selected groups of patients (chapter 13). Surgery is performed in order 1) to replace or debride infected and/or poorly functioning prosthetic valves, 2) to eliminate resistant or difficult to treat microorganisms, 3) to eliminate sources of emboli, 4) to drain persistent foci of infection including periannular and myocardial abscesses, and probably most importantly, 5) to restore hemodynamic stability.

Several important principles have evolved regarding the surgical management of PVE. First, the risk of recurrent or persistent endocarditis following valve replacement for treatment of endocarditis is low even when there is active infection at the time of operation. Among 35 patients with PVE who were operated at the University of Alabama Medical Center, 50% had positive cultures at the time of surgery.[6] However, there were no episodes of recurrent PVE in the 10 patients who survived reoperation. Other studies have also indicated that an infected prosthesis can be replaced during active PVE with a low risk of recurrent infection.[3,7] Similarly, there are substantial data to show that the risk of developing PVE in patients who have received valve prostheses for treatment of uncontrolled NVE is also low.[61–65] Thus, valve replacement may be performed successfully in patients with active endocarditis even when blood or valve cultures are positive in the immediate perioperative period. The low risk of persistent or recurrent endocarditis following valve replacement allows the hemodynamic status of a patient with endocarditis to be the major determining factor in the timing of reoperation as opposed to considerations about the activity of infection or the length of preoperative antibiotic therapy.

Second, the operative mortality per valve replacement in patients with endocarditis is approximately the same as that in patients without endocarditis, when the degree of cardiac disability is similar at the time of surgery for both groups of patients.[6] Furthermore, outcome appears to be worse when surgical intervention is delayed and performed at a time when the endocarditis has progressed to a catastrophic state due to multiple complications, e.g., refractory heart failure, renal insufficiency, major emboli, pneumonia, and/or uncontrolled sepsis.[5–7]

Controversy exists about the optimal time for operation. Valve replacement probably should be delayed until a patient has received an appropriate antimicrobial treatment regimen for a minimum of 5 to 7 days. But, in patients who present with marked hemodynamic instability secondary to paravalvular leak and heart failure, emergency surgical intervention should be performed, carries an acceptable risk and may be life saving.

For example, among thirty-five PVE patients in whom reoperation was required, the in-hospital mortality of the three surgical groups was as follows: elective (next convenient operative date), 29%, urgent (next day), 40%, and emergency (immediate), 62%.[6] In contrast, patients who are stable but require elective reoperation for valve dysfunction secondary to paravalvular leak probably should receive a complete course of antibiotic therapy prior to surgery.

The usual situations in which surgery should be considered in the management of patients with PVE are listed in Table 6. Detailed consideration will be given to only two of the possible indications, namely, heart failure, and infection caused by specific microorganisms. References for discussions of the other possible indications are provided in the table.

Since refractory or progressive heart failure has consistently been shown to be a poor prognostic factor, this complication of PVE has become the most commonly accepted indication for operative intervention. Richardson et al reported that reoperation reduced mortiality in PVE patients with moderate to severe heart failure from 100% in the medically treated group to 44% in the surgically treated group.[6] The mortality in the group with moderate to severe heart failure, regardless of mode of therapy, was 58% and in the group with mild to no failure, 36%. Among 43 patients with late PVE and refractory heart failure reported by Karchmer and colleagues, mortality was 100% in the medically treated group and 75% in the surgically treated group.[5] In the latter study, among the 9 patients with moderate or severe heart failure who died despite reoperation, 4 died within 24 hours of surgery. Perhaps more importantly, in these four, antibiotics had been administered for 6, 11, 26, and 49 days prior to reoperation with resulting delay in surgery and progressive multiorgan deterioration. Among these patients with late PVE, the mortality rate in those with both paravalvular leak and moderate to severe heart failure was 81%. The authors of both of these studies 1) concluded that the combination of dehiscence or dysfunction of the prosthesis and significant heart failure carries a poor prognosis and 2) argued for more aggressive surgical management with early surgical intervention in patients with these complications. The results of numerous other studies of both NVE and PVE patients corroborate that survival is improved after surgical intervention for heart failure.[3,4,7,15,16,23,63–70]

Table 6. Indications for Operative Intervention in Prosthetic Valve Endocarditis*

Hemodynamic complications

1. Heart failure, moderate to severe, or rapidly progressive, caused by valvular insufficiency (tissue valves) or valve dehiscence with paravalvular leak (mechanical valves) [3–7,23,64,66,68]
2. Acute decrease in cardiac output, caused by an obstructed valve [24,30,68,72]

Emboli

1. Recurrent or single major emboli, such as coronary or cerebral emboli [3–6,23,64,68]
2. Echocardiographic evidence of vegetations [24,29–31]

Extension of valve infection resulting in annular abscess, myocardial abscess, mycotic aneurysm, or pericarditis.[5–7,25,26,34,68]

Uncontrolled infection, manifested by persistent fever, or persistent positive blood cultures on therapy, and caused by ineffective or unavailable antimicrobial therapy[3–5,7,23,64,68]

Fungal endocarditis[6,35,68]

Relapse after apparently successful treatment with an appropriate antibiotic regimen [5]

Staphylococcal endocarditis, especially in patients with any of the above indications.[5–6,64,68,71] Management of each patient must be individualized.

*Adapted from Dismukes, W.E.: Management of Infective Endocarditis, in Cardiovascular Clinics, 11/3, Critical Care Cardiology, F.A. Davis Co., Philadelphia, 1981, pp 189–208.

Whereas heart failure has become an accepted indication for early reoperation, surgical intervention for treatment of a particular causative microorganism remains a more controversial issue. While there is universal agreement that fungal PVE should always be managed by early operation plus appropriate antifungal therapy,[35] the timing of reoperation for staphylococcal PVE continues to be debated. Richardson and colleagues reported an overall mortality rate of 62% in staphylococcal PVE, compared with a significantly lower mortality of 27% in streptococcal PVE.[6] Wilson and co-workers in their series of 45 PVE patients, reported a mortality in patients with infection due to *S. aureus* of 90%, *S. epidermidis,* 50%; viridans streptococci, 25%, enterococci, 75%, and gram negative bacilli, 47%[23] Among patients with staphylococcal late PVE reported by Karchmer et al, the mortality rate was 80%[5] In addition, the mortality rate was 39% among patients with streptococcal late PVE, compared with a mortality of 64% among patients in whom the infection was caused by bacteria other than streptococci. With regard to mode of therapy Richardson and colleagues reported an 80% mortality in patients treated with a combined medical-surgical regimen.[6] More specifically, the mortality for *S. aureus* in the medically treated group was 100%, and in the surgically treated group, 50%; for *S. epidermidis,* the mortality in the medically treated group was 75%, and in the surgically treated group, 60%, although the numbers of patients in the various groups by specific staphylococcal type were small.

Besides the high mortality rate, a significant number of patients with staphylococcal PVE had annular and/or myocardial abscesses. The same authors noted a mortality rate of 44% among staphylococcal NVE patients treated medically, compared with a mortality rate of 13% in patients treated with a combined medical-surgical regimen.[6] These data led Richardson et al, to recommend early operation of all patients with staphylococcal NVE and PVE. Other studies have also suggested that the high mortality rate in staphylococcal endocarditis might be favorably altered by early surgical intervention.[5,69] However, there is no unaminous endorsement of this approach at the present time.

Rapaport has critically summarized the data with regard to the surgical management of staphylococcal endocarditis.[71] While acknowledging a trend toward improved survival in surgically treated patients, Rapaport has emphasized that not every patient with staphylococcal endocarditis requires operation for cure. He has suggested that medical therapy should be initially utilized in patients who are hemodynamically and otherwise stable and urges that urgent or emergency valve replacement be reserved for patients with hemodynamic deterioration. He also emphasized that staphylococcal NVE in the addict population carries a much better overall prognosis than staphylococcal NVE and PVE in the non-addict population and rarely requires operative intervention. Until more definitive data are brought to bear on the issue, I agree with Rapaport that therapy in a patient with staphylococcal PVE should be individualized and based not solely on identification of a Staphylococcus species as the infecting agent, but also on the multiple other considerations depicted in Table 6.

As a consequence of the results of several of the studies cited above and in the references in Table 6, prompt surgical intervention has been increasingly employed in the management of PVE. As shown in Table 5, among 105 cases of PVE observed at the University of Alabama Hosptials and the Massachusetts General Hospital over the past four years, 66 or 63% were managed by a combined medical-surgical approach including early surgical intervention. In most cases, progressive heart failure was the indication for reoperation. This high percentage of surgically managed patients differs greatly from findings in earlier studies. Saffle et al,[4] reviewed three large series of PVE cases extending over the years, 1960–1974.[7,23,73] Among 115 patients who survived at least one week after diagnosis, only 22 or 19% were treated by a medical-surgical regimen. Similarly, in another series of 43 cases of late PVE, only 14 or 33% were managed by a combined approach.[5]

The overall survival rate of 71% among PVE patients in the recent Alabama-MGH series is also impressive (Table 5), especially when compared with the lower survival rates ranging from 26% to 56% reported in the review of PVE by Watanakunakorn.[8] Among the 49 patients with staphylococcal PVE in this series, 32 were managed by a combined medical-surgical regimen and 17 medically. The survival rate in the former group was 63% and 53% in the medically treated group. More importantly, the overall survival rate of 73% among 48 patients treated by antibiotics plus early reoperation compares very favorably with the survival figures among comparably managed but smaller patient groups in earlier studies. In the review by Saffle, the overall survival rate was 59% (17 of 29) for patients treated by valve replacement plus antibiotics [compared with a survival rate of 38% (39 of 102) for patients treated medically.][4] When these authors analyzed the subgroup of patients who survived at least one week after diagnosis, the survival rate in surgically treated patients was even higher, 77%. Similarly, in the 47 PVE patients studied by Richardson et al, overall survival was significantly better in patients treated surgically (55% vs. 25%, $p < 0.05$).[6] In contrast, among the 43 patients with late PVE reported by Karchmer and colleagues, medical-surgical therapy did not produce an improvement in survival compared with medical therapy (36% versus 52% $p < 0.32$).[5] Outcome in this group of patients managed by a medical-surgical regimen was adversely biased by a delay of surgery until major complications of PVE had developed, and reflects the subsequent risk of operation in very hemodynamically unstable and seriously ill patients.

Anticoagulation

Whereas anticoagulation is generally not recommended in NVE patients, anticoagulant therapy is usually continued in patients with PVE, especially in patients with mechanical prostheses, since anticoagulants are routinely required to prevent valve thrombosis. Wilson and co-workers reported the results of anticoagulation in a retrospective study of 52 cases of PVE; adequate anticoagulation therapy was given to 38 patients and anticoagulants were discontinued or given in subtherapeutic dosage to 14.[74] The incidence of major clinical central nervous system complications was considered to be the primary cause of 5 of the 8 deaths in this "nonanticoagulated" group. These data led Wilson et al, to recommend temporarily discontinuing anticoagulant therapy in PVE patients who develop cerebral emboli, observing the patient for evidence of intracranial hemorrhage, and if none occurs, reinstituting anticoagulants within 48 to 72 hours after the onset of the embolic event. However, the use of anticoagulants in patients with PVE will remain a controversial issue until more definitive data become available.

REFERENCES

1. Watanakunakorn, C.: Infective endocarditis as a result of medical progress, Am. J. Med. 64:917–919, 1978.
2. Kloster, F.E.: Diagnosis and management of complications of prosthetic heart valves, Am. J. Cardiol. 35:872–885, 1975.
3. Okies, J.E., Viroslav, J., and Williams, T.W.: Endocarditis after cardiac valvular replacement, Chest 59:198-202, 1971.
4. Saffle, J.R., Gardner, P., Schoenbaum, S.C., et al: Prosthetic valve endocarditis: the case for prompt valve replacement, J. Thorac. Cardiovas. Surg. 73:416–420, 1977.
5. Karchmer, A.W., Dismukes, W.E., Buckley, M.J., et al: Late prosthetic valve endocarditis: clinical features influencing therapy, Am. J. Med. 64:199–206, 1978.
6. Richardson, J.V., Karp, R.B., Kirklin, J.W., et al: Treatment of infective endocarditis: a 10-year comparative analysis, Circulation 58:589–597, 1978.
7. Dismukes, W.E., Karchmer, A.W., Buckley, M.J., et al: Prosthetic valve endocarditis: analysis of 38 cases, Circulation 48:365–377, 1973.
8. Watanakunakorn, C.: Prosthetic valve infective endocarditis, Prog. Cardiovas. Dis. 22:181–192, 1979.
9. Kaplan, E.L., Rich, H., Gersony, W., et al: A collaborative study of infective endocarditis in the 1970s: emphasis on infections in patients who have undergone cardiovascular surgery, Circulation 59:327–335, 1979.
10. Rossiter, S.J., Stinson, E.B., Oyer, P.E., et al: Prosthetic valve endocarditis: comparison of heterograft tissue valves and mechanical valves, J. Thorac. Cardiovas. Surg. 76:795–803, 1978.
11. Magilligan, D.J., Quinn, E.L., Davila, J.C.: Bacteremia, endocarditis, and the Hancock valve, Ann. Thorac. Surg. 24:508–518, 1977.
12. Downham, W.H. and Rhoades, E.R.: Endocarditis associated with porcine valve xenografts, Arch. Intern. Med. 139:1350–1352, 1979.
13. Clarkson, P.M. and Barratt-Boyes, B.G.: Bacterial endocarditis following homograft replacement of the aortic valve, Circulation 42:987–991, 1970.
14. Karchmer, A.W. and Swartz, M.N.: Infective endocarditis in patients with prosthetic heart valves, in Kaplan E.L., Taranta, A.V. (eds.): Infective Endocarditis: An American Heart Association Symposium, Monograph No. 52 (Dallas: American Heart Association, 1977) pp 58–61.

15. Garvey, G.J. and Neu, H.C.: Infective endocarditis--an evolving disease: a review of endocarditis at the Columbia-Presbyterian Medical Center, 1968–1973, Med. 57:105–127, 1978.
16. Pelletier, L.L. and Petersdorf, R.G.: Infective endocarditis: a review of 125 cases from the University of Washington Hosptials, 1963–72, Med. 56:287–313, 1977.
17. Delgado, D.G. and Cobbs, C.G.: Infections of prosthetic valves and intravascular devices, in Mandell, G.L., Douglas, R.G., Bennett, J.E. (eds.): Principles and Practice of Infectious Diseases (New York: John Wiley and Sons, 1979), pp 690–700.
18. Blakemore, W.S., McGarrity, G.J., Thurer, R.J., et al: Infection by air-borne bacteria with cardiopulmonary bypass, Surg. 70:830–837, 1971.
19. Ankeney, J.L. and Parker, R.F.: Staphylococcal endocarditis following open heart surgery related to positive intraoperative blood cultures, in Brewer, L.A. III (ed.): Prosthetic Heart Valves (Springfield, Ill.: Charles C. Thomas, 1969) pp 719–30.
20. Kluge, R.M., Calia, F.M., McLaughlin, J.S., et al: Sources of contamination in open heart surgery, J.A.M.A. 230:1415–1418, 1974.
21. Sande, M.A., Johnson, W.D., Hook, E.W., et al: Sustained bacteremia in patients with prosthetic cardiac valves, N. Engl. J. Med. 286:1067–1070, 1972.
22. Dismukes, W.E., and Karchmer, A.W.: The diagnosis of infected prosthetic heart valves: bacteremia vs. endocarditis, in Duma, R.J. (eds): Infections of Prosthetic Heart Valves and Vascular Grafts (Baltimore: University Park Press, 1977) pp 61–80.
23. Wilson, W.R., Jaumin, P.M., Danielson, G.K., et al: Prosthetic valve endocarditis, Ann. Intern. Med. 82:751–756, 1975.
24. Brodie, B.R., Grossman, W., McLaurin, L., et al: Diagnosis of prosthetic mitral valve malfunction with combined echophonocardiography, Circulation, 53:93–100, 1976.
25. Arnett, E.N., and Roberts, W.C.: Prosthetic valve endocarditis: Clinicopathologic analysis of 22 necropsy patients with comparison of observations in 74 necropsy patients with active endocarditis involving natural left-sided cardiac valves, Am. J. Cardiol. 38:281–292, 1976.
26. Madison, J., Wang, K., Gobel, F.L., et al: Prosthetic aortic valvular endocarditis, Circulation 51:940–949, 1975.
27. Roy, P., Tajik, A.J., Giuliani, E.R., et al: Spectrum of echocardiographic findings in bacterial endocarditis, Circulation 53:474–482, 1976.
28. Stewart, J.A., Silimperi, D., Harris, P., et al: Echocardiographic documentation of vegetative lesions in infective endocarditis: clinical implications, Circulation 61:374–380, 1980.
29. Schapira, J.N., Martin, R.P., Fowles, R.E., et al: Two dimensional echocardiographic assessment of patients with bioprosthetic valves. Am. J. Card. 43:510–519, 1979.

30. Strunk, B.L., London, E.J., Fitzgerald, J., et al: The assessment of mitral stenosis and prosthetic mitral valve obstruction, using the posterior aortic wall echocardiogram, Circulation 55:885–891, 1977.
31. Wann, L.S., Hallam, C.C., Dillon, J.C., et al: Comparison of M-mode and cross-sectional echocardiography in infective endocarditis, Circulation 60:728–733, 1979.
32. Ellis, K., Jaffe, C., Malm, J.R., et al: Infective endocarditis: roentgenographic considerations, Radiol. Clin. North Am. 11:415–442, 1973.
33. Welton, D.E., Young, J.B., Raizner, A.E., et al: Value and safety of cardiac catheterization during active infective endocarditis, Am. J. Card. 44:1306–1310, 1979.
34. Anderson, D.J., Buckley, B.H., Hutchins, G.M.: A clinicopathologic study of prosthetic valve endocarditis in 22 patients: morphologic basis for diagnosis and therapy, Am. Heart Jo. 94:325–332, 1977.
35. McLeod, R. and Remington, J.S.: Postoperative fungal endocarditis, in Duma, R.J. (ed.): Infections of Prosthetic Heart Valves and Vascular Grafts (Baltimore: University Park Press, 1977) pp 163–236.
36. Sande, M.A. and Scheld, W.M.: Combination antibiotic therapy of bacterial endocarditis, Ann. Intern. Med. 92:390–395, 1980.
37. Bryant, R.E., and Kimbrough, R.C.: Treatment of infective endocarditis, in Rahimtoola, S.H. (ed.): Infective Endocarditis (New York: Grune and Stratton, 1978) pp 327–360.
38. Sande, M.A. and Courtney, K.B.: Nafcillin-gentamicin synergism in experimental staphylococcal endocarditis, J. Lab. Clin. Med. 88:118–124, 1976.
39. Watanakunakorn, C. and Glotzbecker, C.: Enhancement of the effects of anti-staphylococcal antibiotics by aminoglycosides, Antimicrob. Agents Chemother. 6:802–806, 1974.
40. Watanakunakorn, C. and Baird, I.M.: Prognostic factors in staphylococcus aureus endocarditis and results of therapy with a penicillin and gentamicin, Am. J. Med. Sci. 273:133–139, 1977.
41. Abrams, B., Sklaver, A., Hoffman, T., et al: Single or combination therapy of staphylococcal endocarditis in intravenous drug abusers, Ann. Intern. Med. 90:789–791, 1979.
42. Sande, M.A., and Korzeniowski, O.M., Endocarditis Collaborative group: Comparison of nafcillin with nafcillin plus gentamicin in the treatment of addicts with S. aureus endocarditis, Abstract #362, 19th Interscience Conference on Antimicrobial Agents and Chemotherapy, October, 1979.
43. Cook, F.V. and Farrar, W.E.: Vancomycin revisited, Ann. Intern. Med. 88:813–818, 1978.
44. Sabath, L.D., Laverdiere, M., Wheeler, N., et al: A new type of penicillin resistance of Staphylococcus aureus, Lancet I:443–447, 1977.

45. Licht, J.H.: Penicillinase-resistant penicillin/gentamicin synergism: effect in patients with Staphylococcus aureus bacteremia, Arch. Intern. Med. 139:1094–1098, 1979.
46. Massanari, M., and Donta, S.T.: The efficacy of rifampin as adjunctive therapy in selected cases of staphylococcal endocarditis, Chest 73:371–375, 1978.
47. Faville, R.J., Zaske, D.E., Kaplan, E.L., et al: Staphylococcus aureus endocarditis: Combined therapy with vancomycin and rifampin, J.A.M.A. 240:1963–1965, 1978.
48. Sabath, L.D., Garner, C., Wilcox, C., et al: Susceptibility of Staphylococcus aureus and Staphylococcus epidermidis to 65 antibiotics, Antimicrob. Agents Chemother. 9:962–969, 1976.
49. Tuazon, C.U., Lin, M.Y.C., and Sheagren, J.N.: In vitro activity of rifampin alone and in combination with nafcillin and vancomycin against pathogenic strains of S. aureus, Antimicrob. Agents Chemother. 13:759–761, 1978.
50. Mandell, G.L. and Vest, T.K.: Killing of intraleukocytic S. aureus by rifampin: in vitro and in vivo studies, J. Infect. Dis. 125:486–490, 1972.
51. Lobo, M.C. and Mandell, G.L.: Treatment of experimental staphylococcal infection with rifampin, Antimicrob. Agents Chemother. 2:195–200, 1972.
52. Karchmer, A.W., Dismukes, W.E., Johnson, W.D., et al: Staphylococcus epidermidis prosthetic valve endocarditis, in Nelson, J.D., Grassi, C. (eds.): Current Chemotherapy and Infectious Disease (Washington, D.C.: Am. Soc. Microbiology, 1980) pp 904–906.
53. Archer, G.L., Karchmer, A.W., Dismukes, W.E.: Antibiotic susceptibility of S. epidermidis isolates from patients with prosthetic valve endocarditis. Abstract 603, 19th Interscience Conference on Antimicrobial Agents and Chemotherapy, October, 1979.
54. Ein, M.E., Smith, N.J., Aruffo, J.F., et al: Sensitivity and synergy studies of methicillin-resistant Staphylococcus epidermidis, Abstract A56, Annual Meeting of the American Society for Microbiology, May, 1979.
55. Lowy, F.D., Wexler, M.A., and Steigbigel, N.H.: Therapy of experimental methicillin-resistant Staphylococcus epidermidis endocarditis, in Nelson, J.D., and Grassi, C. (eds.): Current Chemotherapy and Infectious Disease (Washington, D.C.: American Society for Microbiology, 1980) pp 913–915.
56. Laverdiere, M., Peterson, P.K., Verhoef, J., et al: In vitro activity of cephalosporins against methicillin-resistant, coagulase negative staphylococci, J. Infect. Dis. 137:245–250, 1978.
57. Archer, G.L., Tenenbaum, M.J., and Haywood, H.B.: Rifampin therapy of Staphylococcus epidermidis, J.A.M.A. 240:751–753, 1978.

58. Vazquez, G.J., and Archer, G.L.: Antibiotic therapy of experimental Staphylococcus epidermidis endocarditis, Antimicrob. Agents Chemother. 17:280–285, 1980.
59. Van Scoy, R.E., Cohen, S.N., Geraci, J.E., et al: Coryneform bacterial endocarditis: difficulties in diagnosis and treatment, presentation of three cases, and review of literature, Mayo Clin. Proc. 52:216–219, 1977.
60. Murray, B.E., Karchmer, A.W., Moellering, R.C., Jr., et al: Diphtheroid prosthetic valve endocarditis: clinical presentation and therapy based on susceptibility to antimicrobial agents alone or in combination, Abstract 275, 18th Interscience Conference on Antimicrobial Agents and Chemotherapy, October, 1978.
61. Wilson, W.R., Danielson, G.K., Giuliani, E.R., et al: Valve replacement in patients with active infective endocarditis, Circulation 58:585–588, 1978.
62. Young, J.B., Welton, D.E., Raizner, A.E., et al: Surgery in active infective endocarditis, Circulation 60:I–77–I–81, 1979.
63. Utley, J.R., Mills, J., Hutchinson, J.C., et al: Valve replacement for bacterial and fungal endocarditis: a comparative study, Circulation 47–48:III–42–III–47, 1973.
64. Boyd, A.D., Spencer, F.C., Isom, O.W., et al: Infective endocarditis: an analysis of 54 surgically treated patients, J. Thorac. Cardiovas. Surg. 73:23–30, 1977.
65. Jung, J.Y., Saab, S.B. and Almond, C.H.: The case for early surgical treatment of left-sided primary infective endocarditis, J. Thorac. Cardiovas. Surg. 70:509–516, 1975.
66. English, T.A.H., and Ross, J.K.: Surgical aspects of bacterial endocarditis, Brit. Med. J. 4:598–602, 1972.
67. Wilson, W.R., Danielson, G.K., Giuliani, E.R., et al: Cardiac valve replacement in congestive heart failure due to infective endocarditis, Mayo Clin. Proc. 54:223–226, 1979.
68. Stinson, E.B., Griepp, R.B., Vosti, K., et al: Operative treatment of active endocarditis, J. Thorac. Cardiovas. Surg. 71:659–665, 1976.
69. Lowes, J.A., Williams, G., Tabaqchali, S., et al: Ten years of infective endocarditis at St. Bartholomew's Hospital: analysis of clinical features and treatment in relation to prognosis and mortality, Lancet I:133–136, 1980.
70. Baron, D.W., and Hickie, J.B.: Changing concepts in management of infective endocarditis, Med. J. Aust. 1:767–772, 1977.
71. Rapaport, E.: Editorial: The changing role of surgery in the management of infective endocarditis, Circulation 58:598–599, 1978.
72. Copans, H., Lakier, J.B., Kinsley, R.H., et al: Thrombosed Bjork-Shiley mitral prostheses, Circulation 61:169–174, 1980.
73. Slaughter, L., Morris, J.E., and Starr, A: Prosthetic valvular endocarditis: A 12 year review, Circulation 47:1319–1326, 1973.

74. Wilson, W.R., Geraci, J.E., Danielson, G.K., et al: Anticoagulant therapy and central nervous system complications in patients with prosthetic valve endocarditis, Circulation 57:1004–1007, 1978.

Bruce A. Reitz, M.D.
William A. Baumgartner, M.D.
Philip E. Oyer, M.D., Ph.D.
Edward B. Stinson, M.D.

13

SURGICAL TREATMENT OF INFECTIVE ENDOCARDITIS

In the pre-antibiotic era infective endocarditis was almost universally fatal. At the present time cure is achieved in approximately 80% of patients with medical management alone, with five-year survival rates approaching 75%.[1–7] It is apparent, however, that certain subgroups of patients with infective endocarditis continue to have an unfavorable prognosis. These are characterized by development of severe myocardial failure during the course of antibiotic therapy, infections due to antibiotic-resistant or highly virulent organisms, infections with extensive involvement of surrounding muscle or cardiac conduction system, infections of prosthetic heart valves, and infections associated with aneurysms, cerebral emboli, or renal failure. When severe myocardial failure complicates infective endocarditis, mortality approaches 90% in patients treated with antibiotics alone.[7–11] Similarly poor survival rates and increased morbidity are associated with the other subgroups mentioned.

When operative therapy was initially introduced, it was used to treat the residual valvular dysfunction following cure of infective endocarditis by antibiotics. The pioneering efforts of several surgeons in the 1960's established the validity of operation during the active phase of endocarditis in those patients who exhibited clinical findings presaging a poor outcome.[12,13] Following this work, numerous centers have advocated early operation for the management of complicated cases of endocarditis.[14–50] The primary indication in the majority of these cases (approximately 95%) is severe congestive heart failure.

It is the purpose of this review to examine the objectives of surgical management of complicated infective endocarditis and to define the efficacy of this modality of treatment. One hundred and twenty three consecutive patients undergoing valve replacement at Stanford University Medical Center since 1964 because of endocarditis diagnosed within one year of operation form the primary basis for this discussion. Based on this analysis, those subgroups of patients with a poor prognosis using antibiotic therapy alone will be identified and the improved results that can be expected with early surgical intervention emphasized.

Definitions and Patient Characteristics

Infective endocarditis involving native heart valves, whether previously normal or abnormal, is considered *primary,* distinguishing it from infection of previously inserted *prosthetic* heart valves. Further classification, determined by the duration of antibiotic administration prior to operative intervention, is useful. *Healed* endocarditis refers to those patients who completed a planned course of antibiotic therapy. Operations performed prior to completion of such a course is defined as *active* endocarditis. This latter distinction, although not signifying a direct index of the activity of the infectious process itself, correlates with both the operative mortality rates and the pathological and microbiological findings at operation. This classification is useful for clinical decision making and establishment of prognosis.

Selected clinical characteristics of patients in our series are summarized in Table 1. The average age for 66 patients with primary endocarditis was 47 years (range 14–85 years); for the 57 patients with prosthetic infection it was 54 years (range 21–78 years). The ratio of men to women

Table 1. Patient Characteristics

	PRIMARY ACTIVE	PRIMARY HEALED	PROSTHETIC ACTIVE	PROSTHETIC HEALED
Number	39	27	46	11
Average Age (Range/yrs)	49 (22–85)	43 (14–78)	54 (21–78)	55 (34–78)
Sex Male/female	23/16	23/4	30/16	8/3

was greater than 2:1, reflecting the predominance of aortic valve involvement in patients with advanced endocarditis requiring operation, combined with the overall predominance of men in the population at greatest risk after heart valve replacement.[3,51–53]

Factors Prediposing to Infection and Sites of Infection

A summary of predisposing factors in the Stanford series is shown in Table 2. The most common antecedent event in both primary and prosthetic groups was recent dental manipulation, usually without antibiotic prophylaxis. Other events included addiction, other infections, non-cardiac operation, and hemodialysis, although one-half of patients gave no history of an antecedent event. It is also noteworthy that 47% of all patients with primary endocarditis had no diagnosis of prior valvular heart disease, as established by history or at operation.

Table 2. Preoperative Factors in Patients Undergoing Operation for Infective Endocarditis

	PRIMARY ACTIVE	PRIMARY HEALED	PROSTHETIC ACTIVE	PROSTHETIC HEALED
Antecedent Event Identified	21 (55%)	11 (41%)	20 (43%)	5 (45%)
Pre-existent Heart Disease	17 (44%)	18 (67%)	—	—
Site of Infection				
Aortic Valve	27 (69%)	21 (78%)	31 (67%)	6 (55%)
Mitral Valve	9 (23%)	3 (11%)	9 (20%)	4 (36%)
Aortic & Mitral Valves	3 (8%)	3 (11%)	6 (13%)	1 (9%)
Indications for Operation				
CHF*	29 (74%)	24 (89%)	37 (81%)	8 (73%)
CHF and Emboli	8 (20%)	3 (11%)	2 (4%)	3 (7%)
Recurrent Emboli	1 (3%)	0	5 (11%)	0
Persistent Sepsis	1 (3%)	0	2 (4%)	0

*CHF, Congestive Heart Failure

The valvular site most commonly involved in cases of both primary and prosthetic endocarditis requiring surgery (71% and 65% respectively) was the aortic position. Analysis of valvular abnormalities in primary endocarditis revealed the most common to be a bicuspid congenital malformation of the aortic valve (20 patients), followed by rheumatic valvular disease (eight patients), mitral valve prolapse (five patients), subaortic stenosis (one patient), and degenerative aortic valve disease (one patient).

Among patients with prosthetic valve endocarditis, the majority had previous insertion of a mechanical valve prosthesis (Starr-Edwards or other type), with the next most common prosthesis being a porcine aortic valve xenograft.

Indications for Operation

Severe congestive heart failure was the predominant indication for operation in both primary and prosthetic endocarditis (80% and 79%, respectively) (Table 2). Systemic arterial emboli constituted another important indication, both in association with congestive heart failure (13%) and as an isolated factor. Healed and active categories showed similar percentages of patients requiring operation for congestive heart failure. However, the severity and rate of progression of hemodynamic deterioration were greater in the active group (primary and prosthetic).

Bacteriological and Histopathological Findings

Organisms responsible for infection and their correlation with operative mortality are outlined in Table 3. Streptococcal organisms were most frequently encountered, with the viridans streptococci predominating, followed by *Staphylococcus aureus* and *epidermidis.* The remainder of causative infecting organisms were relatively uncommon and were responsible mostly for isolated cases. Agents in this latter group were primarily associated with prosthetic endocarditis. A specific agent responsible for infection was not identified in 27% of the primary group and 21% of the prosthetic group ("abacteremic" endocarditis). All patients had characteristic gross and microscopic pathological findings of endocarditis confirmed at operation.

Four patients with documented *Candida* fungal endocarditis were operated upon in the active stage, with survival of all. No pre-existent valvular disease was evident in two of these patients who had primary infection. Various other fungi have been responsible for both primary as well as prosthetic endocarditis and the operative treatment of this particular subpopulation will be emphasized below.

Microscopic examination by gram stain and/or culture of excised valves was performed in 95% of patients classified as having healed endocarditis (27 primary, 11 prosthetic). Three patients (8%) had one or both tests positive. The average time from completion of antibiotic therapy to operation was 8.8 months. In contrast, patients categorized as having active endocarditis had one or both tests positive in 45% of cases. Discordancy was present in 36% of cases (see Table 4), with the major category being culture-negative/stain-positive, indicating that gram stain may be the more sensitive indicator of recent active disease.

An analysis of the relationships between the duration of preoperative antibiotic therapy, the presence of residual organisms in excised valve tissue, and operative survival revealed no significant correlation for either primary or prosthetic infections (Fig. 1).

Table 3. Relationship Between Etiology and Operative Mortality*

ORGANISM	PRIMARY ACTIVE	PRIMARY HEALED	PROSTHETIC ACTIVE	PROSTHETIC HEALED
Viridans streptococcus	10 (10%)	11 (0%)	8 (13%)	2 (0%)
Anaerobic streptococcus	1 (0%)	—	2 (0%)	1 (0%)
Beta-hemolytic streptococcus	5 (20%)	—	1 (0%)	1 (0%)
Streptococcus, unclassified	1 (20%)	—	—	—
Enterococcus	2 (0%)	—	4 (25%)	—
Group D streptococcus not enterococcus	—	—	3 (33%)	—
Diplococcus pneumoniae	1 (0%)	—	—	—
Staphylococcus aureus	9 (56%)	5 (0%)	—	—
Staphylococcus epidermidis	2 (0%)	—	7 (29%)	2 (0%)
Diphtheroids	—	—	1 (100%)	1 (0%)
Pseudomonas	1 (100%)	—	3 (67%)	—
Escherichia coli	—	—	1 (100%)	—
Serratia marcescens	—	—	1 (0%)	—
Listeria monocytogenes	—	—	1 (100%)	—
Hemophilus influenzae	1 (100%)	—	—	—
Peptococcus magnus	—	—	1 (0%)	—
Eikenella corrodens	—	—	1 (0%)	—
Candida	2 (0%)	—	2 (0%)	
Unknown	4 (0%)	11 (9%)	10 (20%)	4 (25%)
TOTAL	39 (23%)	27 (3.7%)	46 (24%)	11 (9%)

*Numbers represent total patients in each category. Percentages in parentheses represent mortality rate.

Table 4. Relationship Between Valve Culture and Stain in Active Endocarditis 56 Cases (Both Tests Performed)

	NUMBER	(Percent)
Concordant		
Culture (—)/Stain (—)	31	(55%)
Culture (+)/Stain (+)	5	(9%)
Discordant		
Culture (—)/Stain (+)	15	(27%)
Culture (+)/Stain (—)	5	(9%)

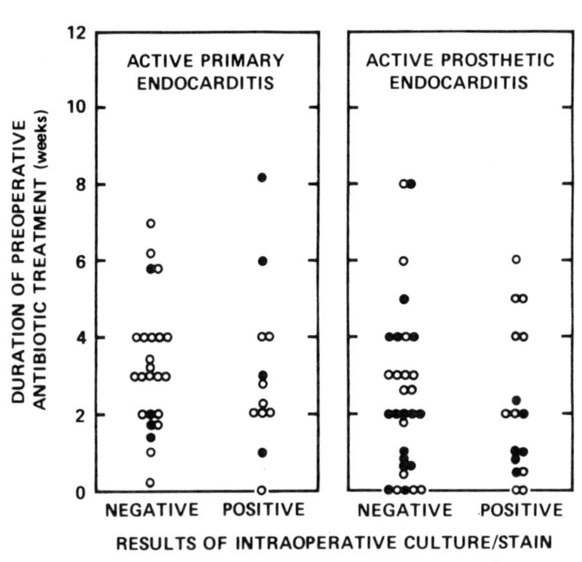

Operative Findings and Procedures

Pathological findings at the time of operation for both primary and prosthetic active endocarditis are summarized in Table 5. The principle features were those manifested by destructive changes, including leaflet

Table 5. Pathologic Findings Encountered in Patients with Active Endocarditis

	PRIMARY		PROSTHETIC	
Vegetations	26	(67%)	33	(72%)
Leaflet Destruction	36	(92%)	6	(13%)
Gross Perivalvular Abscess	16	(41%)	24	(52%)
Prosthesis Dehiscence	—		27	(59%)

perforation, commissural detachment and chordal rupture, as well as the presence of vegetations. Patients with healed primary endocarditis usually exhibited leaflet perforation or destruction and little perivalvular involvement or other anatomic sequelae. Patients with prosthetic valve endocarditis had a high incidence of valvular dehiscence. This latter entity, often associated with prosthetic endocarditis, is due to perivalvular necrosis caused by infection at the interface between prosthetic material and natural tissue. It is frequently associated with abscess formation and sinus tracts extending into the interventricular septum, left ventricular free wall, or border of the fibrous continuity between the aortic and mitral valves.

The goals of operation for infective endocarditis include removal of all infected tissue, restoration of valvular function by valve replacement, and correction of any structural or mechanical defects including aortic aneurysms, fistulae, septal perforations or conduction abnormalities.

All operations in our patients were performed through a median sternotomy incision, and standard techniques for cardiopulmonary bypass were employed. Special precautions were observed in reopening previous sternotomy incisions.[54] In patients with active infection, areas of necrotic tissue were debrided as thoroughly as possible, including the interior of perivalvular abscess cavities or sinus tracts. Generally, the orifices of such lesions were not obliterated by patch or suture closure, but left in communication with the bloodstream, except in cases of extensive tissue loss presaging extracardiac or intracardiac rupture. Special precautions were observed during aortic valve replacement. Anteriorly, in the region of the right coronary cusp, deeply-placed sutures may result in heart block. Posteriorly, in the area near the union of the non-coronary and left coronary cusps and anterior leaflet of the mitral valve, attempts to obliterate abscess cavities can result in distortion of the anterior leaflet of the mitral valve sufficient to cause mitral regurgitation.

Mitral valve excision and replacement has its own inherent hazards. Extensive tissue debridement in the posterior annular area may lead to an atrioventricular groove hematoma or rupture.

Special operative techniques are sometimes necessary because of extensive perivalvular necrosis, particularly in patients with prosthetic valve endocarditis.[23,25,31,36,41] These include buttressing of individual sutures or entire suture lines with synthetic material, insertion of sutures from outside the aorta, graft replacement of the ascending aorta, and in cases when suture placement in the annular region is impossible, translocation of the aortic valve to the ascending aorta.[41,55] This latter procedure is accomplished by resecting aortic valve and supravalvular aorta, ligating both native coronary arteries, insertion of a valve-containing conduit, and the insertion of two or three saphenous vein aortocoronary bypass grafts into the coronary circulation.

Three types of valvular prostheses were employed in our patients. Starr-Edwards ball-valve prostheses, porcine xenografts, and aortic valve allografts. Since 1975, porcine xenografts have been used almost exclusively.

Morbidity and Mortality

Causes of early deaths are summarized in Table 6. The overall operative mortality rate for active endocarditis (primary and prosthetic)

Table 6. Causes of Early Postoperative Mortality

	PRIMARY ACTIVE		PROSTHETIC ACTIVE	
	Number (%Mortality)			
Multiple (Cardiac, renal, pulmonary, and sepsis)	4	(44%)	1	(10%)
Myocardial Failure	2	(22%)	6	(60%)
Technical	1	(11%)	2	(20%)
Arrhythmia	1	(11%)	—	
Suture Line Infection	1	(11%)	—	
Cerebrovascular Accident	—		1	(10%)
Total Operative Mortality	9	(23%)	10	(22%)

was 23%. This represents a salvage rate that approximates 77%, since the majority of these patients underwent urgent or emergent operation because of progressive heart failure. Additional risk factors included peripheral emboli, metastatic abscess, renal failure, and arrhythmias. Considering these features, the survival rates obtained represent a substantial improvement over projected outcome with medical therapy alone.

Operation in the group of patients with active prosthetic endocarditis resulted in a survival rate of 78%, similar to the group with primary endocarditis. This compares favorably with previously reported survival rates of patients with prosthetic endocarditis from other centers.[51–53,56]

In both the primary and prosthetic groups, early postoperative deaths were due to multiple factors including heart failure, renal dysfunction, pulmonary insufficiency, and sepsis. These factors represented in each case a continuance of pre-existing failure antedating operation. The most frequent underlying factor responsible for ensuing complications was severe congestive heart failure, and this constitutes the predominant risk factor in operative treatment of endocarditis.

Operative survival rates for healed primary and prosthetic endocarditis were 96.3% and 91%, respectively, confirming the observation that patients with healed endocarditis generally display stable or slowly deteriorating cardiac function. The overall rate of residual endocarditis was 4%. Another cause of significant morbidity was the development of periprosthetic leaks in 16 of the 123 operative survivors, requiring subsequent reoperation in seven patients.

Correlation of the operative outcome with etiologic agent is summarized in Table 3. Staphylococal organisms were associated with elevation of operative risk when endocarditis was active, in comparison to the streptococcal disease. The small numbers of gram negative and fungal infections do not permit firm conclusions to be drawn, but it would appear that these infectious agents are also associated with increased operative risk.[13,48,49,50,52,53,57]

At the present time 72 of 123 operative survivors (59%) are living, with the average postoperative interval being four years (range 4 months to 14.9 years). Five-year actuarial survival rates of patients discharged from hosptial, separated into categories of active primary, healed primary, and active prosthetic endocarditis, were 66 ± 11%, 72 ± 10%, and 49 ± 15%, respectively. Five late deaths occurred as a result of recurrent or relapsing endocarditis. Cardiovascular deterioration with congestive heart failure was implicated in the majority of the remaining late deaths.

Principles of Therapy

Antibiotic therapy offers a probability of cure for the majority of patients with infective endocarditis.[1–7] However, there are certain groups of patients who continue to sustain low cure rates despite intensive medical management.[7–11] The most common underlying risk factor is the development of progressive cardiac failure, usually in conjunction with aortic valve destruction.[58–61]

Operative intervention in this subgroup of patients has previously been allocated to the role of a salvage procedure, following marked deterioration of clinical status and firm realization of failure of medical management. Validity of the concept of earlier operation is well illustrated in those patients with fungal endocarditis, in whom survival without operation is almost negligible; a satisfactory outcome with early operation, however, was achieved in the four patients of our series, and has been reported by others.[48–50]

The argument for earlier operation, when dealing with patients whose endocarditis is associated with a poor prognosis, is further supported by the low incidence of continuing valvular infection following valve replacement. The concept that insertion or reinsertion of a prosthetic valve at the site of infection will lead to almost certain recrudescence of endocarditis has not been borne out by experience in the large number of patients reported here. The risk of residual endocarditis in the presence of active infection is in the range of 4%. Furthermore, there was little correlation in our patient series between the duration of preoperative antibiotic treatment and operative mortality and late outcome. Continuing medical therapy alone for patients who develop complications during treatment is not warranted, since operative risk is based primarily on the number of pre-existing complications.

From analysis of the results presented here, as well as previously reported experience, two important points can be advanced. First, operative mortality for patients with active endocarditis (primary and prosthetic) is directly related to the status of the cardiovascular system, namely, severity of congestive heart failure. Secondly, there is a low incidence of residual endocarditis following valve replacement in these patients.[37,42,57,62] Even a simplistic application of these two basic tenets yields a strong argument in favor of prompt valve replacement for all cases of infective endocarditis that have an unfavorable prognosis. Certainly, those patients in whom survival with medical treatment is highly likely, characterized by infection with a gram positive coccus that is sensitive to bactericidal antibiotics and by the absence of any serious intracardiac or extracardiac complication upon initial presentation and throughout the period of antimicrobial therapy, should continue with medical therapy alone pending the development of complications. Patients with prosthetic valve endocarditis may be similarly characterized, with the qualification that early postoperative (less than two months) endocarditis of any etiology, imposes a distinctly higher risk.

We would suggest that valve replacement should be considered and performed in the majority of cases of endocarditis that do not fulfill these criteria. This recommendation is based upon both the unsatisfactory results that may be expected with medical therapy and the already documented efficacy of surgical management, even when undertaken only after the appearance of traditional indications, such as intractable heart failure, mulitple macroemboli, persistent sepsis, or relapsing infection. It is reasonable to assume that earlier operation in patients identified to be at high risk from the standpoint of medical treatment alone would result in survival rates superior to those presently achieved, since, in general, the state of hemodynamic deterioration would be less severe. This strategy has been validated by Saffle and coworkers,[62] who reported six consecutive cases of active prosthetic valve endocarditis that were managed successfully by early valve replacement; none of the patients had uncontrolled congestive heart failure before operation.

In our own series of 85 patients with active primary or prosthetic endocarditis, operative intervention was based on the commonly accepted guidelines noted above; nonetheless, the overall survival rate was 77% and almost unquestionably would have been higher had operation been undertaken before the development of severe left ventricular dysfunction that was responsible for the majority of deaths.

We would re-emphasize that, since there is little correlation between the duration of preoperative antibiotic therapy and either intraoperative bacteriologic findings or operative outcome, early operation during the course of antibiotic therapy when sepsis continues or early indicators of progression of disease develop, should result in improved overall patient survival.[63] The theoretical benefit of prolonged antibiotic administration in the hope of achieving bacteriologic "cure" under such circumstances does not seem to be justified. This policy seems to impose greater jeopardy in that surgical intervention applied late in the course of deterioration is associated with important augmentation of operative morbidity and mortality.

The following considerations are therefore offered as guidelines for more aggressive and appropriate application of operative treatment in the management of infective endocarditis: 1) initial presentation with severe heart failure caused by valvular dysfunction (defined as pulmonary edema, systemic congestion, or pulmonary hypertension resulting from left-sided lesions), or heart failure requiring bedrest, digitalis, and diuretics for control; 2) the development of moderate to severe heart failure at any time after initiation of a course of antibiotic treatment, especially in association with a newly appearing murmur of aortic regurgitation or evidence of rupture of the supporting structures of the mitral valve apparatus; 3) more than one clinically evident arterial embolus or a single cerebral embolus which, if exacerbated by any additional embolic insult, would eventuate in sufficient neurologic damage to preclude rehabilitation; 4) lack of any improvement in the clinical state of systemic toxicity after one week of appropriate antibiotics; 5) failure to achieve bloodstream sterility after two to three days of therapy; 6) evidence of progressive spread of intracardiac infection, as manifested by conduction system disturbances, aneurysm, or fistula formation; 7) progressively severe renal dysfunction, especially that due to diffuse immune complex glomerulonephritis; 8) in the case of prosthetic heart valves, any degree of dehiscence (disruption of fixation) or interference with mechanical poppet movement; 9) any patient with the established diagnosis of infection caused by organisms not easily treated by antibiotics, including gram negative bacteria, or fungi, should be considered a probable operative candidate. Especially with fungal endocarditis, delay for the purposes of beginning chemotherapy is not warranted, since early operation is the most effective means of cure in this type of infection.

The major conclusion of this review, therefore, is that the role of surgical treatment of infective endocarditis may be legitimately expanded to include not only repair of mechanical dysfunction, but also removal of the infective lesion itself. Operation, in combination with an appropriately individualized antibiotic regimen, offers hope of a successful outcome in the majority of cases and should be performed at any time during the course of infective endocarditis complicated by an unfavorable etiology or by events associated with a poor prognosis.

REFERENCES

1. Kerr, A., Jr.: *Subacute Bacterial Endocarditis.* (Springfield,Ill.: Charles C. Thomas, Publisher, 1955).
2. Blount, J.G.: Bacterial endocarditis, Am. J. Med. 38:909–922, 1965.
3. Lerner, P.I., and Weinstein, L.: Infective endocarditis in the antibiotic era, New Eng. J. Med. 274:199, 1966.
4. Finland, M., and Barnes, M.W.: Changing etiology of bacterial endocarditis in the antibacterial era, Ann. Int. Med. 72:341, 1970.
5. Cherubin, C.B., and Neu, H.C.: Infective endocarditis at the Presbyterian Hospital in New York City from 1938–1967, Am. J. Med. 51:83, 1971.
6. Kaye, D.: Changes in the spectrum, diagnosis and management of bacterial and fungal endocarditis. Med. Clin. N. Am. 57:941, 1973.
7. Pelletier, L.L., Jr., and Petersdorf, R.G.: Infective endocarditis: A review of 125 cases from the University of Washington Hosptials, 1963–72, Medicine 56:287, 1977.
8. Watanakunakorn, C., Tan, J.S., and Phair, J.P.: Some salient features of *Staphylococcus aureus,* Am. J. Med. 54:473, 1973.
9. Rubinstein, B., Noriega, E.R., Simberkoff, M.S., et al: Fungal endocarditis: Analysis of 24 cases and review of the literature, Medicine 54:331, 1975.
10. McLeod, R., Remington, J.S.: Fungal Endocarditis, in Rahimtoola, S.H. (ed.): *Infective Endocarditis* (New York: Grune & Stratton, 1977, pp. 211–291).
11. Simberkoff, M.S.: Narcotic Associated Infective Endocarditis, in Kaplan, E.L., Taranta, A.V. (eds): *Infective Endocarditis* (Dallas, American Heart Association, 1977, pp. 46–50).
12. Kay, J.H., Bernstein, S., Feinstein, B., et al: Surgical cure of *Candidaa albicans* endocarditis with open-heart surgery, New Eng. J. Med. 264:907, 1961.
13. Wallace, A.G., Young, W.G., Jr., Osterhaut, S.: Treatment of acute bacterial endocarditis by valve excision and replacement, Circulation 31:450, 1965.

14. Braniff, B.A., Shumway, N.E., Harrison, D.C.: Valve replacement in active bacterial endocarditis, New Eng. J. Med. 276:1464, 1967.
15. Kaiser, G.C., Willman, V.L., Thurmann, M., et al: Valve replacement in cases of aortic insufficiency due to active endocarditis, J. Thorac. Cardiovasc. Surg. 54:491, 1967.
16. Wilcox, B.R., Proctor, H.J., Rackley, C.E., et al: Early surgical treatment of valvular endocarditis. J.A.M.A. 200:820, 1967.
17. Robicsek, F , Payne, R.B., Daugherty, H.K., et al: Bacterial endocarditis of the mitral valve treated by excision and replacement, Ann. Surg. 166:854, 1967.
18. Windsor, H.M., Shanahan, M.X.: Emergency valve replacement in bacterial endocarditis, Thorax 22:25, 1967.
19. Hurley, E.J., Eldridge, F.L., Hultgren, H.N.: Emergency replacement of valves in endocarditis, Am. Heart J. 73:798, 1967.
20. Scott, S.M., Fish, R.G., Crutcher, J.C.: Early surgical intervention for aortic insufficiency due to bacterial endocarditis, Ann. Thorac. Surg. 3:158, 1967.
21. Stason, W.B., DeSanctis, R.W., Weinberg, A.M., et al: Cardiac surgery in bacterial endocarditis, Circulation 38:514, 1968.
22. Kretschmer, K.P., and Lawrence, G.H.: Valve replacement in patients with bacterial endocarditis, Am. J. Surg. 118:273, 1969.
23. Hatcher, C.R., Symbas, P.N., Logan, W.D., et al: Surgical aspects of endocarditis of the aortic root, Am. J. Cardiol. 23:192, 1969.
24. Braimbridge, M.V.: Cardiac surgery and bacterial endocarditis, Lancet 1:1307, 1969.
25. Gonzalez-Lavin, L., Scappatura, E., Lise, M., et al: Mycotic aneurysms of the aortic root, a complication of aortic valve endocarditis, Ann. Thorac. Surg. 9:551, 1970.
26. Killen, D.A., Collins, H.A., Koening, M.G., et al: Prosthetic cardiac valves and bacterial endocarditis, Ann. Thorac. Surg. 9:238, 1970.
27. Manhis, D.R., Hessel, E.A., Winterscheid, L.C., et al: Open heart surgery in infective endocaridits, Circulation 41:841, 1970.
28. Sarot, I.A., Weber, D., Schechter, D.C.: Cardiac surgery in active, primary infective endocarditis, Chest 57:58, 1970.
29. Wilson, L.C., Wilcox, B.R., Sugg, W.L., et al: Valvar regurgitation in acute infective endocarditis: Early replacement, Arch. Surg. 101:756, 1970.
30. Hancock, E.W., Shumway, N.E., Remington, J.S.: Valve replacement in active bacterial endocarditis (editorial), J. Infect. Dis. 123:106, 1971.
31. Buckley, M.J., Mundth, E.B., Daggett, W.M., et al: Surgical management of the complications of sepsis involving the aortic valve, aortic root, and ascending aorta, Ann. Thorac. Surg. 12:391, 1971.
32. Hatcher, C.R., Symbas, P.M., Logan, W.D., Jr., et al: Surgical management of complications of bacterial endocarditis, Ann. Surg. 173:1045, 1971.

33. Neville, W.E., Magno, M., Foxworthy, D.T., et al: Emergency aortic valve replacement in bacterial endocarditis, J. Thorac. Cardiovasc. Surg. 6:916, 1971.
34. Crosby, I.K., Carrell, R., Reed, W.A.: Operative management of valvular complications of bacterial endocarditis, J. Thorac. Cardiovasc. Surg. 64:235, 1972.
35. English, T.A.H., and Ross, J.K.: Surgical aspects of bacterial endocarditis, Brit. Med. J. 4:598, 1972.
36. Shumacker, H.B., Jr.: Aneurysms of the aortic sinuses of Valsalva due to bacterial endocarditis, with special reference to their operative management, J. Thorac. Cardiovasc. Durg. 63:896, 1972.
37. Manhas, B.R., Mohri, H., Hessel, E.A., et al: Experience with surgical management of primary infective endocarditis: A collective review of 139 patients, Am. Heart J. 84:738, 1972.
38. Windsor, H.M., Golding, L.A., Shanahan, M.X.: Cardiac surgery in bacterial endocarditis, J. Thorac. Cardiovasc. Surg. 64:282, 1972.
39. Yacoub, M., Pennacchio L., Ross, D., et al: Replacement of mitral valve in active infective endocarditis, Brit. Heart J. 34:758, 1972.
40. Okies, J.E., Bradshaw, M.W., Williams, T.W., Jr.: Valve replacement in bacterial endocarditis, Chest 63:898, 1973.
41. Danielson, G.K., Titus, J.L., DuShane, J.W.: Successful treatment of aortic valve endocarditis and aortic root abscesses by insertion of prosthetic valve in ascending aorta and placement of bypass grafts to coronary arteries, J. Thorac. Cardiovasc. Surg. 67:443, 1974.
42. Jung, J.Y., Saab, S.D., Almond, C.H.: The case for early surgical treatment of left-sided primary infective endocarditis, J. Thorac. Cardiovasc. Surg. 70:509. 1975.
43. Alstrup, P., Froysaker, T.: Immediate and longterm results of emergency aortic valve replacement in acute bacterial endocarditis, Acta Med. Scand 200:373, 1976.
44. Palafox, B.A., Gazzaniga, A.B., Thrupp, L.D., et al: Surgical treatment of infective valvular endocarditis. Arch. Surg. 111:707, 1976.
45. Parrott, J.C.W., Hill, J.D., Kerth, W.J., et al: The surgical management of bacterial endocarditis: A review, Ann. Surg. 183:289, 1976.
46. Stinson, E.B., Griepp, R.B., Vosti, K., et al: Operative treatment of active endocarditis, J. Thorac. Cardiovas. Surg. 71:659, 1976.
47. Wilcox, B.R., Murray, G.F., Starek, P.J.K.: The longterm outlook for valve replacement in active endcarditis, J. Thorac. Cardiovasc. Surg. 74:860, 1977.
48. Kay, J.H., Bernstein, S., Psuji, H.K. et al: Surgical treatment of *Candida* endocarditis, J.A.M.A. 203:621, 1968.
49. Utley, J.R., Mills, J., Hutchinson, J.C., et al: Valve replacement for bacterial and fungal endocarditis. A comparative study, Circulation 57, 58 (Suppl. III):42–47, 1973.
50. Utley, J.R., Mills, J., Roe, B.B.: The role of valve replacement in the treatment of fungal endocarditis, J. Thorac. Cardiovasc. Surg. 69:255, 1975.

51. Slaughter, L., Morris, J.E., Starr, A.: Prosthetic valvular endocarditis, a twelve year review, Circulation 47:1319, 1973.
52. Dismukes, W.E., Karchmer, A.W., Buckley, M.J., et al: Prosthetic valve endocarditis, analysis of 38 cases, Circulation 48:365, 1973.
53. Wilson, W.R., Jauman, P.M., Danielson, G.K., et al: Prosthetic valve endocarditis, Ann. Int. Med. 82:751, 1975.
54. Oyer, P.E., Shumway, N.E.: Again, via the median sternotomy (editorial), Arch. Surg. 109:604, 1974.
55. Reitz, B.A., Stinson, E.B., Watson, D.C., et al: Translocation of the aortic valve for prosthetic valve endocarditis, J. Thorac. Cardiovasc. Surg. 81:212, 1981.
56. Masur, H., and Johnson, W.D.: Prosthetic valve endocarditis, J. Thorac. Cardiovasc. Surg. 80:31, 1980.
57. Boyd, A.D., Spencer, F.C., Isom, O.W., et al: Infective endocarditis. An analysis of 54 surgically treated patients, J. Thorac. Cardiovasc. Surg. 73:23, 1977.
58. Wilson, W.R., Jaumin, P.M., Dainelson, G.K., et al: Cardiac valve replacement in patients with congestive heart failure caused by infective endocarditis, Proc. Mayo Clin. 54:223, 1979.
59. Wigle, E.D., Labrosse, C.J.: Sudden, severe aortic insufficiency, Circulation 32:708, 1965.
60. Wise, J.R., Oakley, C.M., Goodwin, J.F.: Acute aortic reguirgitation in patients with infective endocarditis. The distinctive clinical features and the role of premature mitral valve closure, J. Maine Med. Assoc. 63:273, 1972.
61. Mann, T., McLaurin, L., Grossman, W., et al: Assessing the hemodynamic severity of acute aortic reguirgitation due to infective endocarditis, New Eng. J. Med. 293:108, 1975.
62. Saffle, J.R., Gardner, P., Schoenbaum, S.C., et al: Prosthetic valve endocarditis. The case for prompt valve replacement, J. Thorac. Cardiovasc. Surg. 73:416, 1977.
63. Stinson, E.B.: Surgical Treatment of Infective Endocarditis, Progress in Cardiovascular Disease, Vol. XXII, No. 3 (November/December), 1979.

John E. Erffmeyer, M.D.
Phil Lieberman, M.D.

14

MANAGEMENT OF PENICILLIN ALLERGY IN PATIENTS WITH BACTERIAL ENDOCARDITIS

Incidence

Although it is impossible to ascertain the true incidence of allergic reactions to penicillin,[1] estimates of the frequency of such reactions range from 1 to 10% of patients treated.[2] Penicillin is the most common cause of anaphylaxis.[3] Several reviews concerned with the incidence of anaphylaxis to penicillin have been published.[4,5,6] Based upon these studies, anaphylactic reactions occur with a frequency of one to five per 10,000 patient courses of treatment.[5] It has been estimated that penicillin may be responsible for as many as 75% of anaphylactic deaths in the United States[7] and cause 400 to 800 deaths per year.[8]

Anaphylactic reactions to penicillin occur most commonly in adults between the ages of 20 and 49.[5] However, neither extreme of the age spectrum is exempt. Anaphylactic reactions, though rare in children under 12 years of age,[5] have occurred in both infants[3,9,10] and the elderly.[9]

Another factor, besides that of age, that may effect the incidence of reactions to penicillin is the route of administration. Though allergic reactions may occur following any route of administration, attacks seem to be more frequent and more severe when penicillin is injected.[11,12]

Additionally, the interval between the original episode of anaphylaxis and the subsequent readministration of penicillin is an important variable. The chances of another anaphylactic episode decrease as the time interval between the original attack and readministration increases.

Whether the presence of atopy is a predisposing factor in penicillin anaphylaxis is controversial.[13] Early investigations found that anaphylaxis to penicillin was more common in atopic individuals.[14,15] However, recent evidence has not confirmed this observation.[16] In a multi-center cooperative study of penicillin allergy by the American Academy of Allergy there was no correlation between penicillin reactivity and a personal or familial history of allergy.[17] In 1973, a study involving 1,043 individuals reported no difference in the incidence of positive skin tests to penicillin between nonatopics and atopics.[18] Most deaths from penicillin anaphylaxis have occurred in persons with no history of allergy.[2]

However, anaphylaxis to foods, an antigen to which exposure is mucosal, does appear to occur more frequently in allergic individuals.[19] This is consistent with experimental data showing that atopics are more prone to develop an IgE antibody response when the antigen is administered topically, but show no predisposition to do so when it is administered by injection.[20] Thus, anaphylaxis to oral penicillin could conceivably be more common in the atopic.

Sex, race, and HLA phenotype do not appear to effect the incidence of penicillin allergy. Although some authors have found that the incidence of allergic reactions to penicillin is greater in males than in females,[21] others have found the opposite.[22] There appears to be no significant correlation between any specific HLA phenotype and penicillin allergy.[23] As is the case with other antigens,[24] there is no correlation between penicillin anaphylaxis and race.

Penicillin as an Antigen

Penicillin (benzylpenicillin, crystalline penicillin, penicillin G) produces a heterogeneous immunologic response in man[25,26] and can cause several immunopathologic states[27] including serum sickness, immune hemolytic anemia, urticaria, and anaphylaxis.[28,29] Only the latter two are of acute concern in the administration of penicillin to the penicillin allergic patient. Therefore, this discussion will be limited to those reactions.

Penicillin, like most drugs, is of low molecular weight (333).[30] It is therefore a hapten[31] and not, by itself, immunogenic. Haptens can induce an immune response only by irreversibly combining with tissue macromolecules--usually a protein or oligopeptide.[32] The actual immunogen is the product formed when the drug (hapten) combines with protein. The specificity of the antibody formed includes the drug itself in its altered protein-bound state and certain determinants on the tissue protein (carrier).[33]

The molecular nucleus of penicillin is 6-aminopenicillanic acid (6-APA). Its major components are a β-lactam ring and a thiazolidine ring

(Figure 1). In actuality, it is the metabolic products of penicillin rather than penicillin itself that form the allergenic haptenic moieties. This is due to their greater biochemical reactivity and propensity to bind tissue proteins. This occurs as the ring structures of penicillin are opened.

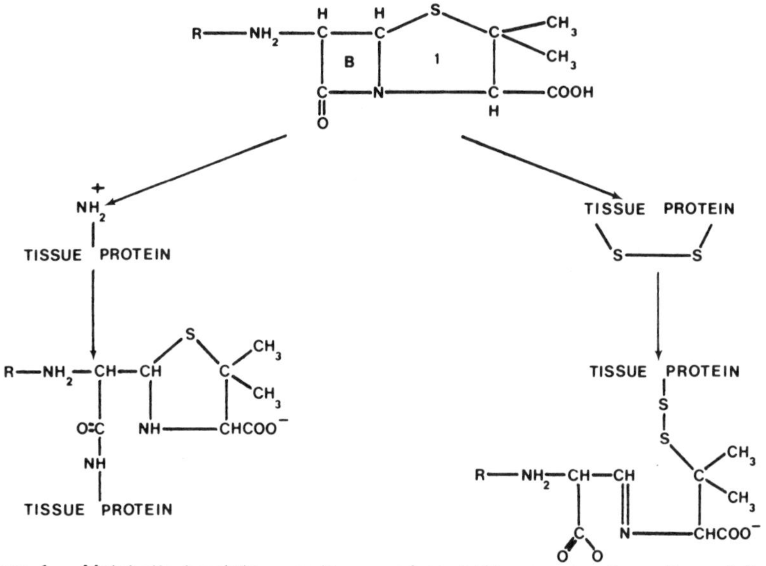

Figure 1: Metabolic breakdown pathways of penicillin showing formation of the antigenic determinants thought to be important in penicillin allergy. The major determinant is formed by the binding of tissue protein with the opened β-lactam ring (B). The minor determinants are formed by the reaction of tissue protein with the opened thiazolidine ring. (1)

The penicilloyl group is the major metabolic product. For this reason, it is referred to as the "major determinant".[26] This antigenic determinant is formed by the reaction of the β-lactam ring with tissue protein amino acids, such as lysine.[34,35] The precise mechanism that leads to the formation of protein-bound penicilloyl has been a subject of debate. It is possible that penicillin may rearrange *in vivo* to form a highly reactive compound, penicillenic acid, and then proceed to the penicilloyl haptenic group.[36,37,38,39] An alternative route of formation is the reaction of the β-lactam ring directly with protein.[40,41,42]

A small amount of penicillin, perhaps 5% or less, is metabolized by several other pathways. The fact that these metabolites are formed in such small quantities has lead to their designation as the minor haptenic determinants or just "minor determinants."[26] The structures of the minor determinants are not entirely known.[43,44] The minor determinant mixture (MDM) is composed of crystalline penicillin and its hydrolysis product, sodium penicilloate, plus other simple chemical products derived from penicillin degradation[43] such as sodium-alpha-benzylpenicilloyl-amine.[45]

The majority of antibodies formed in penicillin allergy are specific for the penicilloyl group.[34,36,46] The discovery that penicilloyl-specific antibodies were important in the generation of a Type I response in man was demonstrated by the fact that they could be detected using direct skin testing[34,36,47] and passive transfer techniques.[48]

The presence of IgE antibodies specific for the minor determinants can also be demonstrated by performing skin tests using the MDM. A standardized, commercially manufactured minor determinant mixture is not available at present. Alternative means for skin testing for the minor determinants are possible and will be discussed later.

Human Immune Response to Penicillin

Penicillin will produce an immune response in nearly every person who receives the drug.[26,49] In fact, if sensitive enough assays are performed, evidence of an immunologic response can be detected in virtually everyone, including individuals who deny ever having received the drug.[49] Presumably enough exposure to the drug is gained through the environment to induce this response.[50,51] Antibodies of all the major classes (IgE, IgA, IgM, IgG, IgD) are formed.

It is the IgE antibody that is responsible for the acute allergic reaction, (the Type I response) with which this discussion is concerned. IgG antibody may play a protective role in preventing allergic reactions, as discussed later.

Penicillin reactions have been classified according to their clinical manifestations. They are immediate and accelerated.[26] Both of these are IgE mediated. Immediate reactions, cutaneous or anaphylactic, occur within the first 30 minutes after administration of penicillin. Accelerated reactions which are usually urticarial in nature, occur within the first 48 hours after initiation of penicillin therapy.[26,52]

The major determinant (penicilloyl) is felt to be the antigen responsible for the causation of accelerated reactions, but not anaphylaxis.[26] It is believed that this occurs because protective IgG antibodies of penicilloyl specificity (blocking antibodies) are synthesized in conjunction with IgE of penicilloyl specificity.[26,52] IgG blocking antibodies are capable of competing with IgE for the antigen (the pencilloyl determinant) and thereby prevent anaphylaxis.

IgE of minor determinant specificity is thought to be responsible for most episodes of penicillin anaphylaxis and other immediate systemic reactions (generalized urticaria, rhinitis, laryngeal edema).[26,45,49] The minor determinants are less likely to induce the concomitant production of blocking antibody, because relatively large amounts of antigen are required to induce IgG antibody synthesis.[53] Consequently, the IgE of minor determinant specificity is capable of reacting with the minor determinants without having to compete with clinically significant amounts of blocking antibody. Anaphylaxis can thus occur.

Detection of the Allergic Patient

The ability to predict which individual might be at risk of experiencing a potentially serious allergic reaction is clearly desirable. For this reason, there have been a number of attempts to devise useful in vitro tests. These include: the Prausnitz-Küstner (passive transfer) reaction;[54] the direct[55] and indirect[56] basophil degranulation test; the fluorometric assay of histamine release;[57] passive cutaneous anaphylaxis in guinea pigs and rabbits;[58] the bacteriophage neutralization test;[59] histamine release from leukocytes;[60] the rat mast cell degranulation test;[61,62] sensitization of monkey ileum (Schultz-Dale reaction);[63] in vitro sensitization of human and monkey lung;[64] and the enzyme-linked immunosorbent assay (ELISA).[65] For various reasons ranging from the technical difficulty involved in performing the test to the lack of reproducibility, these tests have not been found clinically useful as of this time.

Another in vitro test which has been employed clinically with some success is the radioallergosorbent test (RAST).[66] The RAST is a solid phase radioimmunoassay which measures circulating allergen-specific IgE antibody. It is capable of detecting very small quantities of drug specific IgE. Currently, there is no other clinically available in vitro assay for IgE which can match the sensitivity, accuracy, and precision of the RAST.[67] Since it is an in vitro assay, it is devoid of the inherent risks that accompany the administration of any allergy skin test, namely the development of an allergic reaction.

The RAST test has been employed in the investigation of certain aspects of penicillin allergy, i.e., the detection of penicilloyl-specific IgE.[68] These results have correlated with skin tests to penicilloyl-polylysine (PPL).[68,69,70] It has not been as easy to develop successfully a RAST assay for the minor determinants, because some of them are chemically unstable[71] and others unknown.[43,44] Consequently, there is a RAST test for the major determinant, but not for the minor.

The RAST does, however, have certain disadvantages which make it unsuitable for clinical application at the present time. It may take as long as three days for the results of testing to return. In addition, the RAST is not as sensitive as intradermal tests; thus there is a slightly greater risk of a false-negative result. This fact is clinically important when evaluating an individual for potential anaphylactic sensitivity to penicillin.[67,72]

Skin testing has stood the test of time and is the most valuable and convenient method for the clinician to use to evaluate penicillin hypersensitivity. Tests employing multivalent penicilloyl haptens, such as penicilloyl-polylysine (PPL)[34] allow the clinical detection of penicilloyl IgE antibodies, as manifested by a wheal and flare reaction in the skin.[34,47] Additional tests with the minor determinant mixture increase the predictive value of skin testing.[26,45,52,73,74]

A positive skin test for the major determinant (PPL) is associated with an increased risk for developing an accelerated reaction.[26,52] A positive skin test for the MDM detects individuals at risk of developing an immediate systemic reaction or anaphylaxis.[26,45,49]

Nevertheless, episodes of anaphylaxis have occurred on rare occasions upon administration of penicillin to individuals who exhibited only a positive PPL skin test.[49,75,76,77]

Various studies[17,34,45,78–81] have demonstrated and confirmed[82,83,84] the safety and reliability of using penicillin skin tests to predict which individual may be at increased risk of developing an allergic reaction if given penicillin. Skin testing is of value in both adults and children.[85] As already mentioned, in order to detect the maximum number of potential reactors, both penicilloyl-polylysine (PPL) and the minor determinant mixture, or an appropriate substitute such as a fresh solution of penicillin G, must be utilized. Indeed, it has been stated that using both PPL and penicillin when skin testing should detect 90% to 95% of potential anaphylactic reactors.[86] This figure might approach 100% if the MDM were readily available.[86]

Depending upon the particular study, the nature of the patient population, and the skin test reagents used, the incidence of positive skin tests in patients with a history to penicillin allergy has ranged from 10.6% [85] to 91%.[80] The fact that a relatively low incidence of positive skin tests has been found in some studies may indicate that individuals with an invalid history of penicillin allergy were tested or that a long period of time had passed between the reaction and the performance of the skin test. The incidence of positive skin tests decreases as the interval of time since the reaction occurred increases.[81]

False-positive and false-negative skin tests are uncommon, but do occur. The incidence of positive skin tests occurring among history-negative patients is low: 7% or less.[83,87,88] The incidence of significant immediate or accelerated reactions occurring in history-positive, skin test-negative patients (false-negatives) is probably less than 1%.[45,88] When patients with positive histories and skin tests have been given penicillin the incidence of significant allergic reactions reported from two separate studies was 67%[83] and 73%.[45]

The value of skin testing can easily be appreciated. Negative results, when both skin test reagents are used, clearly indicate that the risk of developing an immediate or accelerated reaction is small. Negative results to both reagents are strong evidence that previous penicillin hypersensitivity has diminished or has ceased to exist.[83] Negative results do not, however, absolutely exclude the possibility of a significant allergic reaction occurring. A positive test to either reagent indicates that IgE antibodies are present to either the major or minor determinants and definitely places the individual at increased risk for the development of an immediate or accelerated allergic reaction.[45,83]

Cross-allergenicity of Penicillin, Penicillin Derivatives, and Cephalosporins

It will be recalled that 6-aminopenicillanic acid is the nucleus of the penicillin molecule. It is antigenic.[89,90] Since this nucleus is present in all semi-synthetic penicillins, it is not surprising that cross-allergenicity between penicillins does exist,[91] albeit to various degrees.[92] Though exceptions may occur,[87,93] if a person reports a history of an allergic response to "penicillin", the assumption must be made that the individual is allergic to all penicillins.[2,87,94]

In the patient with a history of penicillin allergy, cephalosporins cannot be considered a uniformly safe substitute for penicillin.[87,95,96,97,98] The basic structures of the penicillins and cephalosporins are similar in several respects (Figure 2). Whereas penicillins consist of a β-lactam ring and a five membered sulphur-containing thiazolidine ring; cephalosporins contain a β-lactam ring and a six-membered sulphur-containing dihydrothiazine ring. Degradation pathways and the subsequent antigenic determinants formed are threfore similar to those of penicillin.[53] It appears that a cephaloyl group[44,99] analagous to the penicilloyl group, may be formed. Whether or not cephalosporin equivalents of the minor determinant haptenic group are formed is uncertain.[44]

Definitive experimental work in animals has demonstrated varying degrees of cross-reactivity between antibodies to cephalosporins and penicillin.[100,101] Immunologic cross-reactivity between cephalothin and penicillin in humans has been shown.[102] Cross-allergenicity in man has also been studied and confirmed via measurement of the release of histamine from sensitized human leukocytes.[103]

A recent study demonstrated that patients treated with a cephalosporin exhibited changes in IgE, IgM, and IgG after therapy, not only to the cephalosporin, but also to penicillin.[104] This was interpreted to indicate that cephalosporin administration induced synthesis of antibodies to penicillin.[104]

In a study of 15,708 patients[105], 701 had a history of penicillin allergy and 57 (8.1%) of these had an allergic reaction upon administration of cephalosporins. There were 15,007 with no history of penicillin allergy. Only 285 (1.9%) of these individuals had an allergic reaction to cephalosporins. On the basis of these data it appears that an individual is approximately four times more likely to have allergic reaction to a cephalosporin if he has a history of penicillin allergy than if he does not.[105] This figure is in agreement with the findings from another study.[106] It has been stated that the risk to a penicillin allergic patient of developing an allergic reaction (excluding anaphylaxis) upon administration of a cephalosporin is 5% to 16%[97] with a mean rate of approximately 8.2%.[107]

THE PENICILLIN NUCLEUS

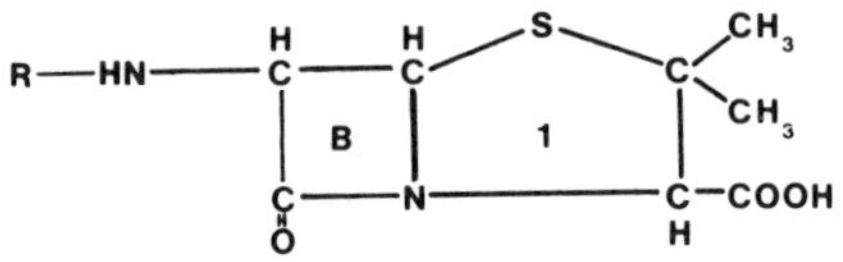

THE CEPHALOSPORIN NUCLEUS

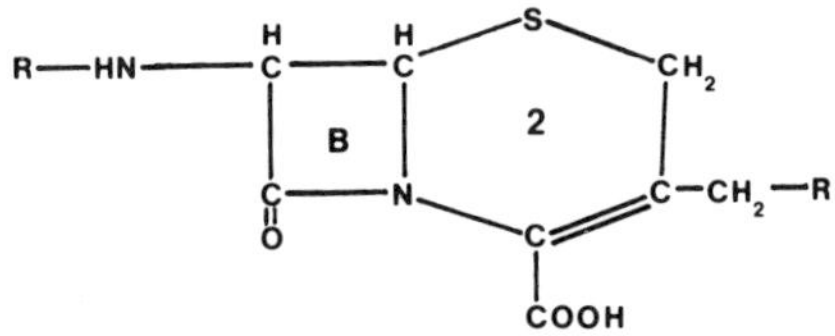

B BETA LACTAM RING
1 THIAZOLIDINE RING
2 DIHYDROTHIAZINE RING

Figure 2: Chemical structures of penicillin and a cephalosporin showing the shared β-lactam ring (B) and similarities of the thiazolidine ring (1) and the dihydrothiazine ring (2).

Only a limited number of studies have been performed using cephalosporins as skin test reagents. However, these investigations have demonstrated that when care is taken to ensure that positive cutaneous reactions are not secondary to nonspecific irritation, cross-allergenicity with penicillin can be shown.[103,108–110] It has also been found in individuals with a history of penicillin allergy and a positive PPL skin test that the incidence of allergic reactions to cephalothin is 50%.[106] In view of these data, it is not surprising that anaphylaxis has occurred in penicillin allergic patients who have been given cephalosporins.[109,111,112,113]

The authors believe that there is allergic cross-reactivity between penicillins and cephalosporins. The degree of cross-allergenicity may not be extensive and probably varies from individual to individual.[44] However, the potential of a life-threatening allergic reaction developing as a result of the administration of a cephalosporin to a patient with a history of penicillin allergy does exist. Thus, cephalosporins cannot be considered a uniformly safe alternative drug in such an individual.

The Approach to the Patient with Penicillin Allergy

When confronted with the endocarditis patient who gives a history of allergy to penicillin, it should be strongly emphasized that each individual's case is unique. Consequently, when one discusses the management of such a patient, especially with regard to the aspect of penicillin allergy, it must be realized that a rigidly defined approach is not appropriate. Instead, only suggested guidelines for the management of such a patient can be made. It is hoped that these guidelines will establish fundamental principles and yet be flexible enough for adaptation to any given situation.

It is of crucial importance to authenticate the clinical history of an allergic reaction to penicillin. Significant aspects of the history to be investigated include the following: the age of the patient at the time of the reaction; the nature of the illness for which the penicillin was given; the type of penicillin used; the route of administration that elicited the reaction; the amount of time that elapsed between the administration of the drug and the onset of the reaction; the nature, extent, and manifestation of the allergic response; whether the patient has received penicillin since the reaction – if so, at what age, and whether a second reaction occurred. Obviously, when the patient's history consists of the statement that he is "allergic to penicillin", and he cannot be more precise than that, it will be impossible to investigate the matter any further. However, if resource persons (e.g., a parent) are available who may be able to give insight to the history, it may prove helpful to query these sources.

Possibilities to be included in the differential diagnosis of an immediate reaction occurring after an injection include a vasovagal episode and an acute anxiety reaction. In addition, intramuscular administration of procaine penicillin can result in pseudo-anaphylaxis.[114] This nonallergic reaction, which resembles anaphylaxis, may be due to inadvertent intravenous injection of procaine.[115]

In discussing skin testing and further management of the patient, reference is made to Figure 3. The drug of choice for the penicillin-allergic patient is a non-β-lactam antibiotic which exerts a bactericidal effect against the infecting bacterium. When clinical judgement indicates that alternative drugs would either be ineffective or associated with unacceptable side effects, the use of penicillin or a cephalosporin must be explored.

In rare instances, the decision to give penicillin to the endocarditis patient with a history of penicillin allergy is made with relative ease, e.g., the infecting organism is sensitive only to penicillins and/or cephalosporins. Consequently, the patient must receive penicillin. Quite often, however, the decision is much more difficult. Use of ordinarily acceptable alternative drugs may not be possible in a particular individual because of an increased risk of side effects or toxicity associated with the use of the alternative agent, e.g., potential nephrotoxicity occurring in a patient who already suffers from significantly impaired renal function. In these

Figure 3. Guidelines for Patient Management

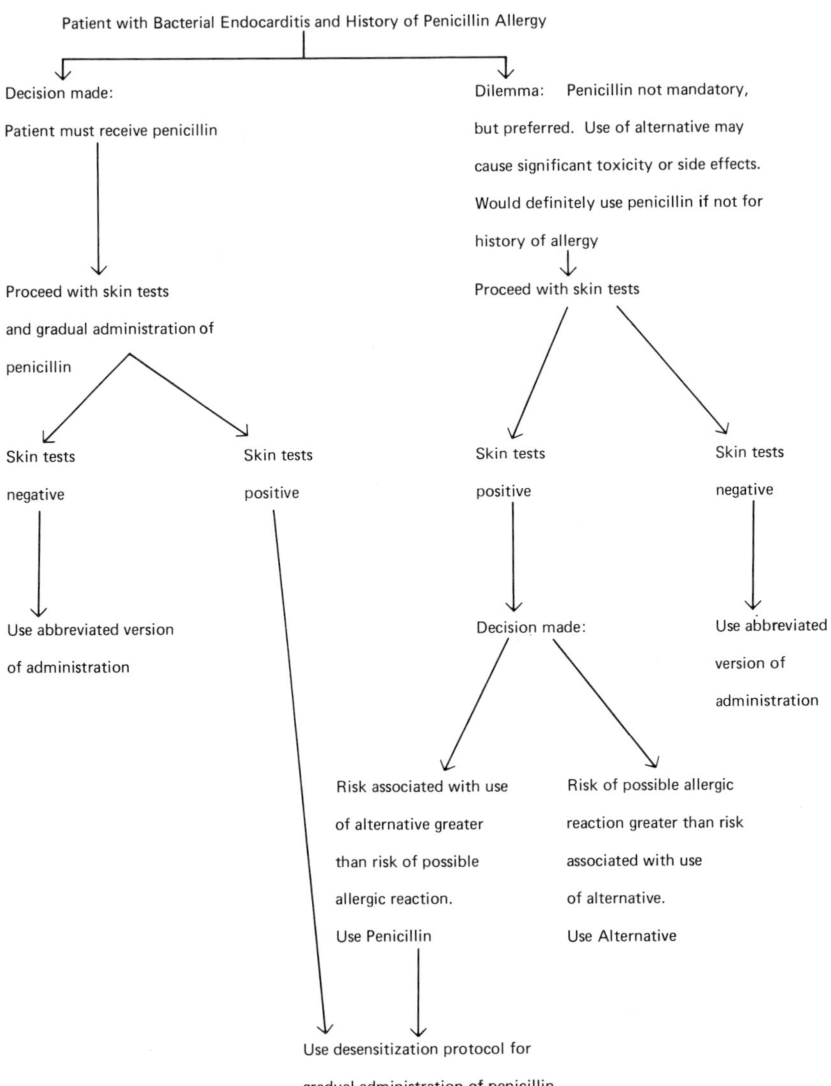

patients, the drug of choice would most certainly be penicillin were it not for the history of penicillin allergy.

Regardless of who will eventually make the decision, the knowledge gained from an allergic evaluation with penicillin skin tests is usually of significant help. If the tests are positive, the patient will be at increased risk of having a significant allergic reaction, and if they are negative, the patient's chances of having a significant allergic reaction will be quite small. Therefore, the skin test results may be of great benefit in aiding the physician who must decide whether to use penicillin or alternative therapy. It may allow the clinician to weigh realistically the risks of a possible allergic reaction against the side effects or toxicity of the alternative drug.

This is not to imply that all patients with a history of penicillin allergy should be routinely skin tested. Skin testing is only indicated when there is an immediate need for penicillin in such a patient and no suitable alternative drug will suffice. It is not to be done to satisfy one's curiosity regarding the current allergic status of the patient. Skin tests are of no value in predicting the occurrence of non-IgE mediated reactions to penicillin such as a delayed exanthem, drug fever, exfoliative dermatitis, hemolytic anemia, or interstitial nephritis.[88]

The reason for the concern expressed above is that the potential, though ever so slight, for a serious allergic reaction occurring as a result of penicillin skin testing does exist. It is known that both non-fatal[116,117] and fatal[118] anaphylactic reactions have occurred as a result of scratch testing with penicillin. Likewise, it is common knowledge that intradermal skin testing with penicillin can cause severe reactions;[119] fatal anaphylactic reactions have occurred.[5,120] It should be mentioned that systemic reactions,[121, 122] including anaphylaxis,[122] have occurred using penicilloyl-polylysine intradermally. However, in each instance either the amount of PPL injected was quite large [122] or the concentration used was excessively strong.[72, 123]

Despite this slight risk of a reaction, multiple studies have shown that penicillin skin testing is an extremely safe procedure when used appropriately by those experienced in the technique. Levine reported no episodes of anaphylaxis in 15 years' experience of penicillin skin testing.[72]

Prior to the performance of penicillin skin testing and the gradual administration of penicillin, it is mandatory that the patient's physician discuss with the patient and, if at all possible, with the patient's family, the reasons why the skin tests are going to be performed. He should mention the possible benefits and risks associated with the skin testing and penicillin administration procedure. The possible manifestations of an allergic reaction should be enumerated, e.g., generalized pruritis, skin rash, urticaria, rhinitis, throat tightness, wheezing, shortness of breath, nausea, vomiting, abdominal pain, diarrhea, light-headedness, and shock. The intent of the above is not to frighten the patient, but to educate him. It should be explained that *if* he were to experience any of these symptoms he should inform the physician *immediately* so that treatment may be initiated.

The fact that such discussions have transpired and the clinical reasoning that led to the decision to perform skin testing and administer penicillin should be documented in the chart.

Before the actual performance of the skin tests, certain precautions should be observed (Table I). An intravenous infusion using a large gauge needle or intravenous catheter should be started. All necessary emergency equipment and medications should be present in the room and easily accessible.

Table 1: Suggested Guidelines for Gradual Administration of Penicillin

A. Preparations of Solutions. Use Crystalline Penicillin G. Each new solution should be made using separate syringes for each dilution.

1. Dilute 20,000,000 unit vial to 20 ml = 1,000,000 units/ml (Solution 1)
2. Add 1 ml of Solution 1 to 9 ml normal saline (NS) = 100,000 units/ml (Solution 2)
3. Add 1 ml of Solution 2 to 9 ml NS = 10,000 units/ml (Solution 3)
4. Add 1 ml of Solution 3 to 9 ml NS = 1,000 units/ml (Solution 4)
5. Add 1 ml of Solution 4 to 9 ml NS = 100 units/ml (Solution 5)

B. Performance of Skin Tests. Use volar (flexor) surface of forearm.

1. Start intravenous infusion. Have all necessary emergency equipment and medications* present in room and readily available. Skin test results (prick and intradermal) are to be interpreted 10 to 15 minutes after performance.
2. Perform prick test using penicilloyl-polylysine** and a control using NS. if negative,
3. Perform intradermal test using penicilloyl-polylysine (0.01—0.02 ml) and a control using NS.
4. Perform prick test using one drop of Solution 3. If negative,
5. Perform intradermal test using Solution 5 (0.01—0.02 ml). If negative,
6. Perform intradermal test using Solution 3 (0.01—0.02 ml).
7. If ALL skin tests are NEGATIVE, proceed with Abbreviated Version of Gradual Administration of Penicillin as outlined in C.
8. If ANY skin test is POSITIVE, proceed with Desensitization Protocol for Gradual Administration of Penicillin as outlined in D.

Table 1: Suggested Guidelines for Gradual Administration of Penicillin (cont'd)

C. Abbreviated Version of Gradual Administration of Penicillin—to be performed only in skin test negative patients.

1. Continue intravenous infusion. Maintain availability of emergency equipment and medications. Initially record blood pressure, pulse, and respiratory rate and auscultate lungs. Monitor vital signs at frequent (15 minute) intervals during course of administration. All doses are to be injected subcutaneously in an extremity at intervals of 15 minutes. Prior to each injection, aspirate to make certain there is no blood return.
2. Initial dose of 500 units (0.5 ml of Solution 4). If no reaction, administer
3. 1000 units (0.1 ml of Solution 3). If no reaction, administer
4. 10,000 units (0.1 ml of Solution 2). If no reaction, administer
5. 100,000 units (1.0 ml of Solution 2). If no reaction,
6. Initiate therapy with full therapeutic dose of penicillin.

---

* Emergency equipment should include: Tourniquets, hypodermic needles, syringes,alcohol, sponges, oxygen with nasal cannula or face mask for administration, laryngoscope, endotracheal tubes, tracheostomy tray, Ambu[R] bag, sphygmomanometer, stethoscope, normal saline for intravenous infusion, and equipment for electrical cardioversion. Medications should include: Epinephrine 1:1000 for subcutaneous injection and 1:10,000 for intravenous injection, a plasma volume expander, levarterenol (Levophed), dopamine (Intropin), diphenhydramine (Benadryl) for parenteral injection, aminophylline, corticosteroids, and sodium bicarbonate.

** Commercially available as Pre-Pen[R] from the Kremers-Urban Co., Milwaukee, Wisconsin 53201

D. Densensitization Protocol for Gradual Administration of Penicillin — to be performed in skin test positive patients.

1. Follow precautions listed in C-1.
2. Administer penicillin as outlined below.

Solution	Penicillin concentration (Units/ml)	Milliliters injected Each 15 Min.	Units per Subcutaneous injection
5	100	0.1	10
		0.2	20
		0.4	40
		0.8	80
4	1,000	0.1	100
		0.2	200
		0.4	400
		0.8	800

Table 1: Suggested Guidelines for Gradual Administration of Penicillin (con't)

D. Continued

3	10,000	0.1	1,000
		0.2	2,000
		0.4	4,000
		0.8	8,000
2	100,000	0.1	10,000
		0.2	20,000
		0.4	40,000
		0.8	80,000
1	1,000,000	0.1	100,000
		0.2	200,000
		0.4	400,000
		0.8	800,000

3. Initiate therapy with full therapeutic dose of penicillin.

Ideally, the patient should not have received any antihistamines during the 24 to 72 hours immediately preceeding the performance of the skin tests. It is conceivable that these medications could prevent a wheal and flare reaction. For similar reasons, the patient should not have received any recent treatment with sympathomimetic drugs such as epinephrine. Corticosteroids do not affect the immediate hypersensitivity skin test.[88]

Skin test results (both prick and intradermal) are to be interpreted 10 to 15 minutes after performance. A skin test is considered positive when the presence of erythema greater than a nickel (21 mm) occurs, provided that the reaction of the test is greater than that of the control. The formation of a wheal, with or without pseudopods, in addition to the erythema, is indicative of a strongly positive test. The same criteria can be applied to evaluating the intradermal skin test.

The authors, as well as others,[12,83] feel that using a fresh solution of crystalline penicillin G is an effective substitute for the minor determinant mixture. Others recommend the use of a mildly alkaline solution of penicillin which has been allowed to stand for several days as a substitute for the MDM.[85, 124, 125] For those who wish to make their own minor determinant mixture, instructions for the synthesis of the various components can be found.[45,73, 82,126]

In patients who give a history of anaphylaxis or who are felt to be especially sensitive to penicillin, it is advisable to initiate prick testing with a solution more dilute than 10,000 units per ml (Solution 3, Table I), e.g., one unit per ml or ten units per ml. If the prick tests with the more dilute solutions are negative, testing with Solution 3 should still be performed before proceeding to intradermal testing. Before the intradermal test using penicillin can be considered negative, a final concentration of 10,000 units per ml must be used.

If the anticipated drug to be used is a penicillin other than penicillin G, or a cephalosporin, skin tests using the anticipated drug, in addition to testing with PPL and penicillin G, should be performed. There is no conversion factor to establish equivalent doses between units of penicillin G and other penicillins or cephalosporins. Therefore, one must empirically test with dilute solutions of the drug to be used. Such a possible skin testing regimen could be performed by doing serial prick tests with solutions of 0.25 mg/ml, 2.5 mg/ml, and 25 mg/ml. If the prick tests were negative, successive intradermal tests using solutions of 2.5 mg/ml and 25 mg/ml could be performed.[127] The detection of positive skin reactors is increased by skin testing with the actual drug to be employed.[128,129]

The interpretation of totally negative skin tests is controversial. Some feel that if the skin tests are negative the patient may receive penicillin with impunity. The authors believe that until a standardized, commercially prepared minor determinant mixture is available for skin testing, even skin test negative patients should be administered penicillin in a gradual manner (See Table I).* Skin test positive patients should receive penicillin via a desensitization protocol. For medicolegal reasons, it is recommended that written informed consent be obtained prior to the administration of penicillin to any patient with a history of penicillin allergy, regardless of the results of skin testing.

The rationale for penicillin desensitization (although as yet unproven) is that the very small incremental doses employed will allow gradual binding of penicillin to IgE antibodies fixed to mast cells or basophils. This in turn would allow gradual rather than massive release of histamine and other mediators of inflammation. When all antibody is bound, penicillin can be given with impunity. Antibody binding is followed, after a lag period of three to four days, by the production of IgG-blocking antibodies which are thought to be protective.

Various methods of penicillin desensitization have been proposed[94,130,131,132] including oral,[12,133,134] subcutaneous,[135] intramuscular,[136] and intravenous administration.[128,137] Non-fatal[76,138,139,140] and fatal[141,142] anaphylaxis has occurred after oral administration of penicillin – sometimes within minutes of ingestion. Fatal anaphylaxis has been reported after as little as 0.01 unit injected intravenously.[5] Therefore, the authors prefer the subcutaneous route of administration. In the event of a reaction, one has the advantage of being able to place a tourniquet promptly on the extremity proximal to the site

* At the time of the writing of this chapter a nationwide, multi-center study, under the auspices of the National Institutes of Allergy and Infectious Diseases, investigating the use of a standardized minor determinant mixture is in progress. Recommendations resulting from this study may alter the procedures suggested above.

of the subcutaneous injection. Epinephrine can also be infiltrated locally at the injection site. Both of these measures are thought to help slow the systemic absorption of the penicillin.

The gradual administration may be performed in the patient's room. A physician must be in attendance during the entire procedure, however.

No pretreatment with antihistamines or corticosteroids is indicated, even in skin test positive patients. If a local reaction occurs, i.e., only at the site of the injection, the procedure should continue. No treatment should be given. If however, any type of systemic reaction occurs, it should be promptly treated with epinephrine, antihistamines and corticosteroids and other measures used to treat anaphylaxis as dictated by the individual situation.[3,12,143,144,145]

Any time a systemic allergic reaction occurs during the course of the procedure, the patient's physician must re-evaluate the situation and once again weigh the benefits of penicillin therapy against the risk of another reaction. If the decision is made to continue the procedure, the patient must first be returned to a stable condition. If the patient had been receiving the abbreviated version of gradual administration, he should receive further penicillin via initiation of the desensitization protocol. If the patient developed anaphylaxis (as opposed to only urticaria or angioedema) during the procedure, he should be transferred to the intensive care unit and be pretreated with epinephrine, antihistamines and corticosteroids prior to the resumption of treatment.[12,139,146]

Once the patient is stable and the appropriate measures discussed above have been taken, reinstitution of the desensitization protocol may begin by dropping back two dilutions from the dose that caused the reaction. If during the second attempt at desensitization another systemic allergic reaction occurs the entire sequence of treatment and thought processes must be repeated. The procedure can be attempted again if all parties involved (patient, the patient's physician, and consultant) agree that there is absolutely no suitable alternative to penicillin therapy.

One may consider at this point, however, performing skin tests to and attempting desensitization with another penicillin or cephalosporin to which the patient may be less sensitive.[12] Despite the fact that cross-allergenicity between penicillins and cephalosporins does exist, it is known that some penicillin allergic patients may be less likely to have an allergic reaction to a cephalosporin than to a penicillin.[129,144] It should be emphasized that in the vast majority of instances penicillin can be administered by desensitization with little or no difficulty.[147] Indeed, the authors have never encountered a situation in a series of approximately 150 patients in which penicillin desensitization could not be completed.

Once the gradual administration procedure has been completed, full therapeutic doses of penicillin should be started immediately. The patient should be observed closely during the 48 to 72 hours after initiation of therapy. Accelerated urticarial reactions can occur.[26,148] These are usually cutaneous and can often be treated successfully with antihistamines alone.[146] The urticaria will usually subside even though the penicillin is continued. This is felt to occur as a result of the production of penicilloyl-specific IgG blocking antibodies.[146,149] However, very rarely, such an allergic reaction can take the form of laryngeal edema and can be fatal.[148]

At the conclusion of therapy the patient should be informed that since the penicillin has been stopped he may once again become "allergic" to penicillin. There are no data to predict how many patients become sensitized or were re-sensitized as a result of their penicillin therapy.

Patients who had an allergic reaction during therapy or who had positive skin tests should be told that penicillin should not be administered in the future without testing. They should be given a medical identification card stating such. They should also be encouraged to consider obtaining medical identification jewelry stating that they are allergic to penicillin.

REFERENCES

1. Stewart, G.T.: Allergy to penicillin and related antibiotics; antigenic and immunochemical mechanism, Annual Rev. Pharmacology. 13:309, 1973.
2. VanArsdel, P.P., Jr.: Allergic Reactions to Penicillin, J.A.M.A. 191:172, 1965.
3. Orange, R.P. and Donsky, G.J.: Anaphylaxis, in Middleton, E. Jr., Reed, C.E. and Ellis, E.F. (eds.): *Allergy: Principles and Practice* (St. Louis: The C.V. Mosby Co. 1978).
4. Rosenthal, A.: Committee on Medicolegal Problems. Follow-up Study of Fatal Penicillin Reactions, J.A.M.A. 167:1118, 1958.
5. Idsoe, O., Guthe, T., Willcox, R.R. et al: Nature and Extent of Penicillin Side-reactions, with Particular Reference to Fatalities from Anaphylactic Shock, Bull. Wld Hlth Org. 38:159, 1968.
6. Parker, C.W.:Editorial: Penicillin Allergy, Am. J. Med. 34:747, 1963.
7. Delage C., and Irey, N.S.: Anaphylactic deaths. A clinical pathologic study of 43 cases, J. Forensic Sci. 17:525, 1972.
8. Valentine, M., Chairman: Allergic Emergencies, in *NIAID Task Force Report: Asthma and Other Allergic Diseases.* Dept. Health, Education & Welfare. Public Health Service NIH Publication 70–387, May 1979, pp 501.
9. Idsoe, O.: Penicillin-sensitivity reactions in Taiwan, Bull, Wld Hlth Org. 18:323, 1958.
10. Matheson, A., and Elegant, L.: Penicillin Reactions in Children. A Study of the Value of the Skin Test in Penicillin Sensitization, J. Allergy, 26:415, 1955.

11. James, L.P., Jr. and Austen, K.F.: Fatal Systemic Anaphylaxis in Man, N. Engl. J. Med. 270:597, 1964.
12. Parker, C.W.: Drug Allergy (three parts), N. Engl. J. Med. 292:511, 732, 957, 1975.
13. Valentine, M., Chairman: Allergic Emergencies, in *NIAID Task Force Report: Asthma and Other Allergic Emergencies.* Dept. Health, Education & Welfare. Public Health Service NIH Publication 79, 387, May 1979, pp 469.
14. Kern, R.A. and Wimberley, N.A., Jr.: Penicillin Reactions: Their nature, growing importance, recognition, management and prevention, Am. J. Med. Sci. 226:357, 1953.
15. Rajka, G. and Skog, E.: On the Relation Between Drug Allergy and Atopy, Acta Allergol. XX:387, 1965.
16. Scanlon, R.T. and Bellanti, J.A.: Immunologically Mediated Disease Involving Exogenous Antigens (Allergy), in Bellanti, J.A. (ed.): Immunology II (Philadelphia: W.B. Saunders Co., 1978)
17. Green, G.R. and Rosenblum, A.: Report of the Penicillin Study Group – American Academy of Allergy, J. Allergy Clin. Immunol. 48:331, 1971.
18. Stember, R.H. and Levine, B.B.: Prevalence of allergic diseases, penicillin hypersensitivity, and aeroallergen hypersensitivity in various populations, J. Allergy Clin. Immunol. 51:100, 1973 (Abst 46).
19. Golbert, T.M., Patterson, R., Pruzansky, J.J.: Systemic allergic reactions to ingested antigens. J. Allergy, 44:96, 1969.
20. Salvaggio, J.E., Cavanaugh, J. J. A., Lowell, F.C. et al: A comparison of the immunologic responses of normal and atopic individuals to intranasally administered antigens, J. Allergy, 35:62, 1964.
21. Smith, J.W., Johnson, J.E. III, and Cluff, L.E.: Studies on the Epidemiology of Adverse Drug Reactions, N. Engl. J. Med. 274:998, 1966.
22. Miller, F.F.: History of drug sensitivity in atopic persons, J. Allergy, 40:46, 1967.
23. Spengler, H. and de Weck, A.L.: Evaluation of Genetic Control of the Immune Response to Penicillin in Man, Monogr, Allergy, 11:116, 1977.
24. Lieberman, P.: Anaphylaxis and anaphylactoid Reactions, in Slavin, R. (ed.): *Clinical Medicine* (Hagerstown, Md,: Harper & Row, in press).
25. Van Dellen, R.G. and Gleich, G.J.: Penicillin Skin Tests as Predictive and Diagnostic Aids in Penicillin Allergy, Med. Clin. N.A. 54:997, 1970.
26. Levine, B.B.: Immunologic Mechanisms of Penicillin Allergy. A Haptenic Model System for the Study of Allergic Diseases of Man, N. Engl. J. Med. 275:1115, 1966.

27. Fellner, M.J.: Penicillin Allergy 1976: A Review of Reactions, Detection and Current Management, Int. J. Derm. 15:497, 1976.
28. Cormia, F.E., Jacobsen, L.Y., and Smith, E.L.: Reactions to Penicillin, Bull. U.S. Army Medical Dept. IV:694, 1945.
29. Waldbott, G.L.: Anaphylactic Death from Penicillin, J.A.M.A. 139:526, 1949.
30. Stewart, G.T., et al: Penicillin allergy: The Nature of the Problem, in Stewart, G.T. and McGovern, J.P. (eds.): *Penicillin Allergy. Clinical and Immunologic Aspects.* (Springfield: Charles C. Thomas Publishers, 1970).
31. Landsteiner, K.: *The Specificity of Serological Reactions* Cambridge, Massachusetts: Harvard University Press, 1945).
32. de Weck, A.L.: Drug Reactions, in Samter, M. (ed.): *Immunological Diseases* (Little, Brown & Company, Inc., 1978), Edition 3.
33. Parker, C.W.: Mechanisms of Penicillin Allergy, Pathobiol. Annual. 2:405, 1972.
34. Parker, C.W., Shapiro, J., Kern, M., et al: Hypersensitivity to penicillenic acid derivatives in human beings with penicillin allergy, J. Exp. Med. 115:821, 1962.
35. Parker, C.W.: The Immunochemical Basis for Penicillin Allergy, Postgr. Med. 40 (Supplement):141, 1964.
36. Levine, B.B. and Ovary, Z.: Studies on the Mechanism of the Formation of the Penicillin Antigen III. The N- (D-α-benzylpenicilloyl) Group as an Antigenic Determinant Responsible for Hypersensitivity to Penicillin G, J. Exp. Med. 114:875, 1961.
37. Levine, B.B.: Studies on the Mechanism of the Formation of the Penicillin Antigen I. Delayed Allergic Cross-Reactions Among Penicillin G and its Degradation Products, J. Exp. Med. 112:1131, 1960.
38. Levine, B.B.: Studies on the Formation of the Penicillin Antigen. II. Some Reactions of D-Benzylpenicillenic Acid in Aqueous Solution at pH 7.5, Arch. Biochem. 93:50, 1961.
39. De Weck, A.L. and Eisen, H.N.: Some Immunochemical Properties of Penicillenic Acid. An Antigenic Determinant Derived from Penicillin, J. Exp. Med. 112:1227, 1960.
40. Levine, B.B.: Immunochemical Mechanisms Involved in Penicillin Hypersensitivity in Experimental Animals and in Human Beings, Postgr. Med. J. 40(Supplement):146, 1964.
41. Schneider C.H. and de Weck, A.L.: A New Chemical Aspect of Penicillin Allergy: The Direct Reaction of Penicillin With E-aminogroups. Nature. 208:57, 1965.
42. Schwartz, M.A. and Wu, G.-M.: Kinetics of Reactions Involved in Penicillin Allergy I. Mechanism of Reaction of Penicillins and 6-Aminopenicillanic Acid with Glycine in Alkaline Solution, J. Pharm. Sci. 55:550, 1966.

43. Valentine, M., Chairman: Allergic Emergencies, in *NIAID Task Force Report: Asthma and Other Allergic Diseases*. Dept. Health, Education & Welfare. Public Health Service NIH Publication 79, 387, May 1979, pp 474.
44. Levine, B.B.: Antigenicity and Cross-Reactivity of Penicillins and Cephalosporins, J. Infec. Dis. 128(Suppl):S364, 1973.
45. Levine, B.B. and Zolov, D.M.: Prediction of penicillin allergy by immunological tests, J. Allergy. 43:231, 1969.
46. De Weck, A.L. and Blum, G.: Recent Clinical and Immunological Aspects of Penicillin Allergy II. Antigenic Specificities of Allergy, Int. Arch. Allergy 27:221, 1965.
47. Levine, B.B. and Price, V.H.: Studies on the Immunological Mechanisms of Penicillin Allergy II. Antigenic Specificities of Allergic Wheal-And-Flare Skin Responses in Patients with Histories of Penicillin Allergy, Immunology. 7:542, 1964.
48. Siegel, B.B. and Levine, B.B.: Antigenic specificities of skin-sensitizing antibodies in sera from patients with immediate systemic allergic reactions to penicillin, J. Allergy 35:488, 1964.
49. Levine, B.B., Redmond, A.P., Fellner, M.J., et al: Penicillin Allergy and the Heterogenous Immune Responses of Man to Benzylpenicillin. J. Clin. Inv. 45:1895, 1966.
50. Siegel, B.B.: Hidden Contacts with Penicillin, Bull. Wld Hlth Org. 21:703, 1959.
51. Welch, H.: Problem of Antibiotics in Foods, J.A.M.A. 170:139, 1959.
52. Voss, H.E., Redmond, A.P. and Levine, B.B.: Clinical Detection of the Potential Allergic Reactor to Penicillin by Immunologic Tests, J.A.M.A. 196:679, 1966.
53. Frick, O.L.: Serum Sickness, in Middleton, E. Jr., Reed, C.E., and Ellis, E.F. (eds.): *Allergy: Prinicples and Practice* (St. Louis: The C.V. Mosby Co., 1978).
54. Waldo, J.F. and Tyson, J.T.: Hypersensitivity to Penicillin, Am. J. Med. 6:396, 1949.
55. Shelley, W.B. and Juhlin, L.: A New Test for Detecting Anaphylactic Sensitivity: The Basophil Reaction, Nature. 191:1056, 1961.
56. Shelley, W.B.: Indirect Basophil Degranulation Test for Allergy to Penicillin and Other Drugs, J.A.M.A. 184:171, 1963.
57. Shelley, W.B. and Comaish, J.S.: New Test for Penicillin Allergy. Fluorometric Assay of Histamine Release, J.A.M.A. 192:122, 1965.
58. Palomeque, F.E., Fulton, J. and Derbes, V.J.: Penicillin Sensitivity, Arch. Dermat. 92:271, 1965.
59. Haimovich, J., Sela, M., Dewdney, J.D., et al: Anti-penicilloyl Antibodies: Detection with Penicilloylated Bacteriophage and Isolation with A Specific Immunoadsorbent, Nature. 214:1369, 1967.
60. Perelmutter, L. and Eisen, A.H.: Studies on Histamine Release from Leukocytes of Penicillin-Sensitive Individuals. Int. Arch. Allergy. 38:104, 1970.

61. Korotzer, J., and Haddad, Z.H.: In vitro detection of human IgE-mediated Immediate hypersensitivity reactions to pollens and penicillin(s) by a modified rat mast cell degranulation technique, J. Allergy. 45:126, 1970 (Abst 58).
62. Lo, C. and Yokoyama, M.M.: The Rat Mast Cell Degranulation Test in Allergy: Review on Principles and Clinical Application, Hawaii Med. J. 133:96, 1974.
63. Kunz, M.L., Reisman, R.E. and Arbesman, C.E.: Evaluation of penicillin hypersensitivity by two newer immunological procedures. J. Allergy. 40:135, 1967.
64. Assem, E.S.K. and Schild, H.O.: Detection of Allergy to Penicillin and Other Antigens by In-Vitro Passive Sensitization and Histamine Release from Human and Monkey Lung, Brit. Med. J. 3:272, 1968.
65. de Haan, P., Boorsma, D.M. and Kalsbeek, G.L.: Penicillin Hypersensitivity, Allergy. 34:111, 1979.
66. Wide, L., Bennich, H. and Johansson, S.G.O.: Diagnosis of Allergy by an In-vitro Test for Allergen Antibodies, Lancet. II:1105, 1967.
67. Adkinson, N.F., Jr.: The radioallergosorbent test: Uses and Abuses, J. Allergy Clin. Immunol. 65:1, 1980.
68. Wide, L., and Juhlin, L.: Detection of penicillin allergy of the immediate type by radioimmunoassay of reagins (IgE) to penicilloyl conjugates, Clin. Allerg. 1:171, 1971.
69. Kraft, D. and Wide, L.: Clinical patterns and results of radioallergosorbent test (RAST) and skin tests in penicillin allergy, Br. J. Derm. 94:593, 1976.
70. Kraft, D., Roth, A., Mischer, P., et al: Specific and total serum IgE measurements in the diagnosis of penicillin allergy. A long term follow-up study, Clin. Allerg. 7:21, 1977.
71. Valentine, M., Chairman: Allergic Emergencies, in *NIAID Task Force Report: Asthma and Other Allergic Emergencies.* Dept. Health, Education, & Welfare. Public Health Service NIH Publication 79,387, May 1979, p. 538.
72. Wide, L.: Clinical significance of measurement of reaginic (IgE) antibody by RAST, Clin. Allerg. 3(Suppl):583, 1973.
73. Levine, B.B., Redmond, A.P., Voss, H.E., et al: Prediction of Penicillin Allergy by Immunological Tests, Ann. N.Y. Acad. 145:298, 1967.
74. Levine, B.B. and Redmond, A.P.: Minor Haptenic Determinant-Specific Reagins of Penicillin Hypersensitivity in Man, Int. Arch. Allergy. 35:445, 1969.
75. Fellner, M.J., Levine, B.B., and Baer, R.L.: Immediate Reactions to Penicillin. Association with Penicilloyl-Specific Skin-Sensitizing Antibodies and Low Titers of Blocking (IgG) Antibodies, J.A.M.A. 202:143, 1967.
76. Parker, C.W.: Screening for penicillin allergy (Letter), N. Engl. J. Med. 293:938, 1975.

77. Rosenblum, A.H.: Penicillin allergy. A report of thirteen cases of severe reactions, J. Allergy. 42:309, 1968.
78. Rytel, M.W., Klion, F.M., Arlander, T.R., et al: Detection of Penicillin Hypersensitivity with Penicilloyl-Polylysine, J.A.M.A. 186:108, 1963.
79. Brown, B.C., Price, E.V., and Moore, M.B., Jr.: Penicilloyl-Polylysine as an Intradermal Test of Penicillin Sensitivity, J.A.M.A. 189:599, 1964.
80. Budd, M.A., Parker, C.W. and Norden, C.W.: Evaluation of Intradermal Skin Tests in Penicillin Hypersensitivity, J.A.M.A. 190:115, 1964.
81. Finke, S.R., Grieco, M.H., Connell, J.T., et al: Results of Comparative Skin Test with Penicilloyl-Polylysine and Penicillin in Patients with Penicillin Allergy, Am. J. Med. 38:71, 1965.
82. Adkinson, N.F., Jr., Thompson, W.L., Maddrey, W.C., et al: Routine Use of Penicillin Skin Testing on an Inpatient Service, N. Engl. J. Med. 285:22, 1971.
83. Green, G.R., Rosenblum, A.H., and Sweet, L.C.: Evaluation of penicillin hypersensitivity: Value of clinical history and skin testing with penicilloyl-polylysine and penicillin G. A cooperative prospective study of the penicillin study group of the American Academy of Allergy, J. Allerg. Clin. Immunol. 60:339, 1977.
84. Warrington, R.J., Simons, F.E.R., Ho, H.W., et al: Diagnosis of penicillin allergy by skin testing: the Manitoba experience, Can. Med. A.J. 118:787, 1978.
85. Bierman, C.W., VanArsdel, P.P., Jr. and Hemphill, B.: Penicillin allergy in children: The role of immunological tests in its diagnosis, J. Allergy. 43:267, 1969.
86. DeSwarte, R.D. and Smith, B.C.: Allergic Reactions to Drugs, in Lockey, R.F. (ed.): *Allergy & Clinical Immunology* (Garden City, N.Y.: Medical Examination Publishing Company, Inc., 1979).
87. Green, G.R.: Antibiotic Therapy in Patients with a History of Penicillin Allergy, in Stewart, G.T. and McGovern, J.P. (eds.): *Penicillin Allergy. Clinical and Immunological Aspects* (Springfield: Charles C. Thomas, 1970).
88. Adkinson, N.F., Jr.: A Guide to Skin Testing for Penicillin Allergy, Resident and Staff Physician. (August):55, 1977.
89. Chisholm, D.R., English, A.R. and MacLean, N.A.: Immunologic Response of Rabbits to 6-Aminopenicillanic Acid, J. Allergy. 32:333, 1961.
90. Wagelie, R.G., Dukes, C.D. and McGovern, J.P.: Antigenicity and Cross-Reactivity of 6-aminopenicillanic Acid and Penicillin G., J. Allergy. 34:489, 1963.
91. Stewart, G.T.: Cross-Allergenicity of Penicillin G and Related Substances, Lancet. I:509, 1962.

92. Van Dellen, R.G., Walsh, W.E., Peters G.A., et al: Differing patterns of wheal and flare skin reactivity in patients allergic to the penicillins, J. Allergy. 47:230, 1971.
93. Luton, E.F.: Methicillin Tolerance After Penicillin G Anaphylaxis, J.A.M.A. 190:39, 1964.
94. Penicillin Allergy, Med. Lett. Drugs and Therapeutics 20:14, 1978.
95. Editorial: Cross-Allergenicity of Penicillins and Cephalosporins, J.A.M.A. 199:495, 1967.
96. Thompson, R.L.: The Cephalosporins, Mayo Clin. Proc. 52:625, 1977.
97. Moellering, R.C., Jr. and Swartz, M.N.: Drug Therapy. The Newer Cephalosporins, N. Engl. J. Med. 294:24, 1976.
98. Penicillin Allergy, Drug and Therapeutics Bull. 13:9, 1975.
99. Batchelor, F.R., Dewdney, J.M. and Gazzard, D.: Penicillin Allergy: The Formation of the Penicilloyl Determinant, Nature. 206:362, 1965.
100. Brandriss, M.W., Smith, J.W. and Steinman, H.G.: Common Antigenic Determinants of Penicillin G , Cephalothin and 6-Aminopenicillanic Acid in Rabbits, J. Immunol. 94:696, 1965.
101. Batchelor, F.R., Dewdney, J.M., Weston, R.D. et al: The Immunogenicity of Cephalosporin Derivatives and their Cross-Reaction with Penicillin, Immunology. 10:21, 1966.
102. Abraham, G.N., Petz, L.D. and Fudenberg, H.H.: Immunohaematological Cross-allergenicity Between Penicillin and Cephalothin in Humans, Clin. Exp. Immunol. 3:343, 1968.
103. Grieco, M.H.: Cross-Allergenicity of the Penicillins and the Cephalosporins, Arch. Intern. Med. 119:141, 1967.
104. Delafuente, J.C., Panush, R.S. and Caldwell, J.R.: Penicillin and Cephalosporin Immunogenicity in Man, Ann. Allergy. 43:337, 1979.
105. Petz, L.D.: Immunologic Cross-Reactivity between Penicillins and Cephalosporins: A Review, J. Infec. Dis. 137(Suppl):S74, 1978.
106. Thoburn, R., Johnson, J.E. III and Cluff, L.E.: Studies on the Epidemiology of Adverse Drug Reactions, J.A.M.A. 198:111, 1966.
107. Petz, L.D.: Immunologic reactions of humans to cephalosporins, Postgr. Med. J. Feb. Suppl.:64, 1971.
108. Assem, E.S.K. and Vickers, M.R.: Tests for Penicillin Allergy in Man II. The Immunological Cross-Reaction Between Penicillins and Cephalosporins, Immunology. 27:255, 1974.
109. Girard, J.-P.: Common Antigenic Determinants of Penicillin G, Ampicillin and the Cephalosporins Demonstrated in Man, Int. Arch. Allergy. 33:428, 1968.
110. Perkins, R.L. and Saslaw, S.: Experiences with Cephalothin, Annals Int. Med. 64:13, 1966.
111. Kabins, S.A., Eisenstein, B. and Cohen, S.: Anaphylactoid Reaction to an Initial Dose of Sodium Cephalothin, J.A.M.A. 193:159, 1965.
112. Rothschild, P.D. and Doty, D.B.: Cephalothin Reaction After Penicillin Sensitization, J.A.M.A. 196:160, 1966.

113. Scholand, J.F., Tennenbaum, J.I., and Cerilli, G.J.: Anaphylaxis to Cepahlothin in a Patient Allergic to Penicillin, J.A.M.A. 206:130, 1968.
114. Batchelor, R.C.L., Horne, G.O. and Rogerson, H.L.: An Unusual Reaction to Procaine Penicillin in Aqueous Suspension, Lancet. 2:195, 1951.
115. Galpin, J.E., Chow, A.W., Yoshikawa, T.T. et al: "Pseudoanaphylactic" Reactions from Inadvertent Infusion of Procaine Penicillin G, Ann. Intern. Med. 81:358, 1974.
116. Coleman, W.P. and Swineford, O., Jr.: Penicillin Hypersensitivity A Brief Review and Report of an Extreme Case, Virginia Medical Monthly. 83:6, 1956.
117. Rosenblum, A.H.: Clinical Experience in Testing Patients with Penicillin Hypersensitivity, in Stewart, G.T. and McGovern, J.P. (eds.): *Penicillin Allergy. Clinical and Immunologic Aspects* (Springfield: Charles C. Thomas, 1970).
118. Dogliotti, M.: An Instance of Fatal Reaction to the Penicillin Scratch-Test, Dermatolog. 136:489, 1968.
119. ____: Tests for Penicillin Allergy, Med. Lett. Dr. 17:54, 1975.
120. Boger, W.P., Sherman, W.B., Schiller, I.W., et al: Allergic Reactions to Penicillin. A Panel Discussion, J. Allergy 24:383, 1953.
121. Ettinger, E., and Kaye, D.: Systemic Manifestations After a Skin Test With Penicilloyl-Polylysine, N. Engl. J. Med. 271:1105, 1964.
122. Resnik, S.S. and Shelley, W.B.: Penicilloyl-Polylysine Skin Test: Anaphylaxis in Absence of Penicillin Sensitivity, J.A.M.A. 196:152, 1966.
123. Levine, B.B., Redmond, A.P., and Voss, H.E.: Penicilloyl-Polylysine Skin Tests and Allergies (Letter), J.A.M.A. 197:131, 1966.
124. Bierman, C.W.: Skin testing for Penicillin Allergy (Letter), Pediatrics. 52:302, 1973.
125. VanArsdel, P.P., Jr.: Adverse Drug Reactions, in Middleton E., Jr., Reed, C.E., and Ellis, E.F. (eds.): *Allergy: Principles & Practice* (St. Louis: The C.V. Mosby Company, 1978).
126. Mozingo, R., and Folkers, K.: The Penilloic and penicilloic acids and their derivatives and analogs, in Clarke, H.T., Johnson, J.R. and Johnson, Sir R. (eds.): *The Chemistry of Penicillin* (Princeton University, 1949).
127. DeSwarte, R.D.: Drug Allergy, in Patterson, R. (ed.): *Allergic Diseases Diagnosis and Management* (Philadelphia: J.B. Lippincott Company, 1972).
128. Gorevic, P.D. and Levine, B.B.: Desensitization for anaphylactic hypersensitivity to penicilloate derivative of carbenicillin, J. Allergy Clin. Immunol 61:147, 1978 (Abst 62).
129. Solley, G.O., Van Dellen, R.G. and Gleich, G.J.: Evaluation of skin tests in patients with penicillin allergy, J. Allergy Clin. Immunol. 63:184, 1979 (Abst 170).

130. Peck, S.M., Siegal, S. and Bergamini, R.: Successful Desensitization in Penicillin Sensitivity, J.A.M.A. 134:1546, 1947.
131. Peck, S.M., Siegal, S., Glick, A.W. et al: Clinical Problems in Penicillin Sensitivity, J.A.M.A. 138:631, 1948.
132. O'Driscoll, B.J.: Desensitization of Nurses Allergic to Penicillin. Br. Med. J. 20:473, 1955.
133. O'Donovan, W.J., and Klorfajn, I.: Sensitivity to Penicillin Anaphylaxis and Desensitization, Lancet. 2:444, 1946.
134. Sullivan, T.J., Wedner, H.J., and Parker, C.W.: Desensitization of patients allergic to penicillin using oral penicillin, J. Allergy Clin. Immunol. 65:195, 1980 (Abst 105).
135. Green, G.R., Peters, G.A. and Geraci, J.E.: Treatment of Bacterial Endocarditis in Patients with Penicillin Hypersensitivity, Ann. Intern. Med. 67:235, 1967.
136. Reisman, R.E., Rose, N.R., Witebsky, E., et al: Penicillin Allergy and Desensitization, J. Allergy. 33:178, 1962.
137. Gilmore, N.J., Yang, W.H. and Del Carpio, J.: Penicillin allergy: A simple, rapid intravenous method of "desensitization," J. Allergy Clin. Immunol. 63:185, 1979 (Abst 171).
138. Batson, J.M.: Anaphylactoid Reactions to Oral Administration of Penicillin, N. Engl. J. Med. 262:590, 1960.
139. Krapin, D.: Anaphylaxis with Orally Administered Penicillin, N. Engl. J. Med. 267:820, 1962.
140. Geyman, J.P.: Anaphylactic Reaction to Oral Penicillin, California Medicine. 114:87, 1971.
141. Levine, M.I., Perri, J. and Anthony, J.J.: A Fatal Anaphylactic Reaction to Oral Penicillin, J. Allergy. 31:487, 1960.
142. Spark, R.P.: Fatal Anaphylaxis Due to Oral Penicillin, Amer. J. Clin. Path. 56:407, 1971.
143. Valentine, M.D. and Sheffer, A.L.: The Anaphylactic Syndromes. Med. Clin. N.A. 53:249, 1969.
144. Austen, K.F. and Sheffer, A.L.: Vascular Responses, in Fitzpatrick, T.B. et al (eds.): *Dermatology in General Medicine* (New York: McGraw-Hill, 1971).
145. Lockey, R.F. and Bukantz, S.E.: Allergic Emergencies, Med. Clin. N. A. 58:147, 1974.
146. Levine, B.B.: Immunochemical Mechanisms of Drug Allergy, in Miescher, P. A. and Müller-Eberhard, H.J. (eds.): *Textbook of Immunopathology* (New York: Grune & Stratton, 1976).
147. Parker, C.W., Wessler, S., and Avioli, L.V.: Enterococcal Endocarditis, J.A.M.A. 204:164, 1968.
148. Grieco, M.H., Dubin, M.R., Robinson, J.L. et al: Penicillin Hypersensitivity in Patients with Bacterial Endocarditis, Ann. Intern. Med. 60:204, 1964.
149. Fellner, M.J., Van Hecke, E., Rozan, M. et al: Mechanisms of clinical desensitization in urticarial hypersensitivity to penicillin, J. Allergy. 45:55, 1970.

L. Barth Reller, M.D.

15

LABORATORY PROCEDURES IN THE MANAGEMENT OF INFECTIVE ENDOCARDITIS

The clinical microbiology laboratory is crucial in the care of patients with infective endocarditis. The presenting features of infective endocarditis (Table 1) are notoriously nonspecific.[1–9] Even classic findings, such as subungual splinter hemorrhages, have no clinical meaning in the face of negative blood cultures.[10] With rare exceptions, the diagnosis of infective endocarditis depends on the finding of persistently positive blood cultures. Results of blood cultures can not be overemphasized, not only for diagnosis but also for proper subsequent management of the patient. The selection of initial antimicrobial therapy, *in-vitro* susceptibility testing, and monitoring the adequacy of medical treatment all require the isolation of the causative microorgansim. The decision to use single-

Table 1. Common Presenting Features of Infective Endocarditis

Symptoms	Signs	Laboratory Abnormalities
Anorexia	Fever	Anemia
Malaise	Heart murmur	Elevated erythrocyte sedimentation rate
Sweats and chills	Petechiae	Microscopical hematuria
Weight loss	Splenomegaly	Proteinuria
Arthralgias	Neurological findings	Positive rheumatoid factor
Myalgias	Emboli	Immune complexes

antibiotic therapy for penicillin-sensitive streptococci or combination antibiotic therapy for enterococci requires having the patient's isolate.[11–14] Even the duration of therapy for endocarditis due to viridans streptococci may depend on *in-vitro* susceptibility testing.[15] Moreover, a number of the indications for surgical treatment of infective endocarditis (e.g., fungal infections, refractory bacterial infections) hinge on the microbiological findings.[16–20]

Microbiological Diagnosis of Infective Endocarditis

Pattern of Bacteremia in Endocarditis

A cardinal feature of intravascular infection is continuous bacteremia.[21,22] In addition to acute and chronic bacterial endocarditis, other causes of continuous bacteremia include suppurative thrombophlebitis and infected aneurysms, arteriovenous fistulas, and intravenous or intraarterial devices. Clues to these causes of continuous bacteremia usually are obvious. Only two other important bacterial diseases, brucellosis and typhoid fever, result in bacteremia that lasts for weeks if untreated.[23,24] *Brucella abortus, suis,* and *melitensis* as well as *Salmonella typhi* are facultatively intracellular bacteria that may be isolated more readily from cultures of bone marrow rather than of blood, especially in patients who have received antibiotics.[23–26] *Brucella* spp. and *S. typhi,* however, are rare causes of bacterial endocarditis.[27,28] Therefore, most patients with fever, a heart murmur, and persistently positive blood cultures without an obvious source do have infective endocarditis.

Collection, Number, and Timing of Blood Cultures

Since the normal bacterial flora of the skin may cause bacterial endocarditis, especially on prosthetic heart valves, the risk of contamination of blood cultures during collection must be reduced to a minimum, ideally less than 3%.[29] After palpation the venipuncture site should be cleansed with 70% alcohol followed by 1–2% tincture of iodine or povidone-iodine. For maximum effectiveness, the disinfectant should be allowed to dry (1–2 minutes) before blood is aspirated. If further palpation of the vein is necessary during aspiration, the finger must be disinfected or a sterile glove should be worn. Blood for culture must never be drawn through an indwelling intravenous or intraarterial catheter.[30–32] For the diagnosis of bacterial endocarditis, arterial blood provides no higher yield than venous blood does.[33] Each sample of blood (minimum of 10 ml from adults and 1–5 ml from children) should be obtained by a separate venipuncture; multiple bottles filled from a single venipuncture should be interpreted as a single blood culture.[1,34]

Although the bacteremia of infective endocarditis is of low magnitude, the number of blood cultures required to establish the diagnosis is small.[22,33–36] In a series of 206 cases of bacterial endocarditis with positive blood cultures reported by Werner, et al.,[36] 95% of 789 blood cultures were positive for the causative microorgansims. The first blood culture obtained was positive in 94% of the cases, and only 4 patients (2%) required 3 or more blood cultures to confirm their bacterial endocarditis. Furthermore, yield of positive blood cultures in patients with streptococcal endocarditis was only reduced from 97% to 91% by taking antimicrobials in the two weeks before blood cultures.

Based on the aforementioned studies, the following number and timing of blood cultures for suspected infective endocarditis are recommended:

1. *Acute.* Obtain 3 blood cultures at 3 separate venipunctures during the first 1 to 2 hours of evaluation and begin therapy.
2. *Subacute.* Obtain 3 blood cultures on first day (ideally 15 or more minutes apart); if all are negative 24 hours later, obtain 2 more. From undiagnosed patients who have received antimicrobials in the week or two before admission, obtain 2 blood cultures on each of 3 successive days. Although prior antimicrobial therapy may cause blood cultures to be negative, it more often causes delayed growth. Therefore, blood cultures from partially treated patients should be incubated at least 14 days.

With optimal culture techniques, positive blood cultures should be obtained in over 95% of cases of infective endocarditis.

Interpretation of Positive Blood Cultures

Even with the most exacting techniques of collection and processing, contamination of blood cultures occurs occasionally.[29] Several criteria have been used for recognizing likely false-positive cultures.[34,37] Pour plates are positive in about 70% of cases of true bacteremia as opposed to about 5% of contaminated blood cultures.[37] The utility of pour plates in distinguishing between true- and false-positive blood cultures is based on the assumption that there are many bacteria per ml of blood with true bacteremia, whereas only a few (less than 1 per ml) microorganisms are picked up during contamination. This may not always be the case. With culture-proved infective endocarditis, for example, pour plates often are negative or show fewer than 10 bacteria per ml of blood.[33,36] Bacterial growth in blood cultures first detected beyond 72 hours of incubation is more commonly associated with contamination than with true bacteremia; however, prior antimicrobials may also delay recognition of positive cultures.[36] Recovery of *Propioni-bacterium acnes, Corynebacterium* spp., *Bacillus* spp., and *Staphylococcus epidermidis* nearly always means contamination, unless these bacteria are present in multiple positive blood cultures obtained by independent venipunctures.[34,37] Infective endocarditis in patients with prosthetic heart valves is caused occasionally by *Corynebacterium* spp. and commonly by *S. epidermidis.*[38–42] Endocarditis caused by *Bacillus* spp. has been reported most often in intravenous drug abusers.[43–45] Whereas the recovery from blood of group A streptococci, pneumococci, *Haemophilus influenzae, Enterobacteriaceae, Bacteroidaceae, Pseudomonas aeruginosa,* and *Candida* spp. is almost always important, the recovery of viridans streptococci or *Staphylococcus aureus* may not be.[34,37,46]

The most reliable way, therefore, to make the distinction between culture-positive infective endocarditis and a contaminated culture is to rely on the results of mulitple blood cultures obtained properly by separate venipunctures (Figure 1). A single blood culture positive for *S. epidermidis* or viridans streptococci is uninterpretable; if followed by two to five negative blood cultures, the initial isolate may be judged confidently a contaminant. Three to six consecutive blood cultures that

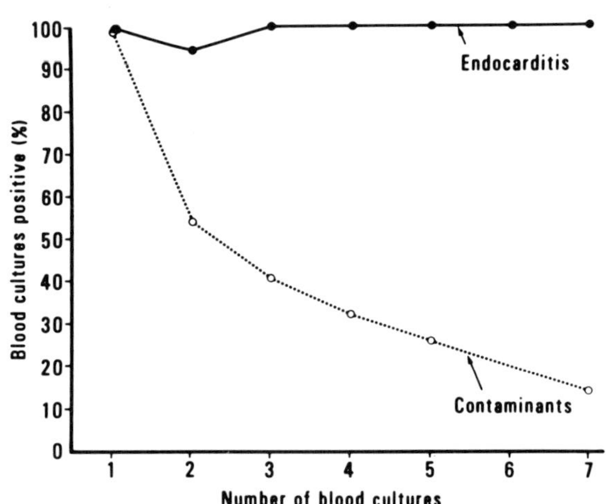

Figure 1: Diagnostic importance of separate serial blood cultures obtained by independent venipuncture for distinguishing between contaminants and the continuous bacteremia of infective endocarditis.

grow *S. epidermidis* from a patient with a prosthetic valve and fever must be interpreted as infective endocaritis. Figure 1 shows the actual results of sequential blood cultures in patients with bacterial endocarditis and contaminated cultures at the University of Colorado Medical Center in 1975–77 (Weinstein, M.P., Reller, L.B., Murphy, J.R., and Lichtenstein, K.A.: unpublished data).

Microbiology of Infective Endocarditis

Many large reviews of the clinical and microbiological findings in infective endocarditis in the antibiotic era have been published.[2–5,36,40–42,47–49] Table 2 summarizes the distribution of microorganisms currently recovered from patients with infective endocarditis on natural and prosthetic heart valves. The microbiology of infective endocarditis within 2 months after valve replacement is characterized by an increased incidence of staphylococci, aerobic gram-negative bacilli, and fungi. After two months, the causes of infective endocarditis on prosthetic heart valves resemble more closely those of

Table 2. Microbiology of Infective Endocarditis on Natural and Prosthetic Valves

Microorganisms	Natural valves (%)	Prosthetic Valves (%) Early (<2 months)	Late (>2 months)
Viridans streptococci	40–65	5	30
Enterococci	5–15	4	6
Staphylococcus aureus	15–20	20	10
Staphylococcus epidermidis	1	30	25
Aerobic gram-negative bacilli	1	15	10
Anaerobic bacteria	1	1	1
Other bacteria	10	8	5
Mixed microorganisms	1	5	5
Fungi	2	9	6

infection on natural valves; however, the risk for staphylococci and gram-negative bacilli remains disproportionately high.[40–42] Moreover, prosthetic valve endocarditis now accounts for about 20% of cases of infective endocarditis in some centers.[47]

A recent review of recurrent infective endocarditis after an interval of 6 months or with a different microorganism showed that this complication is common, especially among chronic drug abusers.[50] The causative organisms were similar with initial and recurrent infections.

Lastly, polymicrobial infective endocarditis is being recognized more often.[51,52] Two groups of patients appear to be at risk. The heart valves of intravenous drug abusers are most often infected with *P. aeruginosa, S. aureus,* enterococci, and fungi. Persons with prosthetic heart valves may also have mixed infections. (Table 2). Although mixed infections are not common, it is essential that bactericidal antimicrobial therapy be provided for all microorganisms isolated.

Culture-negative Endocarditis

A few cases of endocarditis remain culture-negative despite the most strenuous attempts to isolate microorgansims. Table 3 lists the major categories and possible causes of culture-negative endocarditis. The proportion of patients with infective endocarditis whose blood cultures

Table 3. Possible Causes of Culture-negative Endocarditis

Bacterial:	Anaerobes and slow-growing or fastidious bacteria
Mycobacterial:	Tuberculosis
Rickettsial:	Q fever
Chlamydial:	Psittacosis
Fungal:	Candidiasis, histoplasmosis, aspergillosis, and cryptococcosis
Marantic:	Nonbacterial thrombotic endocarditis
Immunological:	Circulating high titer of bactericidal antibodies
Iatrogenic:	Prior antimicrobial therapy
Avoidable:	Inadequate culture techniques

remain negative, however, has been reported to range from 3–41%.[3,53–57] Wherein does the truth lie? The two largest and best studied series in the 1970s, emcompassing 467 episodes of infective endocarditis at the Mayo Clinic and the New York Hosptial, report only 15 (3%) cases with persistently negative blood cultures.[47,49] This is an important issue. Owing to the protean, often vague manifestations of infective endocarditis (Table 1), especially subacute disease with viridans streptococci, it is all too easy to invoke the diagnosis of culture-negative endocarditis in the enigmatic patient with fever of unknown origin. But this is a disservice to the patient and may lead to a delay in the real diagnosis or to an expensive 4–6 week course of antimicrobial therapy in the hospital or to both. Rather the possible causes of culture-negative endocarditis (Table 3) should be sought systematically and alternative diagnoses considered before embarking on a rarely required therapeutic trial.

Bacteria that may be difficult to isolate within the 7 days that many clinical microbiology laboratories retain blood cultures include anaerobes, slow-growing or fastidious gram-negative bacteria, and nutritonal variants of streptococci.[34,49,53,58] Anaerobic bacteria are incriminated infrequently (1% or less) in cases of infective endocarditis.[2–4,59] Their isolation requires incubation in an anaerobic atmosphere or in broth media with a low redox potential (e.g. supplemented peptone broth). Fastidious gram-negative bacteria that cause endocarditis and may be more difficult to isolate include *Brucella* spp., *Cardiobacterium hominis, Actinobacillus actinomycetemcomitans, Haemophilus aphrophilus,* and *Haemophilus parainfluenzae*.[27,58,60–62] Recovery of these bacteria is improved by incubation for at least 2 weeks under 5–10% CO_2 in media containing nicotinamide adenine dinucleotide (NAD) and sufficient blood relative to the volume of broth to provide hemin (X factor).[58] Prolonged incubation (2 weeks or more) also may be required for isolation of *Corynebacterium* spp. from cases of prosthetic valve endocarditis.[38] Finally, a heterogenous group of viridans streptococci that require vitamin B_6 (pyridoxal) for growth now accounts for up to 6% of cases of microbial endocarditis in some centers.[49]

Routine blood culture media fail to grow *Mycobacterium tuberculosis,* rickettsiae, and chlamydiae. Endocarditis is an exceedingly rare complication of miliary tuberculosis.[63] Q fever endocarditis, caused by *Coxiella burnetti,* and chlamydial endocarditis, caused by *Chlamydia psittaci* or *trachomatis,* are best diagnosed by serological tests.[64–71] Q fever endocarditis occurs around the world and accounted for 3 of 7 cases of culture-negative endocarditis in a recent series of 52 patients with proved subacute infective endocarditis reported from England.[48,64–67] Clamydiae are an exceedingly rare, but well-documented, cause of culture-negative endocarditis.[68–71]

Fungal endocarditis can be caused by species of *Candida, Aspergillus, Histoplasma,* and, rarely, *Crytococcus* and other fungi.[72–77] *Candida* spp. account for most cases and are the most common fungi isolated from blood cultures.[3,72] *Aspergillus* endocarditis is only rarely (<5%) diagnosed by positive blood cultures; most cases are recognized first at necropsy.[73] *Aspergillus* spp. may also be recovered from removed heart valves, vegetations, or excised arterial emboli.[72,73] *Histoplasma capsulataum* has caused endocarditis on both natural and prosthetic heart valves.[74–77] As with *Aspergillus* spp., *H. capsulatum* rarely is recovered from blood. Biopsy and culture of bone marrow are the best diagnostic procedures for disseminated histoplasmosis, the setting in which endocarditis usually occurs.[74–77] Since embolic occulsion of major arteries is common in the course of fungal endocarditis, prompt histological examination and culture of any accessible emoblus is crucial.[2,73,77]

Nonbacterial thrombotic endocarditis (NBTE) is associated with wasting diseases, usually malignant neoplasms.[78,79] The malignancies most often complicated by NBTE are carcinomas of the lung, breast, and pancreas.[79] These diseases should be considered in older patients with vegetative endocarditis, arterial emboli, and negative blood cultures.[79]

Perhaps the most common cause of culture-negative endocarditis is iatrogenic, owing to prior antimicrobial therapy for unexplained fever.[2–4,53–55,57] The incidence of culture-negative endocarditis reported in large series in the pre- (10–26%) and post- (5–30%) antibiotic eras is not appreciably different.[3] These upper figures, however, are too high to be acceptable in the 1980s.[47,49] Some reports do not show any marked effect of prior antibiotics on positive cultures.[48,80] It is clear that blood cultures may continue to grow *Staphylococcus aureus* for days to even weeks after therapy for staphylococcal endocarditis.[81] Isolation rates of 97% and 91% were reported for non-treated and treated groups in a large series of endocarditis due to penicillin-sensitive streptococci.[36] Stopping therapy for 24–72 hours may allow return of positive blood culture in patients in whom prior antibiotics may be obscuring a questionable diagnosis of infective endocarditis.[4] Lastly, blood cultures from such patients must be retained for at least 2 weeks.

Before the advent of antimicrobials, Keefer postulated that high titers of circulating bactericidal antibody sterilized the blood of some patients with long-standing subacute bacterial endocarditis caused by viridans streptococci isolated at necropsy from vegetations on heart valves.[56] Prior antibiotic therapy would seem a more frequent cause today for culture-negative endocarditis.[4,57]

The final reason is inadequate culture techniques; this pitfall is avoidable.[53] When done properly, blood cultures should enable a microbiological diagnosis in 95% or more of patients with infective endocarditis.[47,49] In the patient with fever of unknown origin and suspected culture-negative endocarditis, bone marrow cultures may aid detection of brucellosis, typhoid fever, miliary tuberculosis, and histoplasmosis and other disseminated fungal infections. Moreover, infective endocarditis itself rarely may be diagnosed by cultures of bone marrow.[33]

Immunological and Hematological Tests in Infective Endocarditis

Patients with infective endocarditis, especially subacute bacterial endocarditis, often show evidence of immunological chaos that clears after treatment. Serum rheumatoid factor is positive in 25–50% of patients, antinuclear antibodies may be present, and circulating immune complexes and cryoglobulins have been detected in 90% or more of cases in some series.[6,82–85] Serum complement is reduced less frequently[6,86] These immunological aberrations are thought to account for many of the diverse musculoskeletal, renal, and neurological manifestations of infective endocarditis.[6–9,86,87] Consequently, some authors have suggested that tests for circulating immune complexes may be useful in culture-negative, but suspected, infective endocarditis.[82,85] Immunological tests for infective endocarditis, however, lack specificity and fail to provide the microorganism on which rational antimicrobial therapy can be based and followed. Immunological studies are presently of most value in enlarging our understanding of the complex pathophysiology of infective endocarditis.[88,89] As emphasized earlier, blood cultures remain the most sensitive, and certainly the most specific, diagnostic procedure for infective endocarditis.[36,47,49]

Serological tests have been advocated for the differentiation of endocarditis from sepsis caused by *Staphylococcus aureus.*[90,91] The methods depend on detection and quantitation of antibodies directed against teichoic acid antigens in the staphylococcal cell wall. The practical usefulness of tests for detection of antibodies to teichoic acids is not proved. Antibody can not be detected reliably before one to two weeks of illness. Patients with acute staphylococcal endocarditis should be recognized and treated promptly and the diagnosis confirmed retrospectively by multiple positive blood cultures obtained before intense antimicrobial therapy. Even when antibiotics have been given inappropriately before cultures, the blood should eventually grow *S. aureus* in almost all cases.[36,81] Isolation of *S. aureus* enables needed antimicrobial susceptibility testing; serological tests do not.

Nearly all patients with infective endocarditis have anemia and an elevated erythrocyte sedimentation rate.[2–6] Polymorphonuclear leukocytes or histiocytes with ingested bacteria occasionally may be found in the peripheral blood of patients with infective endocarditis.[92,93] The reliability of the procedure, however, has been questioned.[94] Examination of buffy-coat smears for streptococci, the most common cause of bacterial endocarditis, rarely is helpful.[95] Although constant, the bacteremia of endocarditis is of low magnitude.[33,36] The vegetations of bacterial endocarditis are avascular lesions composed of bacteria, fibrin, platelets, and red and white blood cells with more or less necrosis.[88,96] Circulating granulocytes are not actively involved in removal of bacteria from the blood of patients with bacterial endocarditis.[22,94] On balance, the effort and cost of looking for intraleukocytic bacteria in patients with suspected endocarditis are not justified.

Critical Factors in Diagnosis of Endocarditis by Blood Cultures

Volume of Blood Cultured

The majority of patients with infective endocarditis have fewer than 30 microorganisms per ml of peripheral venous blood and some have less than 1.[33,36] Figure 2 shows the relative increase in yield of positive blood cultures per ml of blood cultured in a series of over 1000 episodes of

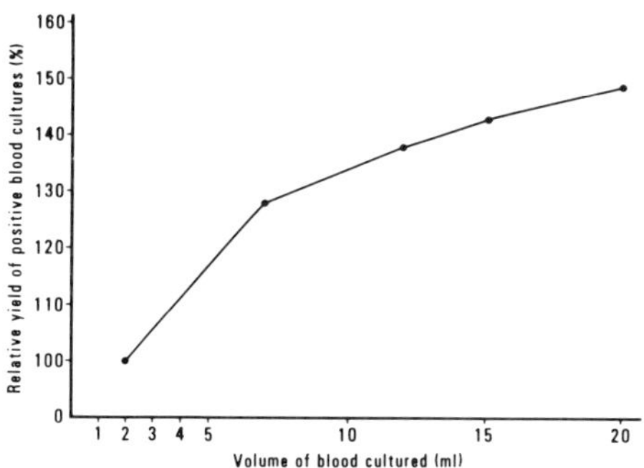

Figure 2: Relative yield of positive blood cultures with increasing volumes of blood cultured between 2 and 20 ml.

sepsis at the University of Colorado Medical Center during 1975–77 (Reller, L.B., Mirrett, S., and Wang, W–L.L.: unpublished data). At least 10 ml of blood should be drawn from adults by separate venipuncture (Figure 1) for each culture.[34] Some centers obtain 20–30 ml of blood for each culture set. Additional amounts of blood are unlikely to increase the yield. In infants and children, collection of 1–5 ml of blood for culture should suffice.[34]

Ratio of Blood to Broth in Blood Cultures

Blood taken from patients with bacterial endocarditis has bactericidal properties and must be diluted in broth.[34,56] In most instances the usual 1:10 or 1:20 dilution of blood in broth is sufficient to protect even a few microorganisms from the lethal activity of human serum. Such dilutions, however, require large volumes of broth if more than 5 ml of blood are cultured. Unless patients are receiving high doses of effective antimicrobials at the time blood cultures are obtained, a 1:5 ratio of blood to broth is as effective as a 1:10 ratio and makes culture of a larger volume of blood more practical. Overall the yield of positive blood cultures has been shown to be greater with 10 ml of blood cultured at a 1:5 ratio of blood to broth than with 5 ml of blood at a 1:10 ratio (Reller, L.B., Lichtenstein, K.A., Mirrett, S. and Wang, W–L.L: Abstr. Annu. Meet. Am. Soc. Microbiol., 1978, CI77, p. 306). At dilutions of 1:5 or greater, the volume of blood cultured appears to be relatively more important than the exact ratio of blood to broth.

Medium Used and Atmosphere and Temperature of Incubation

There have been few published studies in which the volumes of blood cultured have been equal and carefully controlled in the evaluation of different media for blood culture. For the microorganisms that commonly caused endocarditis (Table 2), most media prepared for blood cultures, e.g. brain heart infusion, Brucella, Columbia, supplemented peptone, thioglycollate (thiol), and trypticase (tryptic) soy broths, will perform adequately provided a sufficient volume of blood is cultured. Isolation rates of *Pseudomonas aeruginosa* are significantly less in thioglycollate broth.[34] In a study of 6 strains and 36 cultures from patients with endocarditis, Roberts et al. showed that vitamin B_6 (pyridoxal)-dependent stains of viridans streptococci grow better in brain heart infusion (100%) than in thioglycollate (78%) or trypticase soy (8%) broth.[49] Our own work with 22 strains of nutritionally variant streptococci showed that all grew in supplemented peptone broth and none grew in trypticase soy broth without 1% yeast extract (Reimer, L.G., and Reller, L.B.: J. Clin Microbiol, in press).

Commercially available broth media for blood cultures usually are bottled under vacuum and with 5–10% CO_2. Venting the bottles increases the growth of *Pseudomonas aeruginosa* and yeasts.[34,98,99] The added carbon dioxide as well as routine subcultures to chocolate blood agar are necessary for the maximal yield of fastidious bacteria such as *Actinobacillus actinomycetemcomitans, Brucella* spp., *Cardiobacterium hominis, Eikenella corrodens, Haemophilus aphrophilus, H. paraaphrophilus,* and *H. parainfluenzae.*[34,58,60–62] Although not essential for media with quite low redox potentials, e.g., supplemented peptone broth, an unvented bottle is needed for the best yield of the *Bacteroidaceae,* when Columbia or tryptic soy broth is used.[59,98,99]

The recovery of bacteria from blood is highest when the cultures are incubated at 35° C. Pre-warming of bottles for blood cultures is not necessary.[100] If regular blood cultures are negative and fungal endocarditis is suspected, a biphasic (Castaneda-type) bottle with brain heart infusion agar overlaid with the same broth should be inoculated and incubated in the upright position for 30 days at 30° C.[101] As discussed earlier, biopsy and culture of bone marrow and also indicated in suspected disseminated fungal infections complicated by endocarditis.[74,75]

Anticoagulants for Blood Cultures

Anticoagulant is needed in routine blood cultures to prevent clotting. Sodium polyanetholsulfonate (SPS) is the best anticoagulant now available for blood cultures.[34] Broth media used for direct collection of blood should contain 0.025 to 0.05% SPS. Vacuum collecting tubes for blood to be transported to the laboratory for culture should contain 1 ml of 0.25 to 0.5% SPS per 10 ml of blood. In addition to its anticoagulant properties, SPS also interferes with the function of complement, inhibits phagocytosis, and decreases the activity of aminoglycosides and polymyxins.[34] Although SPS is inhibitory to *Peptostreptococcus anaerobius, Neisseria meningitidis,* and *N. gonorrhoeae,* this effect can be neutralized with 1.2% gelatin, which is present in supplemented peptone broth.[102–104] Moreover, these strains of bacteria only rarely cause endocarditis (Table 2). Sodium amylosulfate (SAS) does not inhibit *P. anaerobius, N. meningitidis,* and *N. gonorrhoeae.*[34] In a controlled clinical trial, however, SAS did slow the growth of some strains of *Staphylococcus aureus* (Reller, L.B. Cox, R.L., Mirrett, S. and Wang, W–L.L.: Abstr. Annu. Meet. Am. Soc. Microbiol., 1979, C12, p.312). Tables 4 and 5 show that SAS slows the growth of *S. aureus* in trypticase soy broth, although it does not decrease the yield of *S. aureus* from blood. There are no important differences between SPS and SAS for other bacteria that commonly cause endocarditis.

Table 4. Effect of Anticoagulant in Blood Culture Media on Speed of Detection of Bacteremia

Bacteria	Same day	SPS earlier	SAS earlier	P
Staphylococcus aureus	30	20	7	<0.02
Staphylococcus epidermidis	13	4	4	NS*
Viridans streptococci	8	3	0	NS
Enterococci	5	0	0	NS
Listeria monocytogenes	3	0	0	NS

*P = >0.1

Note: SPS = sodium polyanetholsulfonate and SAS = sodium amylosulfate

Table 5. Effect of Anticoagulant on Yield of Bacteria in Trypticase Soy Broth

Bacteria	Both SPS and SAS	SPS only	SAS only	P
Staphylococcus aureus	57*	12	13	NS
Staphylococcus epidermidis	21	2	1	NS
Viridans streptococci	11	3	6	NS
Enterococci	5	4	2	NS
Listeria monocytogenes	3	1	1	NS

* Number of bacterial strains isolated

**P = >0.1

Note: SPS = sodium polyanetholsulfonate and SAS = sodium amylosulfate

Role of Hypertonic Media and Beta-lactamases

Blood culture media made hypertonic by the addition of 10% or more sucrose have been advocated to enable isolation of cell-wall defective bacteria from the blood; however, the value of hypertonic media for routine use is doubtful.[34] The only well-controlled published studies failed to show any benefit from the addition of 15% sucrose or sorbitol to tryptic soy broth with SPS.[105,106] In fact, the presence of sucrose or sorbitol diminished the yield of clinically important bacteria. Similarly, addition of 15% sucrose to brain heart infusion broth decreased significantly the recovery of fungi from blood cultures.[107] Hypertonic media were not helpful in one series of culture-negative endocarditis.[108] In another study, stable cell-wall defective variants of *Staphylococcus aureus* failed to cause experimental endocarditis in rabbits; however, *S. aureus* was recovered more readily in hypertonic media, when the animals infected with vegetative *S. aureus* were treated with penicillin G.[109] Table 6 shows the effect of 10% sucrose in supplemented peptone broth on the recovery of bacteria known to cause endocarditis (Weinstein, M.P., Reller, L.B., Mirrett, S., and Wang, W–L.L.: Abstr. Annu. Meet. Am. Soc. Microbiol., 1978, C176, p. 306). Sucrose improved the recovery of *S. epidermidis,* but this was the result of multiple separate blood cultures from a single patient with *S. epidermidis* endocarditis on a bicuspid aortic valve who had relapsed owing to inadequate treatment with oxacillin (Reller, L.B. and Weinstein, M.P.: unpublished data).

Sucrose in supplemented peptone broth decreased significantly the yield of *Neisseria gonorrhoeae* from blood cultures (Table 6). Although

Table 6. Effect of 10% Sucrose on Yield of Bacteria

Bacteria	Both bottles	SPB only	SPB/SUC only	P
Staphylococcus aureus	71*	7	15	NS**
Staphylococcus epidermidis	29	2	22	<0.01
Viridans streptococci	11	1	5	NS
Enterococci	11	2	2	NS
Listeria monocytogenes	9	0	0	NS
Neisseria gonorrhoeae	1	8	0	<0.02

* Number of bacterial strains isolated

**P = >0.1

Note: SPB = supplemented peptone broth and
SUC = 10% added sucrose

less commonly than formerly, *N. gonorrhoeae* still does cause acute bacterial endocarditis.[110] The rare cases occur as a disasterous complication of disseminated gonococcal infection, which most often is caused by strains of *N. gonorrhoeae* that require arginine, hypoxanthine, and uracil for growth.[111,112]

The value of adding penicillinase (β-lactamase) to media for blood cultures has not been critically examined since SPS has been used routinely.[34,113,114] Added penicillinase has resulted in contaminated blood cultures and outbreaks of pseudobacteremia.[115,116] Whenever used, penicillinase requires proper parallel sterility testing to avoid misinterpretations.[34] The effectiveness of incorporating stabilized β-lactamase into blood culture media has not been evaluated in a controlled clinical trial.

Examination of Blood Cultures

Blood cultures should be examined visually twice during the first day of incubation and daily thereafter for 7 days.[34,117] Although the subsequent processing of blood cultures has not been standardized completely, at the University of Colorado Hosptial stained smears and subcultures are done on all bottles after 12 to 24 hours of incubation and at the first sign of visible growth, such as turbidity, hemolysis, or gas. Suspected positive cultures, based on results of visual inspection or gram-stained smears, are subcultured to 5% defibrinated sheep blood, chocolate, and MacConkey agars for aerobic incubation and Brucella blood agar with vitamin K_1 and hemin for anaerobic incubation. All blood culture bottles are incubated for 14 days and are discarded only after results of the terminal subculture are known. Isolates from patients with suspected infective endocarditis should be kept for the inoculum in the serum dilution test for bactericidal activity once treatment is begun. It is wise to keep a subculture stored safely at -70° C in case special tests of antimicrobial susceptibility are required subsequently.

Speciation of Isolates From Blood Cultures

Although often a contaminant in blood cultures, *S. epidermidis* is an important cause of endocarditis on prosthetic heart valves (Table 2).[40–42] *S. epidermidis* is commonly resistant to methicillin and must, therefore, be accurately differentiated from *S. aureus.*[118]

Viridans streptococci that cause endocarditis are almost uniformly killed by concentrations of penicillin that are readily achieved in serum.[119] There are modest differences among species of viridans streptococci in their susceptibility to antibiotics; full identification may be used to corroborate susceptibility tests in selected cases.[119,120] Pyridoxal (vitamin B_6)-dependent streptococci are an important cause of endocarditis and tend to be more resistant to killing by penicillin.[49,121] Nutritionally variant streptococci in general are less sensitive to penicillin than are other strains of viridans streptococci.[122,123] Since *Streptococcus mutans* and other viridans streptococci can be treated with penicillin alone, proper identification is mandatory.[11–13, 124] *S. mutans* endocarditis has been misdiagnosed as enterococcal endocarditis owing to false-positive reactions in commercial media presumed to be selective for enterococci.[125] *S. milleri* may present special problems in management, as it is more likely to be associated with abscess formation.

It is most important to distinguish between enterococcal and nonenterococcal group D streptococci, since enterococci require combined chemotherapy for endocarditis whereas *Streptococcus bovis* can be treated successfully with penicillin alone.[14,126–129] While all group D streptococci give a positive (black) reaction on bile-esculin medium (growth in presence of bile and hydrolysis of esculin), only true enterococci grow in 6.5% NaCl broth.[130] *S. bovis* is the most important nonenterococcal group D streptococcal pathogen for humans. In addition to being an increasingly common cause of endocarditis, bacteremia with *S. bovis* may be an important clue to serious underlying gastrointestingal disease, including carcinoma of the colon.[49,127–129,131,132] *S. faecalis* and *S. faecium* are the most important causes of enterococcal endocarditis.[129] The combination penicillin or ampicillin plus gentamicin is active against almost all strains of enterococci.[14] Strains of *S. faecalis* are also similarly susceptible to penicillin plus tobramycin, whereas strains of *S. faecium* are not.[133,134] Lastly, a novel strain of *S. faecalis* from a patient with enterococcal endocarditis has been reported to be resistant to penicillin (or ampicillin)-gentamicin syngergism but sensitive to penicillin (or ampicillin)-tobramycin synergism (Chapters 6 and 7).[135] These phenomena illustrate the need for isolation, accurate identification, and antimicrobial susceptibility testing of bacteria from the blood of patients with endocarditis.

Importance of Bactericidal Antimicrobial Therapy in Endocarditis

Requisites of Successful Antimicrobial Therapy

Before penicillin virtually everyone with infective endocarditis died, hence the use of the term "malignant endocarditis" by Sir William Osler.[136] Bacteriostatic sulfonamides suppressed symptoms but usually only delayed death. The crucial goal in chemotherapy of infective endocarditis is the killing of all microorganisms in the vegetation.[137] There is now general agreement that antimicrobial therapy of infective endocarditis must be bactericidal or fungicidal, usually parenteral, and prolonged to be successful.[2,3,11–14]

Consequently, antimicrobial susceptibility tests that measure only inhibition of growth do not provide sufficient information to guide the therapy of infective endocarditis.[137] This applies to minimal inhibitory concentrations (MICs) determined by broth or agar dilution testing as well as to direct and standard disk diffusion testing for bacteria isolated from blood cultures.[138,139] What is required is determination of the minimal bactericidal (or fungicidal) concentration (MBC) by subculturing tubes or wells of broth without visible turbidity to media free of antimicrobials.

In-vitro Tests for Selection of Combination Antimicrobial Therapy

Selection of a bactericidal regimen becomes more difficult with microorganisms like the enterococci that require combined chemotherapy.[14] The two usual methods for demonstration of synergy between antimicrobials are the checkerboard titration and the quantitative time-kill curve.[140] Both MICs and MBCs of two antimicrobials diluted serially alone and in all possible combinations (checkerboard titration) can be used to assess synergism, indifference, or antagonism. For practical purposes this method, as well as time-kill curves, is limited to combinations of two, or at most three, antimicrobials.[141] A modified checkerboard technique can be used in which the second antimicrobial is added to all tubes or wells in a constant concentration that is readily obtained in serum but is less than the MBC for that drug. For example, in testing enterococci 6 μg of streptomycin or 2 μg of gentamicin per ml would be added to serial dilutions of penicillin or ampicillin in broth. Time-kill curves, in which the number of surviving organisms are quantitated at varying time periods after exposure to known concentrations of antibiotic agent(s) are laborious and are limited to testing a few fixed concentrations of antimicrobials. The checkerboard and killing-curve techniques measure different phenomena and unfortunately, or perhaps as expected, show a poor correlation in terms of the frequency of bacterial strains showing synergy.[142,143] There is a serious need for standardization of methods used to test for synergy and of criteria for what results constitute synergy.[142] Nonetheless, current methods have been useful in finding successful combinations for the treatment of individual patients.[135,141] These techniques are not widely available, however, nor are they practical for monitoring therapy selected on the basis of likely efficacy, e.g., penicillin plus gentamicin for enterococci.

Value of Tests for Serum Bactericidal Activity

Tests to estimate the bactericidal power of blood antedate the antimicrobial era.[145] The serum dilution test (SDT) or serum bactericidal test (SBT) is a direct method for measuring the inhibitory and bactericidal activity of a patient's serum during antimicrobial therapy against the specific microorgansim causing the infection. Although not everyone agrees with its utility, the serum dilution test is widely used and recommended to guide antimicrobial therapy of infective endocarditis.[14] The serum dilution test is often, but inappropriately, termed the Schlicter test owing to a preliminary report in 1947.[147] In fact Schlicter tested only the inhibitory activity of serum and did not define criteria for determination of bactericidal end points. As emphasized earlier, tests that measure only inhibition of growth may be misleading in the treatment of infective endocarditis.[137]

That bactericidal drugs must be used to treat infective endocarditis is clear from the almost uniform relapse of patients treated with bacteriostatic agents.[137] But how much bactericidal activity over the minimum assessed from *in-vitro* testing of the infecting microorganism is required, when (peak or trough activity in relation to dosage) it needs to be achieved, and how long it must be maintained are not yet clear.[14] Nonetheless, there are many review articles that recommend maintenance of serum bactericidal titers of 1:8 or greater for optimal medical therapy of infective endocaridits.[11,12,14,15,48,146] In some patients, especially those with enterococcal endocarditis, sustained bactericidal activity at a titer of 1:8 or greater is difficult to achieve without appreciable toxicity.[148] There have been cures of infective endocarditis with serum bactericidal titers measured at 1:2 or 1:4.[11,12,15] Although the likelihood of success may be greatest with maintenance of a serum bactericidal titer of at least 1:8 at all times during medical therapy, the importance of this titer at trough is not certain and should not be sought at the cost of unwarranted toxicity. Despite optimal bactericidal activity in serum, surgical intervention may be required for complications of infective endocarditis. However, bactericidal activity in serum at a titer of 1:8 or more is important during and after valve replacement or debridement.[16–20]

There are no large, controlled prospective studies in humans on the value of the serum dilution test in guiding quantitative antimicrobial therapy of infective endocarditis.[14] Nor are such studies likely in the future, given the high rates of success with current regimens.[11–13] There are, however, many case studies of patients with difficult-to-treat microorganisms that provide useful data to support the wisdom of achieving and monitoring bactericidal activity in serum at a titer of 1:8 or greater. A few examples follow. The dramatic title "Deaf or Dead?" was used in the early report of a patient with enterococcal *(Streptococcus faecalis)* endocarditis whose organism was killed successfully only with the combination of penicillin and ototoxic intramsucular neomycin.[149] In 1973 Reller reported a patient with *Bacillus subtilis* endocarditis who remained ill for 12 days with persistently positive blood cultures until an 8-fold or greater margin of bacterial killing by serum was achieved.[43] Successful treatment of *Oerskovia turbata* endocarditis has been achieved with combination chemotherapy that produced adequate (greater than 8 times minimal) bactericidal acitivity in serum.[150] Archer and colleagues have shown the usefulness of combination chemotherapy in achieving adequate bactericidal therapy for prosthetic valve endocarditis with *Staphylococcus epidermidis.*[151] Most patients with *Brucella* endocarditis die, since tetracycline, the most effective antibiotic for brucellosis, is bacteriostatic. A recent patient with endocarditis caused by *Brucella melitensis* was cured with combined antimicrobial therapy and valve replacement.[27] This case illustrated the requisites of successful therapy, since the prosthetic valve did not become infected with *Brucella* as has happened when bactericidal activity was absent or inadequate.[17,27]

The importance of the routine use of the serum dilution test to assess bactericidal therapy in infective endocarditis is being increasingly recognized. "Bactericidal" antimicrobials that inhibit staphylococci can no longer be assumed to kill them.[152–154] The phenomenon of antibiotic-tolerance by *Staphylococcus aureus* has been demonstrated not only with antibiotics that inhibit cell wall synthesis (penicillinase-resistant penicillins, cephalosporins, and vancomycin) but also with the aminoglycosides.[153] Moreover, such antibiotic-tolerant strains of *S. aureus* have been reported to cause endocarditis.[154–158]

Although the phenomenon is real, the true clinical importance and frequency of tolerant staphylococci as causes of endocarditis are not yet known. The finding of tolerance, i.e. a wide divergence between the inhibitory (MIC) and bactericidal (MBC) end points, is dependent in part on both media and methodology.[152,159] Additional problems and uncertanties are lack of agreement on how divergent MICs and MBCs must be to be important clinically and also the inability in one study to correlate *in-vitro* tolerance with failure to respond to therapy in a rabbit model of endocarditis, the limitations of which are well-recognized.[152,153,156–161]

Persistent bacteremia has been most problematical in staphylococcal endocarditis. However, refractory infections with *Streptococcus bovis* that are resistant to the lethal effect of penicillin also have been reported.[162] Strains of viridans streptococci *(S. sanguis)* that exhibit tolerance to penicillin *in vitro* have also been isolated from patients with endocarditis.[163,164] These stains are deficient in endogenous murein hydrolase (autolysin).[163] Tolerant strains of *S. sanguis* are killed much less rapidly than are non-tolerant streptococci in cardiac vegetations in the rabbit model of endocarditis.[164] All these reports suggest that a bactericidal end point must be achieved for successful medical therapy of infective endocarditis.

Standardization of the Serum Dilution Test for Bactericidal Activity

Although the serum dilution test is basically a simple variation of the broth dilution test, there are almost as many methods for the serum dilution test as there are clinical microbiology laboratories that perform the test.[165] This is in contrast to the broth and agar dilution methods recommended by the International Collaborative Study (ICS) sponsored by the World Health Organization (WHO) and the standard disk diffusion method approved by the U.S. Food and Drug Administration (FDA) and National Committee for Clinical Laboratory Standards.[146,166] A critique of methods for the serum dilution test published between 1949 and 1976 has been presented elsewhere.[167] As the test is presently done, there are marked differences from laboratory to laboratory in every major variable in the test, including culture and dilution media, size of bacterial inoculum, cirteria for determination of the bactericidal end point, and stipulation of sufficient details to enable reproducibility.[165–167]

Since inadequate descriptions and variations in test methods among clinical laboratories precluded objective assessment of results from clinical studies, a standardized method for the serum dilution test was developed and proposed.[166,167] The suggested method was based on extensive studies of the critical variables in achieving reproducible results in the serum dilution test for bactericidal activity. Important variables include serum proteins, pH, phosphates, osmolality and salt concentration, and divalent cations.[166–171] Moreover, a practical, quantitative end point for bactericidal activity has been defined.[167] A quantitative end point requires a known initial inoculum and a specified volume for subculture as well as criteria for what constitutes no growth.[171] These factors are spelled out in a proposed standardized serum dilution test that has a bactericidal end point defined as equal to or greater than 99.9% killing of an initial inoculum of 5 x 10^5 colony-forming units (cfu) of the infecting microorganism per ml of the test mixture (Figure 3).[167]

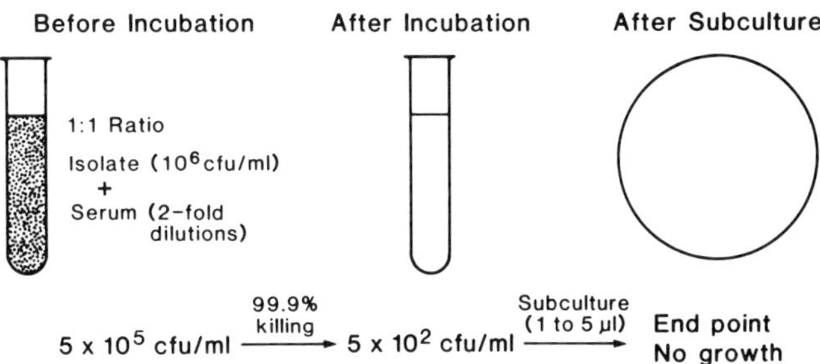

Figure 3: Schema of the serum dilution test for bactericidal activity in patients with infective endocarditis.

The advantages of the serum dilution test (SDT) over antimicrobial assays coupled with determination of minimal inhibitory and lethal concentrations of antimicrobial are that the SDT does not require an analytical balance, standard antimcriobial powders, or the ability to assay combinations of antimicrobials.[146,172,173] In a series of 65 patients with bacteremia the standardized SDT for bactericidal activity correlated well with expected results calculated from antimicrobial assays of serum and MBCs for the infecting microorgansims (Stratton, C.W., Weinstein, M.P., and Reller, L.B.: Unpublished data). For example, serum containing 32 µg/ml of methicillin showed a bactericidal titer of 1:16 against a *S. aureus* with an MBC of 2 µg/ml.

In addition the serum dilution test is a convenient method for evaluating the efficacy of combination antibiotic therapy for endocarditis.[25,150,154] The SDT is easier to do than are checkerboard titrations and time-kill curves.[140–143] The serum dilution test enables evaluations of combinations of antimicrobials for both inhibitory and bactericidal end points with less effort than it takes to do a broth dilution test of susceptibility to a single antimicrobial. Moreover, the effect of elimination of a potentially toxic aminoglycoside from a combination of antimicrobials can be measured by treating the patient's serum with cellulose phosphate to remove aminoglycoside activity.[144,174] If the bactericidal activity of the patient's serum is not reduced appreciably by removal of the aminoglycoside, combined chemotherapy may not be needed.

Lastly, the standardized serum dilution test can be modified readily for fastidious bacteria. Anaerobic bacteria usually can be tested in Schaedler broth.[175,176] Streptococci that do not grow well in Mueller-Hinton broth (MHB) with 50% pooled human serum can be tested in trypticase soy broth with 1% yeast extract or 0.001% pyridoxal.[167] An example of such streptococci are those that require vitamin B_6 (pyridoxal) for growth; these stains are known as to cause infective endocarditis.[49,121] Unless *Psuedomonas aeruginosa* is being tested against serum containing an aminoglycoside, it is not necessary to supplement MHB with calcium and mganesium.[170]

Recommended Macromethod for the Serum Dilution Test

The methodology is shown schematically in Figure 3. The macrotechnique for the serum dilution test is the same method as that used for the broth dilution test recommended by the International Collaborative Study sponsored by the World Health Organization except that the patient's serum is used in place of the double-strength antimicrobial solution in the first tube in a series of dilution steps. The final volume in each tube is 1 ml of which 0.5 ml is the inoculum; these volumes may be doubled as long as the ratio remains the same. The subculture for the bactericidal end point requires transfer of 1 to 5 μl of medium to an antimicrobial-free agar plate that will permit growth of any remaining viable microorganisms. The effect of antimicrobial carry-over is negligible with subcultures of 10 μl or less.[169] Comparison of the macromethod with the micromethod that follows show that both methods give comparable results.[164,165,175]

Recommended Micromethod for Serum Dilution Test

The basic procedure is the same as that for doing a minimal inhibitory (MIC) and minimal bactericidal (MBC) concentration in the microtiter broth dilution test except that the patient's serum is used in place of the double-strength antimicrobial solution.[165] The results are reported in terms of the inhibitory dilution and lethal dilution for the patient's microorganism.

Procedure

1. Drop 0.05 ml of pooled human serum (HS) into wells #2 through #12, rows A and B. Then drop 0.05 ml of supplemented Hinton broth (MHB-S) (see below) into wells #2 through #12, rows C and D.
2. Drop 0.1 ml of the patient's serum into well #1, rows A,B,C, and D.
3. Flame the 50 μl dilutors to a *dull* red, quench in sterile water, and blot on a blotter.
4. Dilute from well #1 through #11. Leave well #12 free of patient's serum.
5. Make a 1:200 dilution of a suspension of the patient's organism that contains 1.5 x 10^8 cfu/ml (0.5 McFarland turbidity standard). Make this dilution in MHB-S according to the detailed directions in Appendix B.
6. Inoculate each of wells with the above.
7. Seal the plate to prevent evaporation and incubate at 35° C for 16–24 hours.
8. Read the inhibitory dilution as the last well in the dilution series that shows no turbidity.
9. Subculture the plate using an inoculum replicator (multipoint inoculator), 1–5 μl micropipette, or 1 μl calibrated loop. Incubate the subculture plate for 16–24 hours at 35° C. A repeat subculture can be done after 48 hours of incubation if the MIC and MBC readings are divergent and tolerant bacteria are suspected.[152] Read the lethal dilution as the greatest dilution showing no growth on the subculture.

Preparation of Supplemented Mueller-Hinton Broth (MBH-S)

Solution 1. Calcium chloride injection 10% w/v (13.6 mmol/10 ml). (Elkins-Sinn, Inc.,Cherry Hill, New Jersey).
Solution 2. Magnesium sulfate injection (USP, 50%) (Eli Lilly and Co., Indianapolis, Indiana).

Calcium Chloride (10%)		Magnesium Sulfate (50%)		MHB
2 ml	+	0.4 ml	+	1000 ml
1 ml	+	0.2 ml	+	500 ml
0.2 ml	+	0.04 ml	+	100 ml

Use sterile technique to add the $CaCl_2$ and $MgSO_4$ to the sterile Mueller-Hinton broth. Be sure to mix well. Adding the calcium and magnesium salts before autoclaving will cause a phosphate precipitate to form.

Preparation of Inoculum for Susceptibility Tests

Serum and Broth Dilution Tests

From a fresh subculture of the organism proceed in one of two ways:

1. Pick 5 isolated colonies to 5 ml of trypticase soy broth with 1% yeast extract. Incubate 2 to 6 hours. Visually adjust to the density of a 0.5 McFarland standard. Make a 1:200 dilution of this suspension in the appropriate broth. This 1:200 dilution is the inoculum.
2. From the above *pure* overnight subculture transfer some of the growth into sterile saline or water to form a smooth suspension. Adjust to the density of the 0.5 standard as in (1.) above or adjust to 70% T at 530 nm on the Spectronic-20 (Bausch and Lomb, Rochester, New York). Dilute this suspension 1:200 with the appropriate broth to get the inoculum.

For a 1:200 dilution, take 0.01 ml (calibrated loop) into 2 ml broth, 20 μl (micropipette) into 4 ml broth, or 50 μl (micropipette) into 10 ml broth.

SUMMARY

The foremost contribution of the clinical microbiology laboratory in the management of patients with infective endocarditis is the isolation and identification of the infecting microorganism in persistently positive blood cultures. This should be possible in over 95% of cases, if an adequate volume of blood is obtained from separate venipunctures and is cultured in a rich broth with sodium polyanetholsulfonate and necessary growth factors. The selection of initial antimicrobial therapy, *in-vitro* susceptibility testing, and monitoring the results of medical therapy all require having the patient's isolate.

Antimicrobial therapy for infective endocarditis must be bactericidal, usually parenteral, and prolonged to be successful. The easiest way to assess adequacy of chemotherapy is with a standardized serum dilution test for bactericidal acitvity. Ideally, the patient's serum should show lethal activity against the infecting microorgansim at a dilution of 1:8 or more at all times; however, the importance of this titer at trough is not established. Most methods to evaluate synergistic activity with combinations of antimicrobials are complex; the serum dilution test offers a simple alternative. Both micro- and macromethods can be used for the serum dilution test, but a standard procedure with a known inoculum size and defined quantitative end point must be used if the results are to be interpretable.

REFERENCES

1. Hutter, A.M., Jr., and Moellering, R.C.: Assessment of the patient with suspected endocarditis. J.A.M.A. 235:1603, 1976.
2. Lerner, P.I., and Weinstein, L.: Infective endocarditis in the antibiotic era. N. Eng. J. Med. 274:199, 259, 323, 388, 1966.
3. Weinstein, L., and Rubin, R.H.: Infective endocarditis – 1973. Prog. Cardiovasc. Dis. 16:239, 1973.
4. Pelletier, L.L., Jr., and Petersdorf, R.G.: Infective endocarditis: a review of 125 cases from the University of Washington Hosptials, 1963–72. Medicine (Baltimore) 56:287, 1977.
5. Wedgewood, J.: Early diagnosis of subacute bacterial endocarditis. Lancet 2:1058, 1955.
6. Churchill, M.A., Jr., Geraci, J.E., and Hunder, G.G.: Musculoskeletal manifestations of bacterial endocarditis. Ann. Intern. Med. 87:754, 1977.
7. Gutman, R.A., Striker, G.E., Gilliland, B.C., and Cutler, R.A.: The immune complex glomerulonephritis of bacterial endocarditis. Medicine (Baltimore) 51:1, 1972.
8. Ziment, I.: Nervous system complications in bacterial endocarditis. Am. J. Med. 47:593, 1969.
9. Jones, H.R., Jr., Siekert, R.G., and Geraci, J.E. Neurologic manifestations of bacterial endocarditis. Ann. Intern. Med. 71:21, 1969.
10. Kilpatrick, Z.M., Greenberg, P.A., and Sanford, J.P.: Splinter hemorrhages - their clinical significance. Arch. Intern. Med. 115:730, 1965.
11. Karchmer, A.W., Moellering, R.C., Jr., Maki, D.G., and Swartz, M.N. Single-antibiotic therapy for streptococcal endocarditis. J.A.M.A. 241:1801, 1979.
12. Malacoff,R.F., Frank, E., and Andriole, V.T.: Streptococcal endocarditis (nonenterococcal, non-group A): single vs. combination therapy. J.A.M.A. 241:1807, 1979.
13. Wolfe, J.C., and Johnson, W.D., Jr.: Penicillin-sensitive streptococcal endocarditis: in-vitro and clinical observations on penicillin-streptomycin therapy. Ann. Intern. Med. 81:178, 1974.
14. Sande, M.A., and Scheld, W.M.: Combination antibiotic therapy of bacterial endocarditis. Ann. Intern. Med. 92:390, 1980.
15. Wilson, W.R., Geraci, J.E., Wilkowske, C.J., and Washington, J.A., II: Short-term intramuscular therapy with procaine penicillin plus streptomycin for infective endocarditis due to viridans streptococci. Circulation 57:1158, 1978.
16. Stinson, E.B.: Surgical treatment of infective endocarditis. Prog. Cardiovasc. Dis. 22(3):145, 1979.
17. Okies, J.E., Bradshaw, M.W., and Williams, T.W., Jr.: Valve replacement in bacterial endocarditis. Chest 63:898, 1973.

18. Richardson, J.V., Karp., R.B., Kirklin, J.W., and Dismukes, W.E.: Treatment of infective endocarditis: a 10-year comparative analysis. Circulation 58:589, 1978.
19. Turnier, E., Kay, J.H., Berstein, S., Mendez, A.M., and Zubiate, P.: Surgical treatment of *Candida* endocarditis. Chest 67: 262, 1975.
20. Utley, J.R., Mills, J., and Row, B.B.: The role of valve replacement in the treatment of fungal endocarditis. J. Thorac. Cardiovasc. Surg. 69:255, 1975.
21. Bennett, I.L., Jr., and Beeson, P.B.: Bacteremia: a consideration of some experimental and clinical aspects. Yale J. Biol. Med. 26:241, 1954.
22. Beeson, P.B., Brannon, E.S., and Warren, J.V.: Observations on the sites of removal of bacteria from the blood in patients with bacterial endocarditis. J. Exp. Med. 81:9, 1945.
23. Schirger, A., Nichols, D.R., Martin, W.J., Wellman, W.E., and Weed, L.A.: Brucellosis: experiences with 224 patients. Ann. Intern. Med. 52:827, 1960.
24. Coleman, W., and Buxton, B.H.: The bacteriology of blood in typhoid fever: an analysis of 1602 cases. Am. J. Med. Sci. 133:896, 1907.
25. Gilman, R.H., Terminel, M., Levine, M.M., Hernandez-Mendoza, P., and Hornick, R.B.: Relative efficacy of blood, urine, rectal swab, bone-marrow, and rose-spot cultures for recovery of *Salmonella typhi* in typhoid fever. Lancet 1:1211, 1975.
26. Guerra-Caceres, J.G., Gotuzzo-Herencia, E., Crosby-Dagnino, E., Miro-Quesda, M., and Carrillo-Paradi, C.: Diagnositc valve of bone marrow culture in typhoid fever. Trans. R. Soc. Trop. Med. Hyg. 73:680, 1979.
27. Pratt, D.S., Tenney, J.H., Bjork, C.M., and Reller, L.B.: Successful treatment of *Brucella melitensis* endocarditis. Am. J. Med. 64:897, 1978.
28. Mokhobo, K.P.: Typhoid cardiac involvement. S. Afr. Med. J. 49:55, 1975.
29. Wilson, W.R., Van Scoy, R.E., and Washington, J.A., II: Incidence of bacteremia in adults without infection. J. Clin. Microbiol. 2:94, 1975.
30. Maki, D.G., Weise, C.E., and Sarafin, H.W.: A semiquantitative culture method for identifying intravenous-catheter-related infection. N. Engl. J. Med. 296:1305, 1977.
31. Band, J.D., and Maki, D.G.: Infections caused by arterial catheters used for hemodynamic monitoring. AM. J. Med. 67:735, 1979.
32. Tonneson, A., Peuler, M., and Lockwood, W.R.: Cultures of blood drawn by catheters vs. venipuncture. J.A.M.A. 235:1877, 1976.
33. Mallen, M.S., Hube, E.L., and Brenes, M.: Comparative study of blood cultures made from artery, vein, and bone marrow in patients with subacute bacterial endocarditis. Am. Heart J. 33:692, 1947.

34. Washington, J.A., II: Blood cultures: principles and techniques. Mayo Clin. Proc. 50:91, 1975.
35. Belli, J., and Waisbren, B.A.: The number of blood cultures necessary to diagnose most cases of bacterial endocarditis. Am. J. Med. Sci. 232:284, 1956.
36. Werner, A.S., Cobbs, C.G., Kaye, D., and Hook, E.W.: Studies on the bacteremia of bacterial endocarditis. J.A.M.A. 202:199, 1967.
37. MacGregor, R.R., and Beaty, H.N.: Evaluation of positive blood cultures: guidelines for early differentiation of contaminated from valid positive cultures. Arch. Intern. Med. 130:84, 1972.
38. Van Scoy, R.E., Cohen, S.N., Geraci, J.E., and Washington, J.A., II.: Coryneform bacterial endocarditis: difficulties in diagnosis and treatment, presentation of three cases, and review of literature. Mayo Clin. Proc. 52:216, 1977.
39. Gerry, J.L., and Greenough, W.B., III.: Diphtheroid endocarditis. Report of nine cases and review of the literature. Johns Hopkins Med. J. 139:61, 1976.
40. Dismukes, W.E., Karchmer, A.W., Buckley, M.J., Austin, W.G., and Swartz, M.N.: Prosthetic valve endocarditis: analysis of 38 cases. Circulation 48:365, 1973.
41. Wilson, W.R., Jaumin, P.M., Danielson, G.K., Giuliani, E.R., Washington, J.A., II, and Geraci, J.E.: Prosthetic valve endocarditis. Ann. Intern. Med. 82:751, 1975.
42. Watankunakorn, C.: Prosthetic valve endocarditis. Prog. Cardiovasc. Disc. 22(3):181, 1979.
43. Reller, L.B.: Endocarditis caused by *Bacillus subtilis.* Am. J. Clin. Path. 60:714, 1973.
44. Weller, P.F., Nicholson, A., and Braslow, N.: The spectrum of *Bacillus* bacteremia in heroin addicts. Arch. Intern. Med. 139:293, 1979.
45. Tuazon, C.V., Murray, H.W., Levy, C., Solny, M.N., Curtin, J.A., and Sheagren, J.N.: Serious infections from *Bacillus* sp. J.A.M.A. 241:1137, 1979.
46. Broome, C.V., Moellering, R.C., Jr., and Watson, B.K.: Clinical significance of Lancefield groups L-T streptococci isolated from blood and cerebrospinal fluid. J. Infect. Dis. 133:382, 1976.
47. Wilson, W.R., and Washington, J.A., II: Infective endocarditis - a changing spectrum? Mayo Clin. Proc. 52:254, 1977.
48. Lowes, J.A., Hamer, J., Williams, G., Houang, E., Tobaqchali, S., Shaw, E.J., Hill, I.M., and Rees, G.M.: 10 years of infective endocarditis at St. Bartholomew's Hosptial: analysis of clinical features and treatment in relation to prognosis and mortality. Lancet 1:133, 1980.
49. Roberts, R.B., Krieger, A.G., Schiller, N.L., and Gross, K.C.: Viridans streptococcal endocarditis: the role of various species, including pyridoxal-dependent streptococci. Rev. Infect. Dis. 1:955, 1979.

50. Welton, D.E., Young, J.B., Gentry, W.D., Raizner, A.E., Alexander, J.K., Chahine, R.A., Miller, R.R.: Recurrent infective endocarditis: analysis of predisposing factors and clinical features. Am. J. Med. 66:932, 1979.
51. Child, J.A., Darrell, J.H., Rhys Davies, N., and Davis-Dawson, L: Mixed infection endocarditis in a heroin addict. J. Med. Microbiol. 2:293, 1969.
52. Saravolatz, L.D., Burch, K.H., Quinn, E.L., Cox, F., Madhavan, T., and Fisher, E.: Polymicrobial endocarditis: an increasing clinical entity. Am. Heart J. 95:163, 1978.
53. Cannady, P.B., and Sanford, J.P.: Negative blood cultures in infective endocarditis: a review. South. Med. J. 69:1420, 1976.
54. Hampton, J.R., and Harrison, M.J.G.: Sterile blood cultures in bacterial endocarditis. Q. J. Med. 36:167, 1967.
55. Hall, B., and Dowling, H.F.: Negative blood cultures in bacterial endocarditis: a decade's experience. Med. Clin. North Am. 50:159, 1966.
56. Keefer, C.S.: Subacute bacterial endocarditis: active cases without bacteremia. Ann. Intern. Med. 11:714, 1937.
57. Pesanti, E.L., and Smith, I.M.: Infective endocarditis with negative blood cultures: an analysis of 52 cases. Am. J. Med. 66:43, 1979.
58. Ellner, J.J., Rosenthal, M.S., Lerner, P.I., and McHenry, M.C.: Infective endocarditis caused by slow-growing, fastidious, gram-negative bacteria. Medicine (Baltimore) 58:145, 1979.
59. Nastro, L.J., and Finegold, S.M.: Endocarditis due to anaerobic gram-negative bacilli. Am. J. Med. 54:482, 1973.
60. Beiger, R.C., Brewer, N.S., and Washington, J.A., II: *Haemophilus aphrophilus:* a microbiologic and clinical review and report of 42 cases. Medicine (Baltimore) 57:345, 1978.
61. Geraci, J.E., Wilkowske, C.J., Wilson, W.R., and Washington, J.A., II: *Haemophilus* endocarditis: report of 14 patients. Mayo Clin. Proc. 52:209, 1977.
62. Chunn, C.J., Jones, S.R., McCutchan, J.A., Young, E.J., and Gilbert, D.N.: *Haemophilus parainfluenzae* infective endocarditis. Medicine (Baltimore) 56:99, 1979.
63. Wainright, J.: Tuberculous endocarditis: a report of 2 cases. S. Afr. Med. J. 56:731, 1979.
64. Wilson, H.G., Neilson, G.H., Galea, E.G., Stafford, G., and O'Brien, M.F.: Q fever endocarditis in Queensland. Circulation 53:680, 1976.
65. Rosman, M.S., Lubbe, W.F., Hayden, M., Basson, N., and Uys, C.J.: Q fever endocarditis: a report of 2 cases. S. Afr. Med. J. 53:296, 1978.
66. Applefeld, M.M., Billingsley, L.M., Tucker, H.J., Fiset, P.: Q fever endocarditis: a case occurring in the United States. Am. Heart J. 93:669, 1977.

67. Kimbrough, R.C., III, Ormsbee, R.A., Peacock, M., Rogers, W.R., Bennetts, R.W., Raaf, J., Krause, A., and Gardner, C.: Q fever endocarditis in the United States. Ann. Intern. Med. 91:400, 1979.
68. Birkhead, J.S., and Apostolov, K.: Endocarditis caused by psittacosis agent. Br. Heart J. 36:728, 1974.
69. Dick, D.C., McGregor, C.G.A., Mitchell, K.G., Sommerville, R.G., and Wheatley, D.J.: Endocarditis as a manifestation of *Chlamydia* B infection (psittacosis). Br. Heart J. 39:914, 1977.
70. Van der Bel-Kahn, J.M., Watanakunakorn, C., Menefee, M.G., Long, H.D., Dicter, R: *Chlamydia trachomatis* endocarditis. Am. Heart J. 95:627, 1978.
71. Regan, R.J., Dathan, J.R.E., and Treharne, J.D.: Infective endocarditis with glomerulonephritis associated with cat chlamydia *(C. psittaci)* infection. Br. Heart J. 42:349, 1979.
72. Rubinstein, E., Noriega, E.R., Simberkoff, M.S., Holzman, R., and Rahal, J.J., Jr.: Fungal endocarditis: analysis of 24 cases and review of the literature. Medicine (Baltimore) 54:331, 1975.
73. Kammer, R.B., and Utz, J.P.: *Aspergillus* species endocarditis: the new face of a not so rare disease. Am. J. Med. 56:506, 1974.
74. Smith, J.W., and Utz, J.P.: Progressive disseminated histoplasmosis: a prospective study of 26 patients. Ann. Intern. Med. 76:557, 1972.
75. Davies, S.F., McKenna, R.W., and Sarosi, G.A.: Trephine biopsy of the bone marrow in disseminated histoplasmosis. Am. J. Med. 67:617, 1979.
76. Alexander, W.J., Mowry, R.W., Cobbs, C.G., and Dismukes, W.E.: Prosthetic valve endocaridits caused by Histoplasma *capsulatum.* J.A.M.A. 242:1399, 1979.
77. Goodwin, R.A., Jr., Shaprio, J.L., Thurman, G.H., Thurman, S.S., and Des Prez, R.M.: Disseminated histoplasmosis: clinical and pathologic correlations. Medicine (Baltimore) 59:1, 1980.
78. MacDonald, R.A., and Robins, S.L.: The significance of nonbacterial thrombotic endocarditis: an autopsy and clinical study of 78 cases. Ann. Intern. Med. 56:255, 1957.
79. Rosen, P., and Armstrong, D.: Nonbacterial thrombotic endocarditis in patients with malignant neoplastic diseases. Am. J. Med. 54:23, 1973.
80. Pedersen, F.K., and Petersen, E.A.: Bacterial endocarditis at Blegdamshospitalet in Copenhagen 1944–1973. Scand. J. Infect. Dis. 8:99, 1976.
81. Reymann, M.T., Holley, H.P., Jr., and Cobbs, C.G.: Persistent bacteremia in staphylococcal endocarditis. Am. J. Med. 65:729, 1978.
82. Bayer, A.S., Theofilopoulos, A.N., Tillman, D.B., Dixon, F.J., and Guze, L.B.: Use of circulating immune complex levels in the serodifferentiation of endocarditic and nonendocarditic septicemias. Am. J. Med. 66:58, 1979.

83. Williams, R.C., Jr., and Kunkel, H.G.: Rheumatoid factor, complement, and conglutinin aberrations in patients with subacute bacterial endocarditis. J. Clin. Invest. 41:666, 1962.
84. Hurwitz, D., Quismorio, F.P., and Friou, G.J.: Cryoglobulinaemia in patients with infective endocarditis. Clin. Exp. Immunol. 19:131, 1975.
85. Miller, M.H., and Casey, J.I.: Infective endocarditis: new diagnostic techniques. Am. Heart J. 96:123, 1978.
86. Boulton-Jones, J.M., Sissons, J.G.P., Evans, D.J., and Peters, D.K.: Renal lesions of subacute infective endocarditis. Br. Med. J. 2:11, 1974.
87. Pruitt, A.A., Rubin, R.H., Karchmer, A.W., and Duncan, G.W.: Neurologic complications of bacterial endocarditis. Medicine (Baltimore) 57:329, 1978.
88. Weinstein, L. and Schlesinger, J.J.: Pathoanatomic, pathophysiologic and clinical correlations in endocarditis. N. Engl. J. Med. 291:832, 1122, 1974.
89. Phair, J.P., and Clarke, J.: Immunology of infective nedocarditis. Prog. Cardiovasc. Dis. 22(3):137, 1979.
90. Crowder, J.G., White, A.: Teichoic acid antibodies in staphylococcal and nonstaphylococcal endocarditis. Ann. Intern. Med. 77:87, 1972.
91. Nagel, J.G., Tuazon, C.U., Cardella, T.A., Sheagren, J.M.: Teichoic acid serologic diagnosis of staphylococcal endocarditis: use of gel diffusion and counterimmunoelectrophoretic methods. Ann. Intern. Med. 82:13, 1975.
92. Powers, D.L., and Mandell, G.L.: Intraleukocytic bacteria in infective endocarditis patients. J.A.M.A. 227:312, 1974.
93. Engle, R.L., Jr., and Koprowski, I.: The appearance of histiocytes in the blood in subacute bacterial endocarditis. Am. J. Med. 26:965, 1959.
94. Carlson, B.E., and Andersen, B.R.: Value of granulocyte examination for bacteria. J.A.M.A. 235:1465, 1976.
95. Brooks, G.F., Pribble, A.H., and Beaty, H.N.: Early diagnosis of bacteremia by buffy-coat examination. Arch. Intern. Med. 132:673, 1973.
96. Allen, A.C.: nature of vegetations of bacterial endocardidis. Arch. Pathol. 27:661, 1939.
97. Eyster, E., and Bernene, J.: Nosocomial anemia. J.A.M.A. 223:73, 1973.
98. Blazevic, D.J., Stemper, J.E., and Matsen, J.M.: Effect of aerobic and anaerobic atompsheres on isolation of organisms from blood cultures. J. Clin. Microbiol. 1:154, 1975.
99. Harkness, J.L., Hall, M., Ilstrup, D., and Washington, J.A., II: Effects of atmosphere of incubation and of routine subcultures on detection of bacteremia in vacuum blood culture bottles. J. Clin. Microbiol. 2:296, 1975.

100. Model, D.G., and Peel, R.N.: The effect of temperature of the culture medium on the outcome of blood culture. J. Clin. Pathol. 26:529, 1973.
101. Roberts, G.D., and Washington, J.A., II: Detection of fungi in blood cultures. J. Clin. Microbiol. 1:309, 1975.
102. Wilkins, T.D., and West, S.E.H.: Medium-dependent inhibition of *Peptostreptococcus anaerobius* by sodium polyanetholsufonate in blood culture media. J. Clin. Microbiol. 3:393, 1976.
103. Eng, J. and Iveland, H.: Inhibitory effect in vitro of sodium polyanethol sulfonate on the growth of *Neisseria meningitidis.* J. Clin. Microbiol. 1:444, 1975.
104. Rintala, L., and Pollock, H.M.: Effects of two blood culture anticoagulants on growth of *Neisseria meningitidis.* J. Clin. Microbiol. 7:332, 1978.
105. Washington, J.A., II, Hall, M.M., and Warren, E.: Evaluation of blood culture media supplemented with sucrose or with cysteine, J. Clin. Microbiol. 1:79, 1975.
106. Hall, M.M., Mueske, C.A., Ilstrup, D.M., and Washington, J.A., II: Evaluation of vented blood culture media with sorbitol. J. Clin. Microbiol. 10:690, 1979.
107. Roberts, G.D., Horstmeier, C.D., and Ilstrup, D.M.: Evaluation of a hypertonic sucrose medium for the detection of fungi in blood cultures. J. Clin. Microbiol. 4:110, 1976.
108. Phair, J.P., Watankunakorn, C., Linnemann, C., Jr., and Carleton, J.: Attempts to isolate well-defective microbial variants from clinical specimens. Am. J. Clin. Pathol. 62:601, 1974.
109. Linnemann, C.C., Jr., Watankunakorn, C., and Bakie, C.: Pathogenicity of stable L-phase variants of *Staphylococcus aureus:* failure to colonize experimental endocarditis in rabbits. Infect. Immun. 7:725, 1973.
110. Williams, R.H.: Gonococcic endocarditis: a study of twelve cases, with ten postmoretem examinations. Arch. Intern. Med. 61:26–38, 1938.
111. Holmes, K.K., Counts, G.W., and Beaty, H.M.: Disseminated gonococcal infection. Ann. Intern. Med. 74:979, 1971.
112. Knapp, J.S., and Holmes, K.K.: Disseminated gonococcal infections caused by *Neisseria gonorrhoeae* with unique nutritional requirements. J. Infect. Dis. 132:204, 1975.
113. Dowling, H.F., and Hirsh, H.L.: The use of penicillinase in cultures of body fluids obtained from patients under treatment with penicillin. Am. J. Med. Sci. 210:756, 1945.
114. Carleton, J.A., and Hamburger, M.: Unmasking of false-negative blood cultures in patients receiving new penicillins. J.A.M.A. 186:157, 1963.
115. Norden, C.W.: Pseudosepticemia. Ann. Intern. Med. 71:789, 1969.
116. Faris, H.M., and Sparling, F.F.: *Mima polymorpha* bacteremia: false-negative cultures due to contaminated penicillinase. J.A.M.A. 219:76, 1972.

117. Blazevic, D.J., Stemper, J.E., and Matsen, J.M.: Comparison of macroscopic examination, routine gram stains, and routine subcultures in the initial detection of positive blood cultures. Appl. Microbiol. 27:537, 1974.
118. Siebert, W.T., Moreland, N., and Williams, T.W., Jr.: Synergy of vancomycin plus cefazolin or cephalothin against methicillin-resistant *Staphylococcus epidermidis.* J. Infect. Dis. 139:452, 1979.
119. Bourgault, A-M., Wilson, W.R., and Washington, J.A., II: Antimicrobial susceptibilities of species of viridans streptococci. J. Infect. dis. 140:316, 1979.
120. Facklam, R.R.: Physiological differentiation of viridans streptococci. J. Clin. Microbiol. 5:184, 1977.
121. Carey, R.B., Brause, B.D., and Roberts, R.B.: Antimicrobial therapy of vitamin B_6-dependent streptococcal endocarditis. Ann. Intern. Med. 87:150, 1977.
122. Cooksey, R.C., Thompson, F.S., and Facklam, R.R.: Physiological characterization of nutritionally variant streptococci. J. Clin. Microbiol. 10:326, 1979.
123. Cooksey, R.C., and Swenson, J.M.: In vitro antimicrobial inhibition patterns of nutritionally variants streptococci. Antimicrob. Agents Chemother. 16:514, 1979.
124. Baker, C.N., and Thornesberry, C.: Antimicrobial susceptiblity of *Streptococcus mutans* isolated from patients with endocarditis. Antimicrob. Agents Chemother. 5:268, 1974.
125. Neefe, L.I., Chretien, J.H., Delaha, E.C., and Garagusi, V.F.: *Streptococcus mutans* endocarditis: confusion with enterococcal endocarditis by routine laboratory testing. J.A.M.A. 230:1298, 1974.
126. Thornesberry, C., Baker, C.N., and Facklam, R.R.: Antibiotic susceptibility of *Streptococcus bovis* and other group D streptococci causing endocarditis. Antimicrob. Agents Chemother. 5:228, 1974.
127. Watanakunakorn, C.: *Streptococcus bovis* endocarditis. Am. J. Med. 56:256, 1974.
128. Hoppes, W.L., and Lerner, P.I.: Nonenterococcal group-D streptococcal endocarditis caused by *Streptococcus bovis.* Ann. Intern. Med. 81:588, 1974.
129. Moellering, R.C., Jr., Watson, B.K., and Kunz, L.J.: Endocarditis due to group D streptococci: comparison of disease caused by *Streptococcus bovis* and that produced by the enterococci. Am. J. Med. 57:239, 1974.
130. Facklam, R.R.: Recognition of group D streptococcal species of human origin by biochemical and physiological tests. Appl. Microbiol. 23:1131, 1972.
131. Murray, H.W., and Roberts, R.B.: *Streptococcus bovis* bacteremia and underlying gastrointestinal disease. Arch. Intern. Med. 138:1097, 1978.

132. Klein, R.S., Recco, R.A., Catalano, M.T., Edberg, S.C., Casey, J.I., and Steigbigel, N.H.: Association of *Streptococcus bovis* with carcinoma of the colon. N. Engl. J. Med. 297:800, 1977.
133. Moellering, R.C., Jr., Wennersten, C., and Weinstein, A.J.: Penicillin-tobramycin synergism against enterococci: a comparison with penicillin and gentamicin. Antimicrob. Agents Chemother. 3:526, 1973.
134. Moellering, R.C., Jr., Korzeniowski, O.M., Sande, M.A., and Wennersten, C.B.: Species-specific resistance to antimicrobial synergism in *Streptococcus faecium* and *Streptococcus faecalis.* J. Infect. Dis., 140:203, 1979.
135. Moellering, R.C., Jr., Murray, B.E., Schoenbaum, S.C., Adler, J., and Wennersten, C.B.: A novel mechanism of resistance to penicillin-gentamicin synergism in *Streptococcus faecalis.* J. Infect. Dis. 141:81, 1980.
136. Osler, W,: Malignant endocarditis. Lancet 1:415, 1885.
137. Hunter, T.H.: Speculations on the mechanism of cure of bacterial endocarditis. J.A.M.A. 144:524, 1950.
138. Witebsky, F.G., MacLowry, J.D., and French, S.S.: Broth dilution minimum inhibitory concentrations: rationale for use of selected antimicrobial concentrations. J. Clin. Microbiol. 9:589, 1979.
139. Mirrett, S., and Reller, L.B.: Comparison of direct and standard antimicrobial disk susceptibility testing for bacteria isolated from blood. J. Clin. Microbiol. 10:482, 1979.
140. Rahal, J.J., Jr.: Antibiotic combinations: the clinical relevance of synergy and antagonism. Medicine (Baltimore) 57:179, 1978.
141. Berenbaum, M.C.: A method for testing synergy with any number of agents. J. Infect. Dis. 137:122, 1978.
142. Norden, C.W., Wentzel, H., and Kaleti, E.: Comparison of techniques for measurement of in vitro antibiotic synergism. J. Infect. Dis. 140:629, 1979.
143. Moellering, R.C., Jr.: Antimicrobial synergism - an elusive concept. J. Infect. Dis. 140:639, 1979.
144. Parrillo, J.E., Borst, G.C., Mazur, M.H., Iannini, P., Klempner, M.S., Moellering, R.C., Jr., and Anderson, S.E.: Endocarditis due to resistant viridans streptococci during oral penicillin chemoprophylaxis. N. Engl. J. Med. 300:296, 1979.
145. Miles, A.A., and Misra, S.S.: The estimation of the bactericidal power of the blood. J. Hyg. (Camb) 38:732, 1938.
146. Rosenblatt, J.E.: Laboratory tests used to guide antimicrobial therapy. Mayo Clin. Proc. 52:611, 1977.
147. Schlichter, J.G., and MacLean, H.: A method for determining the effect therapeutic level in the treatment of subacute bacterial endocarditis with penicillin: a preliminary report. Am. Heart J. 34:209, 1947.

148. Mandell, G.L., Kaye, D., Levison, M.E., and Hook, E.W.: Enterococcal endocarditis: an analysis of 38 patients observed at the New York Hospital - Cornell Medical Center. Arch. Intern. Med. 125:258, 1970.
149. Havard, C.W.H., Garrod, L.P., and Waterworth, P.M.: Deaf or dead? A case of subacute bacterial endocarditis treated with penicillin and neomycin. Br. Med. J. 1:688, 1959.
150. Reller, L.B., Maddoux, G.L., Eckman, M.R., and Pappas, G.: Bacterial endocarditis caused by *Oerskovia turbata.* Ann. Intern. Med. 83:664, 1975.
151. Archer, G.L., Tenenbaum, M.J., and Haywood, H.B., III: Rifampin therapy of *Staphylococcus epidermidis:* use in infection from indwelling artifical devices. J.A.M.A. 240:751, 1978.
152. Sabath, L.D., Wheeler, N., Laverdiere, M., Blazevic, D., and Wilkinson, B.J.: A new type of penicillin resistance of *Staphylococcus aureus.* Lancet 1:443, 1977.
153. Watanakunakorn, C.: Antibiotic-tolerant *Staphylococcus aureus.* J. Antimicrob. Chemother. 4:561, 1978.
154. Faville, R.J., Zaske, D.E., Kaplan, E.L., Crossley, K., Sabath, L.D., and Quie, P.G.: *Staphylococcus aureus* endocarditis: combined therapy with vancomycin and rifampin. J.A.M.A. 240:1963, 1978.
155. Massanari, R.M., and Donta, S.T.: The efficacy of rifampin as adjunctive therapy in selected cases of staphylococcal endocarditis. Chest 73:371, 1978.
156. Denny, A.E., Peterson, L.R., Gerding, D.N., and Hall, W.H.: Serious staphylococcal infections with strains tolerant to bactericidal antibiotics. Arch. Intern. Med. 139:1026, 1979.
157. Gopal, V., Bisno, A.L., and Silverblatt, F.J.: Failure of vancomycin treatment in *Staphylococcus aureus* endocarditis. J.A.M.A. 236:1640, 1976.
158. Rajashekaraiah, K.R. Rice, T., Rao, V.S. Marsh, D., Ramakrishna, B., and Kallick, C.A.: Clinical significance of tolerant strains of *Staphylococcus aureus* in patients with endocarditis. Ann. Intern. Med. 93:796, 1980.
159. Peterson, L.R., Gerding, D.N., Hall, W.H., and Schierl, E.A.: Medium-independent variation in bactericidal activity of antibiotics against susceptible *Staphylococcus aureus.* Antimicrob. Agents Chemother. 13:665, 1978.
160. Goldman, P.L., and Petersdorf, R.G.: significance of methicillin tolerance in experimental staphylococcal endocarditis. Antimicrob. Agents Chemother. 15:802, 1979.
161. Freedman, L.R., and Valone, J., Jr.: Experimental infective endocarditis. Prog. Cardiovasc. Dis. 22(3): 169, 1979.
162. Savitch, C.B., Barry, A.L., and Hoeprich, P.D.: Infective endocarditis caused by *Streptococcus bovis* resistant to the lethal effect of penicillin G. Arch. Intern. Med. 138:931, 1978.

163. Horne, D., and Tomasz, A.: Lethal effect of a heterologous murein hydrolase on penicillin-treated *Streptococcus sanguis.* Antimicrob. Agents Chemother. 17:235, 1980.
164. Pulliam, L., Inokucki, S., Hadley, W.K., and Mills, J.: Penicillin tolerance in experimental streptococcal endocarditis. Lancet 2:957, 1979.
165. Pien, F.D., and Vosti, K.L.: Variation in performance of the serum bactericidal test. Antimicrob. Agents. Chemother. 6:330, 1974.
166. Stratton, C.W., and Reller, L.B.: Serum dilution test for bactericidal activity. I. Selection of a physiologic diluent. J. Infect. Dis. 136:187, 1977.
167. Reller, L.B., and Stratton, C.W.: Serum dilution test for bactericidal activity. II. Standardization and correlation with antimicrobial assays and susceptibility tests. J. Infect. Dis. 136:196, 1977.
168. Pien, F.D., Williams, R.D., and Vosti, K.L.: Comparison of broth and human serum as the diluent in the serum bactericidal test. Antimicrob. Agents Chemother. 7:113, 1975.
169. Hamilton-Miller, J.M.T.: Towards greater uniformity in sensitivity testing. J. Antimicrob. Chemother. 3:385, 1977.
170. Reller, L.B., Schoenknecht, F.D., Kenny, M.A., and Sherris, J.C.: Antibiotic susceptibliity testing of *Pseudomonas aeruginosa:* selection of a control strain and criteria for magnesium and calcium content in media. J. Infect. Dis. 130:454, 1974.
171. Barry, A.L., and Lasner, R.A.: In-vitro methods for determining minimal lethal concentrations of antimicrobial agents. Am. J. Clin. Pathol. 71:88, 1979.
172. Sabath, L.D.: The assay of antimicrobial compounds. Hum. Pathol. 7:287, 1976.
173. Hewitt, W.L., McHenry, M.C.: Blood level determinations of antimicrobail drugs: some clinical considerations. Med. Cl. North Am. 62:1119, 1978.
174. Stevens, P., and Young, L.S.: Simple method for elimination of aminoglycosides from serum to permit bioassay of other antimicrobial agents. Antimicrob. Agents Chemother. 12:286, 1977.
175. Stalons, D.R., and Thornsberry, C.: Broth-dilution method for determining the antibiotic susceptibility of anaerobic bacteria. Antimicrob. Agents Chemother. 7:15, 1975.
176. Thornesberry, C.: Techniques for anaerobic susceptibility testing. J. Infect. Dis. 135 (Suppl.):S4, 1977.
177. Prober, C.G. Dougherty, S.S., Vosti, K.L., and Yeager, A.S.: Comparison of a micromethod for performance of the serum bactericidal test with the standard tube dilution method. Antimicrob. Agents Chemother. 16:46, 1979.

Amnon Rosenthal, M.D.

16

TREATMENT AND PREVENTION OF INFECTIVE ENDOCARDITIS IN INFANTS AND CHILDREN

Infective endocarditis is a serious complication of heart disease in infants and children. The improvement in medical and surgical therapy of congenital heart disease during the last thirty years has resulted in an increase in number and age of patients susceptible to infective endocarditis.[1] Prevention remains the best hope for decreasing the frequency, severity and adverse complications of endocarditis. This chapter will, therefore, focus on the prevention of infective endocarditis, particularly as it relates to the pediatric population. Specific and supportive therapy once endocarditis is established differs little from that used in adults. Only areas in which management may differ significantly from the adult will be discussed.

Prevention

The high mortality (19–25%),[1,2] increased morbidity and prolonged hospitalization for treatment of endocarditis point to the importance of prevention. Despite the increasing frequency and devastating consequences of the disease, only few studies have been performed on the epidemiology and prevention of endocarditis.[3] Many of our concepts and practices are based on animal experimental models,[4,5] untested hypotheses and inferences.[6]

Abnormalities in Children Leading to Increased Risk for Endocarditis

Infants and children at increased risk of the development of infective endocarditis are predominantly those with clinically apparent or silent structural cardiac disease and to a lesser extent, patients with other abnormalities (Table 1). Children with innocent murmurs such as Stills murmur, venous hum, carotid bruit or physiologic pulmonary ejection murmur are not at increased risk of developing endocarditis. In one large series in children, 91% of patients with endocarditis had congenital heart disease, 3% had rheumatic heart disease, and 6% had no known preexisting heart disease.[1] The frequency of endocarditis varies with the type of cardiac abnormality.[7] The incidence may be as high as 23/1000 patient-years in ventricular septal defect with aortic regurgitation,[8] 3.3/1000 patient-years in patent ductus arteriosus,[9] or 0.2/1000 patient-years in isolated valvar pulmonary stenosis.[2] The incidence of endocarditis in infants with congenital heart disease is similar to that reported for children.[10] In general, all patients with congenital heart disease are at increased risk of endocarditis except for those with isolated atrial septal defect secundum and those with trivial valvar pulmonary stenosis.

Table 1. Abnormalities in Children Resulting in Increased Risk of Infective Endocarditis

1. Congenital Heart Disease
    - clinically apparent
    - silent lesions
        - bicuspid aortic valve
        - prolapsed mitral valve
        - idiopathic hypertrophic subaortic stenosis
2. Systemic Disorders with Cardiac Involvement
    - rheumatic heart disease
    - inherited disorders of metabolism and connective tissue
    - collagen disorders
3. Ventriculoatrial Shunt for Hydrocephalus
4. Long-Term Indwelling Venous or Arterial Lines
5. Drug Addiction

Increased susceptibility to endocarditis continues after surgical repair of most forms of congenital heart disease.[2,11] The possible exceptions are patients with isolated patent ductus arteriosus, isolated atrial septal defect secundum and completely closed ventricular septal defect. Even in those children chemoprophylaxis is advised for six months after surgery, until complete healing has occurred. With most forms of congenital heart disease, an increased risk is to be expected even in the patients with successful hemodynamic repair because of persistent anatomic abnormalities. For example, in postoperative patients with tetralogy of Fallot, residua and sequelae include pulmonary regurgitation (94%), ventricular septal defect (20%), tricuspid regurgitation or peripheral pulmonary stenosis.[12] The less frequent and severe the residual abnormalities, the less likely is endocarditis to occur. The frequency of endocarditis after repair of ventricular septal defect has declined from 2.4/1000 patient-years to 0.6/1000 patient-years.[2] In contrast, patients with aortic stenosis may experience an even higher risk of contracting endocarditis after surgery.[2]

Long-term medical supervision of preoperative and post-operative children with congenital heart disease along with parental counseling and education will lead to appropriate preventive measures in the population at risk. Careful cardiac examination and selective non-invasive studies should be performed in all patients in an attempt to detect silent lesions. For example, mitral valve prolapse in the patient with atrial septal defect secundum[13] or bicuspid aortic valve in a postoperative patient with ventricular septal defect[8] is an indication for continued chemoprophylaxis. In the follow-up examination, the need for chemoprophylaxis at times of predictable risk should be emphasized to the patient and parents. Specific written instructions such as the American Heart Association's card on antimicrobial prophylaxis should be distributed to the parents of patients at risk.

Procedures Associated with Bacteremia

Bacteremia must occur prior to the development of infective endocarditis. Preventive measures must, therefore, focus on an illness or procedure which is associated with significant bacteremia (Table 2). Although many procedures and illnesses have been shown to be associated with a high rate of bacteremia, their effect on the actual risk for the development of infective endocarditis remains unclear. An identifiable event preceding the diagnosis of endocarditis may be recognized in only 21% of patients.[9] In nearly 2/3 of these, the antecedent event prior to endocarditis has been a surgical or dental procedure.

Transient bacteremia occurs in approximatley 50% of children after dental extraction and is less frequent after other dental procedures[14–18] (Table 3). The prevalence of bacteremia after periodental procedures will vary with the age of the patient, type of procedure, severity of the periodontal disease, preoperative preparation of the gingiva and the cultural techniques used. Endontic procedures limited to root canal system are rarely associated with bacteremia. There are, however, few studies in children on procedures other than dental extraction and prophylaxis.

Table 2. Procedures and Diseases in Children Associated with Transient and Significant Bacteremia

PROCEDURES

- Dental procedures
- Tonsillectomy and adenoidectomy
- Open heart surgery
- Gastrointestinal and genitourinary instrumentation
- Abscess incision and drainage
- Intravenous alimentation
- Circumcision[20]

DISEASES

- Severe gingival and periodontal inflammation
- Genitourinary infection
- Impetigo, acne
- Malnutrition
- Third degree burns[1,20]
- Asplenia syndrome
- Omphalitis

Dental procedures as an etiologic factor in endocarditis have been implicated in 19–25% of patients with endocarditis.[1,2] However, since nearly half of all episodes of endocarditis in children are caused by mouth organisms[1,11] (e.g. viridans streptococci) the oropharynx may be a focus for bacteremia even in the absence of any dental procedures. Daily activities, such as chewing,[19] toothbrushing,[19,20] use of dental floss,[21] or oral irrigation devices[20] have all been shown to lead to transient bacteremia. The frequency of bacteremia increases with the increasing severity of gingival and periodontal disease.[20] Optimal dental care and good dietary habits undoubtedly improve oral hygiene and may diminish the frequency of bacteremia. Dental health education of parents and children, use of flouride to prevent caries and reminders by the patient's pediatrician should result in better control of dental and gingival disease. Prompt referral should be made to the family dentist or dental clinic. Many dentists are reluctant to care for infants and children with complex congenital heart disorders and these children should be evaluated and treated in the medical center. Written instructions on antimicrobial prophylaxis should be mailed to the patient's dentist.

Chronic periodontal inflammation is especially common in children with cyanotic congenital heart disease.[7] Gingivitis and dental caries in these children and adolescents are probably the result of chronic hypoxemia and polycythemia. The associated increase in intravascular

Table 3. Bacteremia Associated with Dental Procedures in Children

PROCEDURE	SAMPLE SIZE	PERCENT POSITIVE CULTURE	PREDOMINANT ORGANISMS	REFERENCE #
Extraction	400	49.0	streptococcus	9
Extraction	100	55.0	streptococcus	10
Extraction	80	48.8	streptococcus staphylococcus	11
Dental prophylaxis	32	0.0	-	12
Dental prophylaxis	39	28.0	diptheroids	13

volume and small vessel proliferation[23] renders the patients susceptible to gingival trauma, bleeding and bacteremia. The often peculiar dietary habits of children with cardiac disease and the reluctance of many dentists to treat such patients contribute to the gingival inflammation and poor oral hygiene.

Cardiac Catheterization

Endocarditis following catheterization has been reported in 0.02% of all procedures[24] and estimated to occur in 0.94/1000 patient-years among children with ventricular septal defect, aortic stenosis, and pulmonary stenosis.[2] Cardiac catheterization is an antecedent event in 2% of all children[1] and probably a greater percent of infants.[7] With the widespread use of the percutaneous technique in all pediatric patients, the frequency of bacterial contamination, local infection, endarteritis and endocarditis after catheterization can be expected to diminish further. Because of the rarity of bacteremia and endocarditis after cardiac catheterization, antimicrobial prophylaxis is not routinely administered for this procedure. If contamination or bacteremia is suspected, blood cultures should be obtained and appropriate antibiotics administered. If diaper dermatitis or other local or systemic infection is present, the procedure should be postponed until the infection is cleared.

Cardiac Surgery

Cardiac surgery is an antecedent event in 8–26%[7,25] of infants and children with endocarditis. Endocarditis has been reported in 1.3% of 400 patients operated upon for repair of congenital heart disease.[26] After prosthetic valve replacement in children, the incidence of endocarditis is 4%.[27] The prevalence within 6 months of cardiac surgery for patients with pulmonary stenosis, ventricular septal defect, or aortic stenosis enrolled in the Natural History Study of Congenital Heart Disease has been estimated at 4.3/1000 patient-years.[2] The increased susceptibility to bacterial colonization during and after cardiac surgery has been variously attributed to use of intracardiac foreign body during surgery,[26] multiple indwelling catheters in the perioperative period[28] and failure in aseptic technique. Prevention of endocarditis after cardiac surgery should include meticulous aseptic techniques in the operating room and intensive care unit, and minimal use of implanted foreign materials such as conduits or valves. Indwelling vascular catheters should be removed as early as possible.[28] Despite the temptation to place indwelling catheters in infants in the femoral area, this site should be avoided because the inguinal region is frequently contaminated. We have encountered endocarditis with *Streptococcus fecalis* secondary to an indwelling femoral venous line left in place after cardiac catheterization in anticipation of surgery. Although there are no conclusive studies demonstrating the efficacy of antimicrobial prophylaxis in preventing postsurgical endocarditis, nearly all cardiac surgeons administer antibiotics 12 hours prior to, during and for 5 days after all cardiovascular procedures. We currently give cefazolin.

Extracardiac Anomalies

Extracardiac anomalies occur in approximately 25% of all infants and children with congenital heart disease.[25] The anomalies may lead to infection, bacteremia and subsequent intracardiac or vascular colonization.[29] Genitourinary anomalies present in 5.3%, especially when obstructive, are often associated with inflammatory disease, such as pyelonephritis and cystitis. In such patients, bacteremia may occur spontaneously or in association with a diagnostic or therapeutic genitourinary procedure.[30] Associated extracardiac malformations in the gastrointestinal and genitourinary tract should therefore be routinely excluded.

Infections

Common infections in children, such as pneumonia, acne, impetigo, and pyelonephritis may lead to bacteremia. In the child with a cardiac defect, the risk of bacterial endocarditis is thus increased. Sinusitis, a not infrequent complication of cyanotic congenital heart disease, may also serve as the source of bacteremia and subsequent endocarditis.[31] The asplenia syndrome is almost invariably associated with serious congenital heart disease. Because patients with this syndrome are at increased risk of sepsis, they should be placed on continuous antimicrobial prophylaxis and receive pneumococcal vaccination.[32] The greater prevalence of infective endocarditis in infants with normal hearts may in part be due to the frequent occurrence of sepsis in this age group.[10] Specific factors predisposing infants to bacteremia and endocarditis include omphalitis,[33] intravenous alimentation,[34] cardiac catheterization[7] and ventriculovenous shunt for hydrocephalus.[25,35] Vigorous treatment of all localized pyogenic infections and prompt therapy of sepsis in all infants and children with congenital heart disease should reduce the incidence of infective endocarditis.

Antimicrobial Prophylaxis

General guidelines for chemoprophylaxis are outlined by the American Heart Association recommendations (Chapter 17 and Appendix I). In recommending the choice, route and duration of antibiotic administration for the individual child, one should consider three major factors. These are: the cardiac diagnosis, general health status, and the type of procedure to be performed (Figure 1). Each of these may modify the recommendations for the individual patient. The patient at highest risk for the development of infective endocarditis is one

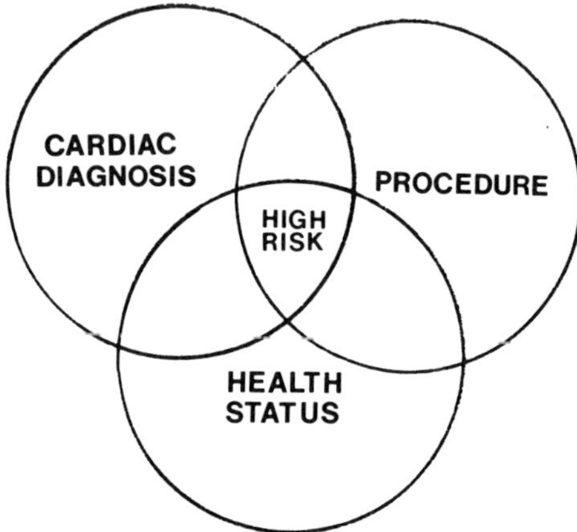

Figure 1: Major factors to be considered in recommending antibiotic prophylaxis for the child susceptible to infective endocarditis.

with a cardiac malformation most likely to be colonized by bacteria, undergoing a procedure associated with marked bacteremia in the presence of a localized or other systemic infection. A few examples serve to illustrate this approach to chemoprophylaxis. The children most vulnerable to endocarditis, such as those with conduits or valve prostheses should receive antimicrobial prophylaxis even for a procedure that usually results in a low frequency of bacteremia such as nasotracheal intubation, or brush biopsy. Parenteral administration of antimicrobial prophylaxis is preferred for high risk patients such as those with aortic valve abnormality or cyanotic congenital heart disease. A postoperative patient with aortic stenosis and severe periodontal disease should receive parenteral rather than oral antibiotics when undergoing dental extraction, because the procedure results in marked bacteremia. If the tooth extracted is abscessed, antibiotic administration should be continued beyond the recommended two days after the procedure. By contrast, the child with valvar pulmonary stenosis or ventricular septal defect, with excellent oral hygiene, undergoing dental prophylaxis may recieve oral penicillin at the recommended regimen. Appropriate recommendation for antimicrobial prophylaxis by the physician should therefore take into account the cardiac diagnosis, type and extent of bacteremia occurring from the procedure and the dental and general health status of the host. When an individual is considered at high risk, recommendations may include more than one antibiotic, to be given parenterally. In many patients, this may require a brief hospitalization.

Treatment

The medical and surgical management of the child with suspected or diagnosed bacterial endocarditis is similar in many respects to the adult with endocarditis and is reviewed elsewhere in this book. For many of the newer drugs, dosage for children is not firmly established, and some drugs are not approved for use in very young infants, for example cefazolin sodium. Dosage in infants and children is calculated on the basis of body weight. The manufacturers, however, should be consulted, especially when newer drugs are used in infants. The concomitant use of diuretics (especially loop diuretics) with aminoglycosides may increase the risk of nephrotoxicity and ototoxicity. These and other drugs should be used with greater caution in neonates because of renal immaturity.[36,37]

In the presence of congestive heart failure, anticongestive therapy may be initiated including digoxin, diuretics, low salt diet and oxygen. In acute onset of pulmonary edema from massive aortic or mitral incompetence, intravenous furosemide and afterload reducing drugs may be life saving, while the patient is awaiting surgery.

Bed rest reduces the workload of the heart and is therefore an important element in the treatment. Younger children should not be restrained since the generated anxiety and struggle may be counterproductive. Ambulation should be gradual, usually after the first or second week, when systemic evidence of infection subsides. Mobility and activity will be limited to some degree by the continued presence of an intravenous line. Sedatives or analgesics are rarely necessary in children. Antipyretic treatment is initiated when elevated temperature causes discomfort or is greater than 103°. Acetaminophen, aspirin, and tepid sponging may be used. Persistent fevers after the first week are often due to drug reaction, phlebitis or continued infection. Anemia should be treated with slow transfusions of packed red blood cells. This is especially crucial in the child with hypoxemia who is dependent on an adequate oxygen carrying capacity for oxygen transport.[23] In acyanotic children, hemoglobin should be maintained at least at 10 grams, and in cyanotic children, it should be greater than 15 grams.

The indications for surgical therapy in endocarditis are described in Chapter 13. In all patients with endocarditis daily observations, frequent examinations and laboratory studies are essential for early detection of complications and appropriate therapy. Psychologic support for the child and family is often neglected, while life saving measures are instituted.

However, it assumes great importance following the first week of hospitalization. Continuity of care by skilled physicians, psychologic support and explanation of the need for prolonged hospitalization will facilitate the child's care and well being. The staff caring for the child should be skilled in performing intravenous punctures and maintenance of IV lines. As the weeks go by, this may be the greatest source of frustration for the child and staff. Contact should be established with the play therapist or hospital school attendant as soon as the child feels well.

The child should preferably remain at the medical center for the entire course of therapy. This will facilitate early detection of any complication and its prompt treatment. A cardiac surgeon should be readily available and consulted early on if surgery is anticipated.

The patient is discharged from the hospital one week after discontinuation of antibiotic therapy, provided blood cultures are sterile and there are no major complications. Return to full activity is usually feasible within a month after discharge. Elective cardiac catheterization, cardiac or noncardiac surgery should be postponed for 6 months to allow sufficient time for the cardiac, renal, pulmonary or other lesions to heal.

REFERENCES

1. Johnson, D.H., Rosenthal, A., Nadas, A.S.: A forty year review of bacterial endocarditis in infancy and childhood. Circulation 51:581, 1975.
2. Gersony, S.M, and Hayes, C.J.: Bacterial endocarditis in pulmonary stenosis, aortic stenosis and ventricular septal defect. Circulation 56: Supp 1, 84–87, 1977.
3. Everett, E.D., Hirschman, J.V.: Transient bacteremia and endocarditis prophylaxis. A review. Medicine 56:61, 1977.
4. Durack, D.T., Petersdorf, R.G.: Chemotherapy of experimental streptococcal endocarditis I. Comparison of commonly recommended prophylactic regimen. J. Clin. Invest. 52:592, 1973.
5. Pelletier, L.L. Jr., Durack, D.T., Petersdorf, R.G.: Chemotherapy of experimental streptococcal endocarditis IV. Further observations on prophylaxis. J. Clin. Invest. 56:319, 1975.
6. Editorial: Prophylaxis of bacterial endocarditis. Faith, Hope and Charitable Interpretations. Lancet 1:519, 1976.
7. Rosenthal, A., and Nadas, A.S.: Infective endocarditis in infants and children. In, Infective endocarditis (ed) Rahimtoola S.H., Grune & Stratton, Inc. 1977.
8. Rosenthal, A.: When to operate on congenital heart disease, In, Controversy in Cardiology, Ed. Chung, E.K., Springer-Verlag Publ.
9. Manning, J.A.: Endocarditis prophylaxis in the child with congenital heart disease after surgery. Presented at the International Symposium on the child with congenital heart disease after surgery, Toronto June 5–7. 1975.

10. Johnson, D.H., Rosenthal, A., Nadas, A.S.: Bacterial endocarditis under two years of age. Am. J. Dis. Child. 129: 183–186, 1975.
11. Kaplan, E.L., Rich, H., Gersony, W.M., and Manning J.A.: A collaborative study of infective endocarditis in the 1970's. Circulation 59:327, 1978.
12. Morris, J.H., McNamara, D.G.: Residua, sequelae and complications of surgery for congenital heart disease in Rosenthal A, Sonnenblich, A.H., Lesch, M., edit: Postoperative congenital heart disease. New York, Grune & Stratton, 1975.
13. Victoria, B.E., Elliot, L.P. and Gessner, I.H.: Ostium secundum atrial septal defect associated with balloon mitral valve in children. Am. J. Cardiol. 33:668, 1974.
14. Taran, L.M.: Rheumatic fever in its relation to dental disease. NY J. Dent. 14:107, 1944.
15. Elliott, R.H. and Dunbar, J.M.: Streptococcal bacteremia in children following dental extraction. Arch. Dis. Child. 43:451, 1968.
16. Petereson, L.J. and Peacock, R.: The incidence of bacteremia in pediatric patients following tooth extraction. *Circulation* 53:676, 1976.
17. Hurwitz, G.A., Speck, W.T., and Keller, B.G.: Absence of bacteremia in children after prophylaxis. Oral Surg. 32:891, 1971.
18. DeLeo, A.A., Schoenknecht, E.D., Anderson, M.W. and Peterson, J.C.: The incidence of bacteremia following oral prophylaxis on pediatric patients. Oral Surg. 37:36, 1974.
19. Cobe, H.M.: Transitory bacteremia. Oral Surgery 7:609, 1954.
20. Silver, J.G., Martin, A.W., and McBride, B.L.: Experimental transient bacteremia in human subjects with varying degrees of plaque accumulation and gingival inflammation. J. Clin. Perio. 4:92, 1977.
21. Lineberger, L.T. and DeMarco, T.J.: Evaulation of Transient bacteremia following routine periodental procedures. P. Perio. 44:757, 1973.
22. Berger, S.A., Weitzman, S., Edberg, S.C. and Casey, J.I.: Bacteremia after use of an oral irrigation device. Ann. Intern. Med. 80:510, 1974.
23. Rosenthal, A., Button, L.N., Nathan, D.G., Miettinen, O.S. and Nadas: Blood volume changes in cyanotic congenital heart disease. Am. J. Cardiol. 27:162–167, 1971.
24. Braunwald, E., Swan, H.J.C., (eds): Cooperative study in cardiac catheterization. Amer. Heart Assoc. Monograph. 20, 1968.
25. Zakrzewski, T.,and Keith, J.D.: Bacterial Endocarditis in Infants and children. J. Pediatr. 67:1179, 1965.
26. Jey, T.J., Ariabtawi, I.N., Cornett, V.E., et al: Bacterial endocarditis following open heart surgery. An. Thorac. Surg. 3:29, 1967.
27. Freed, M.D., Bernhard, W.F.: Prosthetic valve replacement in children. Prog. Cardiovascular Dis. 17:475, 1975.

28. Freeman, R., King, B.: Analysis of results of catheter tip cultures in open heart surgery. Thorax 30:26, 1975.
29. Greenwood, R.D., Rosenthal, A., Parisi, L., Fyler, D.C. and Nadas, A.S.: Extracardiac abnormalities in infants with congenital heart disease, Ped. 55:485, 1975.
30. Sullivan, N.M, Sutter, V.L., Mims, M.M., et al: Clinical aspects of bacteremia after manipulation of the genitourinary tract. J. Infect. Dis. 127:49, 1973.
31. Rosenthal, A., Fellows, K.: Acute infectious sinusitis in cyanotic congenital heart disease. Pediatrics 52: No. 5, 692–696, 1973.
32. Waldman, J.D., Rosenthal, A., Smith, A.L., Shurin, S., Nadas, A.S.: Sepsis and congenital asplenia. J. Ped. 90:555, 1977.
33. Lewis I.C.: Bacterial endocarditis complicating septicemia in an infant. Arch. Dis. Child. 29:144, 1954.
34. Joshi, V.V. and Wang, N.S.: Repeated pulmonary embolism in an infant. Am. J. Dis. Child. 125:257, 1973.
35. Noonan, J.A., Ehmke, D.A.: Complications of ventriculovenous shunts for control of hydrocephalus: Report of three cases with thromboemboli to the lung. N. Eng. J. Med. 269:70, 1963.
36. McCracken, G., Jr., and Nelson, J.: Antimicrobial therapy for newborns: Practical applications of pharmacology to clinical usage. New York. Grune & Stratton, 1977.
37. Griffin, J.P. and D'Arcy, P.F.: A manual of adverse drug interactions. Second Edition. Chicago, Year Book Medical Publishers, Inc, 1979.

Alan L. Bisno, M.D.

17

ANTIMICROBIAL PROPHYLAXIS OF INFECTIVE ENDOCARDITIS

Infective endocarditis is a life-threatening illness which is often dramatic both in its acute clinical manifestations and in its long-term effects on the patient's well-being. As amply documented in the preceding pages of this volume, there are many still unresolved and controversial issues in the therapy of the disease. Fortunately, the incidence of endocarditis remains low enough that the average primary care physician will only rarely be called upon to manage such a patient. In contrast, generalists, pediatricians, cardiologists, surgeons and dentists will, almost without exception, be required with regularity to make decisions regarding the advisability of antimicrobial prophylaxis of bacterial endocarditis, and, if such prophylaxis is deemed necessary, regarding the specific regimen to be employed.

The Committee on Rheumatic Fever and Bacterial Endocarditis of the American Heart Association (AHA), in concert with the Council on Dental Therapeutics of the American Dental Association, publishes a set of official recommendations for prevention of bacterial endocarditis. These recommendations, revised most recently in 1977 (Appendix I) are widely disseminated, published in *Circulation*[1] and quoted in many journal articles and textbook chapters. They are, however, more complicated than the previous AHA recommendations published in 1972, and are based at least in part on data obtained *in vitro* and in experimental animals. For these reasons they have been the subject of considerable debate.[2] In this chapter I shall outline some of the constraints which make any such recommendations regarding prevention of endocarditis somewhat empiric, summarize the facts and assumptions which underlie the current AHA statement, and venture a personal critique. In so doing, I hasten to acknowledge my membership on the committee which formulated the 1977 revision and so accept an appropriate share of responsibility for any defects in the document.

Theoretical Considerations

Antimicrobial prophylaxis of bacterial endocarditis is of course only feasible when one is able to predict the occurrence of a bacteremia. As a practical matter, this limits the use of prophylaxis to a variety of invasive procedures and manipulations of the type performed by physicians (especially surgeons) and dentists. Unfortunately, we approach the subject of prevention of bacterial endocarditis following such procedures from a vantage point of both inadequate knowledge and obvious frustration. Not only do we lack human data indicating the relative efficacy of one or another antibiotic regimen in preventing bacterial endocarditis, we do not even possess firm data indicating that any form of antimicrobial prophylaxis is acutally effective in prevention of this disease in man.

Even if we had at hand an ideal means of prophylaxis, we would be able to prevent only a small proportion of the total number of cases of endocarditis occurring each year. It has been estimated that only about one half of patients undergoing procedures which put them at risk are aware of having underlying heart disease; only about two thirds of cases of endocarditis are due to streptococci of the types against which our prophylactic regimens are ordinarily directed; and only about 20 per cent of patients with endocarditis have had a recognized prior procedure as the initiating event. Using figures such as these, Kaye[3] has calculated that we could at best prevent only about seven per cent of cases of endocarditis by the types of prophylaxis currently recommended.

The risk of endocarditis following a given procedure undoubtledly fluctuates considerably, depending upon the state of hygiene in the bodily area being manipulated and upon the nature of the underlying cardiovascular lesion. Crude estimates of the risk of endocarditis in a susceptible individual undergoing dental extraction range from 1:500 to 1:3000.[4,5] This very low incidence, the unacceptability on ethical grounds of prophylactic trials incorporating placebos, and the extraordinary number of patients required to compare two regimens, both of which are presumably at least partially effective, have so far discouraged any attempts to attack the problem by means of controlled prospective studies. Even case-control studies would be difficult to accomplish due to the large number of variables (e.g., state of periodontal hygiene, cardiovascular lesion, etc.) which would need to be matched.

Unless and until such studies can be organized on a multi-center basis, recommendations regarding endocarditis prophylaxis must be based upon analysis of data derived from four sources: (a) investigations of the frequency of bacteremia and of endocarditis in man following various procedures; (b) clinical studies of the occurrence of endocarditis among patients with different heart lesions; (c) case reports of failures of bacterial endocarditis prophylaxis; and (d) animal models simulating human disease.

Frequency of Bacteremia and Endocarditis Following Various Procedures

Because viridans streptococci are the most frequent causative agents of infective endocarditis, because these organisms comprise a major portion of the normal aerobic flora of the oral cavity, and because of the temporal relationship between dental procedures and onset of endocarditis in many cases, considerable attention has focused upon the incidence of bacteremia after various dental manipulations. Following extractions, bacteremia usually occurs within one to five minutes, lasts only a few minutes and is low grade (10 to 15 colony forming units per milliliter of blood).[6] It has been documented to occur in approximately 50% of children undergoing extraction (chapter 16) and with an even higher frequency (60–80%) in adults.[6,7] Viridans streptococci are the most commonly isolated bacteria, but a variety of other organisms may also be found, including diphtheroids, *Staphylococcus epidermidis,* anaerobic streptococci, gram positive and gram negative anaerobic[7,8] bacilli. Bacteremia has also been documented to occur frequently after a wide range of other dental procedures, such as professional cleaning, gingivectomy, and root planing. To place these observations in proper perspective, it should be noted that bacteria may enter the blood stream after much milder dental trauma, e.g., tooth brushing and flossing, chewing paraffin for prolonged periods and even chewing gum. Most authorities believe that the risk of bacteremia is strongly related to the state of periodontal hygiene, although not all studies have been able to confirm this association.[7]

Surgery or instrumentation of the respiratory, gastrointestinal or genitourinary tracts likewise allows for flora colonizing their respective mucosal surfaces to gain entry into the circulation (Table 1). The range of organisms potentially causing bacteremia following procedures below the diaphragm is broad and includes enterococci and Enterobacteriaceae.

In practice the risk of endocarditis following a given procedure is probably influenced by a number of factors other than the mere occurrence of bacteremia *per se.* Chief among these is undoubtedly the identity of the infecting microorganisms. Viridans streptococci, staphylococci and enterococci account for the great majority of cases of infective endocarditis in virtually all published series, while anaerobes, gram negative aerobic bacteria, and fungi are much less frequent offenders. The intensity and/or duration of bacteremia are still additional factors which might theoretically influence the subsequent occurrence of endocarditis. Thus, data on frequency of bacteremia must be balanced by

Table 1. Selected Studies of Rate of Bacteremia Following Various Procedures*

Author, Year (Ref. number)	Procedure	Patients Studied	Percent Positive	Predominant organism
Elliot, 1939 (9)	Tonsillectomy	100	38.0	Streptococcus, Hemophilus, diphtheroids, other
Burman, 1960 (10)	Bronchoscopy (rigid scope)	52	15.4	Streptococcus, *Staphylococcus epidermidis*, aerobic gram-neg. rods
Pereira et al, 1975 (11)	Bronchoscopy (fiberoptic)	43	0	
Baltch et al, 1975 (12)	Upper gastrointestinal endoscopy	170	12.4	*Staphylococcus epidermidis*, diphtheroids, Streptococcus, Lactobacillus, other
Dickman et al, 1976 (13)	Colonoscopy	52	5.8	*E. coli*, Bacteroides
LeFrock et al, 1975 (14)	Barium enema	175	11.4	Aerobic and anaerobic gram-neg. rods, enterococcus
Marshall, 1961 (15)	Retropubic Prostatectomy			
	Sterile urine	16	12.8	Aerobic gram-neg. rods
	Infected urine	34	82.4	enterococcus
Sullivan et al, 1973 (16)	TUR**	77	31.2	Not tabulated by procedure
	Cystoscopy	81	17.3	Aerobic and anaerobic gram-neg. rods
	Urethral dilation	67	23.9	Enterococcus and other streptococcus
	Urethral catheterization	75	8.0	other
McCormack et al, 1975 (17)	Parturition	327	4.9	Alpha, microaerophilic and anaerobic streptococcus

*Adapted from Everett, E.D., and Hirschmann, J.V.,[7] with permission.
**Transurethral resection of prostate gland

careful consideration of which procedures are known to be epidemiologically associated with infective endocarditis.

Starkebaum et al[18] analyzed 1164 cases of subacute bacterial endocarditis (SBE) collected from a large number of series in the literature. A potential portal of entry was evident in only 38.3% of cases. Dental extractions were implicated in 144 cases, 12.4% of the total. These same authors collected 76 cases of streptococcal SBE in which there was an identifiable procedure preceding onset of symptoms and in which the incubation period was clearly stated. In over 80% of these cases, endocarditis began within two weeks of the implicated procedure. Dental extraction was responsible for 72% of the 60 cases of nonenterococcal streptococcal SBE. Of the 16 enterococcal cases, 50% followed prostatectomy or other urologic procedures, and 37% followed obstetric or gynecologic procedures.

Cardiovascular Lesions Associated with Endocarditis

In the pre-antibiotic era, the great majority of cases of infective endocarditis occurred in patients with congenital or rheumatic valvular heart disease. These two entities still account for a substantial proportion of cases; the relative risks associated with specific congenital lesions are outlined in chapter 16. Because the incidence of acute rheumatic fever and rheumatic carditis has declined dramatically in the U.S. over the past four decades it is to be anticipated that rheumatic heart disease will play a relatively minor role in the future as a precursor of endocarditis. On the other hand, a number of other entities, some of them newly recognized, are now being reported frequently in association with endocarditis. These include idiopathic hypertrophic subaortic stenosis, myxomatous degeneration of cardiac valves, and the syndrome of mitral valve prolapse (MVP). The two auscultatory features of this latter syndrome, mid-systolic click and late apical systolic murmur (LASM), are common among healthy young women.[19–21] Systematic echocardiographic studies of this population group have revealed MVP in from six to 21% of subjects tested.[19,20]

The overall incidence of infective endocarditis in patients with MVP syndrome cannot yet be stated with precision. Two long-term follow-up studies have been published, however. Allen et al[22] followed-up 58 patients who had previously been found to have phonocardiographic evidence of LASM; the average period of follow-up was 14 years. Five patients (8.6%) had developed bacterial endocarditis in the interim. In a similar study, Mills et al[23] followed 53 patients with phonocardiographically proven LASM or systolic click. During a mean follow-up of 13.7 years, three patients (5.7%) developed endocarditis. Analysis of 25 patients with MVP and bacterial endocarditis seen at Stanford Medical Center suggested that MVP was the basis of about one-third of instances of bacterial endocarditis associated with isolated mitral regurgitation at that institution.[24] Eighty-eight per cent of these patients had holosystolic murmurs at the time of presentation, leading the authors to speculate that the risk of endocarditis might be appreciably greater among patients with more severe mitral regurgitation.

In patients over 60 years of age, endocarditis frequently develops in patients with no previously diagnosed heart disease, although many of these may have been told of a heart murmur sometime previously.[25] In these patients, the underlying disorder may consist of degenerative forms of heart disease, including calcific changes in the aortic and mitral valves.[26]

Other groups of patients found prone to develop endocarditis in recent years include dialysis patients with arteriovenous shunts, hospitalized patients requiring indwelling intravenous catheters for fluid therapy or parenteral hyperalimentation, and those with a previous episode of endocarditis for whatever cause. Two groups at very high risk are individuals with prosthetic cardiac valves (chapter 12) and drug addicts. The latter develop endocarditis with a wide variety of organisms (staphylococci, fungi and gram-negative rods), often right-sided and frequently on previously normal valves.

Reports of Failure of Endocarditis Prophylaxis

Case reports of endocarditis failures have been infrequent in the medical literature. Nearly 20 such cases are cited in the recent brief editorial review by McGowan.[27] At least one additional case has appeared subsequently in the literature.[28] Review of these cases[28-34] indicates that, for the most part, they shed very little light on the problem. Cases reported in the older literature generally involved much smaller dosages of penicillin than we are now accustomed to giving. Most of the reports are vague as to the specific regimens employed and the exact timing of doses. In many instances the antimicrobial susceptibility of the endocarditis strain is omitted. It is noteworthy, however, that in virtually every published case in which the preceding event was a dental procedure, it consisted of a single or multiple dental extractions.

Table 2 summarizes the salient features of some seven reported cases in which the antibiotic regimens consisted of doses of penicillin which are in the general range currently recommended. In each of the first four cases cited, loading doses of penicillin were given 30 to 60 minutes prior to the procedure, and penicillin was continued for two or three days thereafter. Nevertheless, three of the patients developed endocarditis with a penicillin-sensitive viridans streptococcus. In the fourth instance the infecting bacterium was not stated. In the latter three cases, prophylaxis was started one to four days prior to the extraction. In two of these cases penicillin-resistant viridans streptococci were the cause of the endocarditis, and in the third, *Eikenella corrodens* infected a prosthetic Starr - Edwards valve. These data, although extremely limited, provide support

Table 2. Selected Cases of Failure of Endocarditis Prophylaxis After Dental Extraction

Author (Reference)	Year	Regimen	Organism	Penicillin sensitivity
Dormer (29)	1958	500,000 u* crystalline penicillin 30 mins. before, then 300,000 u procaine penicillin twice daily for three days	Viridans streptococcus	Sens.
Barnes & Hurley (30)	1963	1,000,000 u crystalline penicillin 1 hr. before, then twice that day, twice next day, once third day	Viridans streptococcus	Sens.
Neutze & Arter (31)	1973	1,000,000 u penicillin G 1 hr. before, oral penicillin three times a day for three days	Not stated	Not stated
Durack & Littler (32)	1974	1,000,000 u penicillin G + 500 mg cloxacillin intramuscularly 1 hr. before, then 1,000,000 u penicillin G intramuscularly every twelve hours for three doses, plus cloxacillin 500 mg every six hours for eight doses	Viridans streptococcus	MIC**.01 μgm/ml
McCarthy et al (28)	1979	Penicillin V 250 mg orally four times a day for 72 hours starting 24 hrs. before	*S. sanguis* 1	MIC 1.6u/ml MBC***6.4u/ml
Garrod et al (33)	1962	500,000 u penicillin every six hours starting two & four days before	Viridans streptococcus	4u/ml
Geraci et al (34)	1974	250 mg erythromycin four times daily starting day before; 1 gm. cephalothin 1 hr. after	*Eikenella corrodens* (Prosthetic valve)	Erythromycin MIC 0.5 μgm/ml

*units
**Minimal inhibitory concentration
***Minimum bactericidal concentration

for the AHA's recommendation that prophylaxis should not be be initiated until shortly before the planned procedure.

In view of the infeasibility of prospective studies of endocarditis prophylaxis and the paucity of published data concerning failures, the AHA's Committee on Rheumatic Fever and Bacterial Endocarditis has recently organized a registry of endocarditis prophylaxis failures and solicited case reports by letters in medical journals and direct mailings to physicians on the rosters of the AHA and Infectious Diseases Society of America. Data are still under analysis and indeed still accumulating, but preliminary results are of interest. Of twenty-five reports received by the committee which meet reasonable criteria for prophylaxis failure, 88% followed dental procedures and 91% of the etiologic agents isolated were viridans streptococci.[35] One of the penicillins had been used in 23%. Oral prophylaxis alone had been administered to 72% with the rest receiving parenteral or combined parenteral-oral regimens. Most of the etiologic agents were sensitive to the antibiotic that had been given.

Interestingly, the most common cardiac lesion underlying these cases of endocarditis was MVP (36%), followed by congenital (32%) and rheumatic (24%) lesions. Twelve percent of cases occurred on combined lesions and 16% of infections were in patients with prosthetic valves. Patients failing oral prophylaxis generally received low-dose regimens rather that the initial loading dose recommended currently by the AHA.

Prevention of Endocarditis in the Rabbit Model

The experimental model of infective endocarditis now in wide use is a modification of the technique described by Garrison and Freedman.[36] As currently employed, a polyethylene catheter is passed into the heart via a jugular vein (right-sided endocarditis) or a common corotid artery (left-sided lesion) and allowed to remain in place for 24 to 72 hours, during which time sterile vegetations develop on the valve in contact with the catheter. In studies of prophylaxis, the desired parenteral regimen is then initiated and, after approximately 30 minutes, a large challenge dose of microorganisms is injected intravenously. Efficacy of the regimens is evaluated by sacrificing the rabbits one or two days later and quantitatively culturing the excised cardiac vegetations. Using this technique, Durack and associates[37–39] have evaluated a number of antibiotic dosages and combinations for prophylactic efficacy against a penicillin - sensitive viridans streptococcus (*S. sanguis,* serotype II) and against a number of enterococcal (*S. faecalis)* strains. Their results may be summarized as follows: (a) bacteriostatic antibiotics were ineffective; (b) penicillin was most effective when administered in schedules which provided for both a high initial blood level and persistence of substantial levels for 12 hours or more; (c) the combination of a penicillin plus an aminoglycoside antibiotic was synergistic against both the viridans streptococcus tested and against enterococci; (d) vancomycin was a highly effective prophylactic agent against the viridans streptococcus and against the enterococci as well. (Data from certain of these experiments are presented in Tables 2 and 3, chapter 2). Based upon these results, a ranking of antibiotics according to relative prophylactic efficacy in the experimental model[40] may be constructed (Tables 3 and 4). Of greatest import for formulation of recommendations in humans is the fact that one of the regimens most widely used for dental prophylaxis - namely, penicillin V without a loading dose - is ineffective in the rabbit model. Moreover, erythromycin, the most widely used form of oral prophylaxis in penicillin-allergic patients, is not highly effective.

There has been considerable debate regarding the relevance of the rabbit model as a guide to selection of prophylactic regimens in humans. On the one hand, the model has many features which mimic endocarditis in man. Organisms most likely to cause endocarditis in humans are most effective in initiating infection in the rabbit model. The resulting infection gives rise to vegetations similar to those seen in man as well as to a constant bacteremia and, eventually, to death. On the other hand, the fact that the bacteria are presented in a single bolus of very high inoculum (usually about 10^8 organisms) raises the question of the comparability of the situation in rabbits to that in humans, particularly when one speaks of experiments designed to test *prophylactic* regimens. The studies of viridans streptococci were performed using only a single bacterial strain. Moreover, the fact that the experiments were performed with a foreign body (the intravascular catheter) left in place during the period of bacterial challenge makes the model somewhat more akin to prosthetic valve endocarditis than to the cases of endocarditis seen most frequently in general medical practice. These observations are not intended to denigrate a highly ingenious and useful series of experiments. Indeed, many of the problems listed above are inherent in the experimental design when one is trying to achieve high enough attack rates to allow statistically meaningful conclusions. They do indicate the need, however, for caution in extrapolating directly data obtained in this model to prevention of disease in humans. Nevertheless, as Dr. Durack[40] has stated, "any regimen that proved effective under these rigorous experimental conditions should provide a margin of safety in clinical use".

AHA Recommendations for Prevention of Infective Endocarditis: A Reappraisal

Given the basic facts set forth above, a number of practical issues immediately present themselves. First of all, is antimicrobial prophylaxis of endocarditis worthwhile at all? It is inconvenient, often expensive, and exposes the patient to the hazards of allergic and toxic reactions; its efficacy in man is unproven; and on theoretical grounds it would be expected, at best, to prevent only a small minority of all cases of

Table 3. Efficacy of Various Antibiotics in Preventing Endocarditis due to a Viridans Streptococcus in Rabbit Model*

Effective
- Penicillin G plus streptomycin
- Repeated penicillin V with large loading dose
- Vancomycin

Partially effective
- Procaine penicillin G
- Repeated erythromycin
- Cefazolin plus streptomycin
- Streptomycin

Ineffective

Ampicillin	Clindamycin
Penicillin G	Erythromycin
Penicillin V without loading dose	Rifampin
	Tetracycline
Cefazolin, cephalexin	Trimethoprim-sulfamethoxazole

*From Durack, D.T. (40)

Table 4. Efficacy of Various Antibiotics in Preventing Enterococcal Endocarditis in the Rabbit Model*

Effective
- Ampicillin plus gentamicin
- Ampicillin plus streptomycin
- Vancomycin (high dose)
- Vancomycin (lower dose) plus streptomycin

Partially effective
- Vancomycin (lower dose)
- Ampicillin
- Streptomycin

Ineffective
- Gentamicin
- Cefazolin
- Cefazolin plus gentamicin

*From Durack, D.T. (40)

endocarditis. Opinions on this question vary widely. Hilson[5] has called for a controlled trial of prophylaxis, with antibiotics omitted in half of the susceptible individuals who undergo dental extractions or similar procedures. Such a trial is most unlikely to occur in the U.S., both because of the many thousands of subjects required for such a study and the ethical issues involved. Oakley and associates[41–43], on the other hand, suggest that prophylaxis should be given before *all* dental procedures associated with bacteremias, even in individuals with normal cardiovascular systems! The consensus of most authorities in the field, with which this author concurs, is that endocarditis prophylaxis is advisable for those individuals whose underlying cardiovascular status places them at increased risk of infective endocarditis and who are undergoing procedures which have been epidemiologically associated with the development of endocarditis.

It is for this reason that the AHA's recommendations, first published in 1965 as a modest statement of just over one printed page, were promulgated. With each revision (1972 and 1977) these recommendations have become more specific, more complex and more controversial. This is particularly true of the 1977 version, which undertook to deal with several major issues, as outlined below.

What types of cardiovascular lesions require prophylaxis? The current AHA recommendations in this regard are summarized in Table 5. They are for the most part straight-forward, although it is impossible to evaluate the need for prophylaxis in every conceivable clinical condition. The term "other acquired valvular heart disease" is necessarily a vague one, which refers primarily to the various calcific and degenerative lesions now being found associated with endocarditis in the elderly, as well as to myxomatous changes seen in patients with Marfan's syndrome. The issue of which elderly patients with heart murmurs deserve further workup to establish the presence of significant valvular pathology is one to be decided at the bedside and goes beyond the scope of a written recommendation.

One of the most significant changes between the 1972 and 1977 statements, reflecting recent clinical experience, was the specific inclusion of MVP as an indication for prophylaxis. The recommendation presents some serious problems. The reportedly high prevalence of MVP in normal individuals[19–21] could result in very large numbers of otherwise healthy persons, who are almost certainly at rather low risk of endocarditis, being subjected to repeated courses of antibiotics. On the other hand, there is certainly adequate documentation in the literature from long-term follow-up studies, individual case reports and collections of cases, that MVP syndrome is a precursor of endocarditis. The dilemma might be resolved if one were able to identify certain subsets of patients falling into this diagnostic category who are at particularly great risk of endocarditis and others who are not. The data of Corrigall et al[24] reviewed above, and our knowledge of the pathophysiology of endocarditis suggest that patients with definite valvular insufficiency might be at considerably greater risk.

Table 5. Antimicrobial Prophylaxis of Bacterial Endocarditis*

A. Prophylaxis required

- Prosthetic heart valve
- Most congenital heart disease, including:
  - Ventricular septal defect
  - Tetralogy of Fallot
  - Aortic stenosis
  - Pulmonic stenosis
  - Complex cyanotic heart disease
  - Patent ductus arteriosus
  - Systemic to pulmonary artery shunts
- Rheumatic valvular heart disease
- Idiopathic hypertrophic subaortic stenosis
- Mitral valve prolapse syndrome with mitral insufficiency
- Other acquired valvular heart disease
- Documented previous episode of infective endocarditis

B. Prophylaxis not required

- Uncomplicated secundum atrial defect
- Six months or more after surgery for:
  - Uncomplicated secundum atrial septal defect repaired by direct suture without a prosthetic patch
  - Ligation and division of patent ductus arteriosus
- Following surgery for coronary artery bypass grafting

C. Need for prophylaxis not established

- Ventriculoatrial shunt for hydrocephalus
- Indwelling transvenous cardiac pacemakers
- Implanted arteriovenous shunt for renal hemodialysis

*Adapted from AHA (1). For complete text of statement see appendix I.

Assessment of MVP may be aided considerably by echocardiography, provided the echocardiographer is both skilled in its performance and highly experienced in interpretation. Its role is limited, however, because of the expense and sophistication of the technique and the large number of individuals potentially requiring evaluation. Thus, in everyday medical practice, the decision frequently faced is: which auscultatory findings qualify a patient for prophylaxis? Is a mid-systolic click alone adequate? Is a LASM indicative of valvular regurgitation necessary? The AHA recommendations imply the latter.

This is a well-nigh insoluble diagnostic dilemma. The exact incidence of click and click-murmur syndromes is difficult to ascertain in the general population because of the subtle and often variable character of the auscultatory manifestations. In the case of patients with endocarditis, one frequently does not know whether the apical systolic murmur is a manifestation of the MVP syndrome or of the endocarditis itself, or both. The author has seen one case of infective endocarditis in an MVP patient with no murmur present on admission; several others are documented in the medical literature. Nevertheless, I agree with the current AHA recommendation in the case of asymptomatic individuals with MVP. It is a conservative one, and this would seem prudent in view of our current state of confusion regarding the actual risk of endocarditis in these patients and considering the prevalence of asymptomatic systolic clicks in otherwise healthy persons. In this as in other aspects of the statement, however, physicians should be cognizant of the fact that committee recommendations are likely to be framed conservatively because they are basically consensus statements and because they must be generalized to large population groups. Practitioners should feel free to make exceptions in those areas wherein the mass of data are clearly inconclusive and controversial.

The above remarks apply with equal force to the items listed in Table 5, category C ("Need for prophylaxis not established"). Kaye,[44] for example, recommends prophylaxis for all patients with intracardiac pacemakers and shunts for hemodialysis.

What procedures require endocarditis prophylaxis? Such data as are available regarding frequency of bactermia and of endocarditis following various procedures (see above) are fragmentary, and it is not possible to make dogmatic pronouncements about the risk of endocarditis associated with every one of the myriad of potential procedures which physicians and dentists perform in care of their patients. The recommendations embodied in Tables 6 and 7 do cover a number of the most frequent procedures and represent at least educated guesses as to the risk-benefit ratios involved in prophylaxis of each. They leave an appropriate degree of responsibility with the individual physician (e.g., the necessity of prophylaxis for fiberoptic bronchoscopy without brushing or biopsy— a procedure associated with a low risk of bacteremia). Many practitioners, this author included would be even more vigorous in patients with

Table 6. Procedures and Conditions Which Require Endocarditis Prophylaxis*

All dental procedures (including routine professional cleaning) likely to cause gingival bleeding

Tonsillectomy

Adenoidectomy

Bronchoscopy—especially with a rigid bronchoscope

Surgical procedures involving the respiratory mucosa

Surgery or instrumentation of the genitourinary tract, especially urethral or prostatic manipulations

Urethral catheterization, whether the urine is infected or not

Surgery and instrumentation of the lower gastrointestinal tract and gall bladder

Obstetrical infections, including septic abortion or peri-partum infection

Surgery on any infected or contaminated tissues, including incision and drainage of abscesses

*Adapted from AHA (1). For complete text see appendix I.

Table 7. Procedures Which Do Not Ordinarily Require Endocarditis Prophylaxis*,**

Spontaneous shedding of deciduous teeth

Simple adjustment of orthodontic appliances

Uncomplicated vaginal delivery

Upper gastrointestinal endoscopy (without biopsy)

Percutaneous liver biopsy

Barium enema

Pelvic examination

Dilatation and curettage of uterus

Uncomplicated insertion or removal of intrauterine contraceptive device

Diagnostic cardiac catheterization and angiography

*Adapted from AHA (1). For complete text of statement see appendix I.

**Prophylaxis should be considered on an individual basis for certain of these procedures in the patient with a prosthetic heart valve. See appendix I.

prosthetic heart valves, because of the increased incidence of endocarditis in these patients[45] and the poor prognosis in such individuals should they become infected. For example, I would routinely give prophylaxis to any such patient undergoing a uterine dilatation and curettage and probably also an upper gastrointestinal endoscopy or normal vaginal delivery, despite the low risk of bacteremia and endocarditis reported for the latter procedures.[12,46]

What specific antibiotic regimens are indicated for prevention of bacterial endocarditis? Significant changes were made in the 1977 revision of the endocarditis prevention statement regarding the antimicrobial regimens recommended for prophylaxis of dental and upper respiratory tract procedures (Table 8). These changes, reflecting data from the rabbit endocarditis model, have proved to be the most controversial aspect of the statement, in part perhaps because dental prophylaxis is such a common and recurring problem in the lives of patients with congential heart disease or acquired valvular lesions.

The statement indicates that "parenteral administration is favored when practical".[1] Such practicality is extremely doubtful for most cases of dental prophylaxis. Few dentists administer parenteral antibiotics in their offices. The logistics of getting the injection administered, presumably in a private physician's office or public clinic, 30 to 60 minutes prior to the procedure are thus quite difficult. Moreover, in order to administer parenteral penicillin as recommended by the AHA, it is necessary for the physician or dentist to mix aqueous crystalline penicillin G (ACPG), 1,000,000 units, with procaine penicillin G, 600,000 units. Many physicians do not maintain office stocks of ACPG. The Committee on Rheumatic Fever and Bacterial Endocarditis of the AHA has contacted major pharmaceutical manufacturers regarding marketing of a single-dose, pre-prepared combination of ACPG-procaine penicillin G in the doses currently recommended for adults, but none has expressed interest in the project.

In terms of specific regimens, the 1977 statement increased the amounts of ACPG and procaine penicillin G to be given intramuscularly, omitted penicillin G from the available choices, and, when oral prophylaxis with penicillin V was to be used, required an initial loading dose. An equally acceptable regimen was so-called "regimen B", a combination of parenteral penicillin *plus streptomycin* followed by oral penicillin V. Thus, practitioners were given a choice of an oral or parenteral-oral form of penicillin therapy, but they also had AHA sanction for using the regimen most effective in animal models, namely, penicillin-streptomycin.

The addition of this penicillin-streptomycin regimen as a recommended alternative for routine dental prophylaxis, even in patients without prosthetic heart valves, has, in the opinion of this author, been a mistake, for the following reasons. (1) There is not yet adequate documentation that the previously recommended regimens are associated with an unacceptably high failure rate. (2) The vast majority of

Table 8. Prophylaxis for Dental Procedures and Surgery of the Upper Respiratory Tract: AHA Recommendations*

Adults with no history of penicillin allergy**

Regimen A

1. Parenteral - oral combined
   Aqueous crystalline penicillin G
   1,000,000 units intramuscularly
   mixed with
   Procaine penicillin G
   600,000 units intramuscularly
   Followed by
   Penicillin V, 500 mg. orally, every 6 hours for 8 doses

2. Oral Penicillin V, 2.0 grams orally 1½ to 2 hours prior to procedure
   followed by
   Penicillin V, 500 mg. orally, every 6 hours for 8 doses

Regimen B: Penicillin plus streptomycin. Same as regimen A1 (parenteral-oral combined) except that streptomycin, 1.0 gram intramuscularly, is given at the same time as the parenteral penicillin injection

Adults who are penicillin allergic**

1. Parenteral - oral combined
   Vancomycin, 1.0 gram intravenously over 30 to 60 minutes. Start initial vancomycin infusion ½ to 1 hour prior to procedure
   Follow with:
   Erythromycin, 500 mg. orally, every 6 hours for 8 doses

2. Oral
   Erythromycin, 1.0 gram orally 1½ to 2 hours prior to the procedure
   followed by
   Erythromycin, 500 mg. orally, every 6 hours for 8 doses

*Adapted from AHA (1). See appendix I for details.

**For children's dosages, see appendix I.

prophylaxis for dental procedures is administered by dentists themselves and is almost certain to consist of penicillin V orally, unless some very hard evidence can be produced to indicate that this is insufficient. (3) Streptomycin is a seldom-used drug today, and many younger physicians and dentists are not comfortable with it. (4) Although rabbit model data indicate that penicillin-streptomycin is the most effective preventative combination (along with vancomycin), such ultimate protection may not be needed in the human situation, in which the magnitude of bacteremia is surely many orders of magnitude lower than in the rabbit model and in which, if the bacterium does reach the heart valve, we are attempting to eradicate the bacterial nidus from an endothelial surface rather than from a polyethylene catheter. (5) The inclusion of the penicillin-streptomycin regimen considerably complicates the recommendation, often leaving the physician or dentist confused as to its aims and priorities.

The insertion of this regimen into the statement may have created a "credibility gap", tending to dilute the effect of the entire document. I do agree that the penicillin-streptomycin regimen is warranted in patients with prosthetic heart valves; it should be reserved for such patients. Individual physicians may also wish to avail themselves of the theoretical advantages of the combination in other special circumstances, e.g., multiple extractions in a patient with significant peridontal disease and a "high risk" heart lesion.

Other authoritative sources also down-play the use of streptomycin for routine dental prophylaxis in patients without prosthetic heart valves.[47] Indeed, Dr. Petersdorf, one of the investigators who has provided us with much of our information regarding endocarditis prevention in the rabbit model, challenges the AHA's emphasis upon parenteral prophylaxis of any kind for routine dental procedures. He asserts that such parenteral prophylaxis for endocarditis due to viridans streptococci "should be reserved for high risk patients, such as those with prosthetic heart valves, and need not be used for patients without such intracardiac devices".[2]

Most patients with prosthetic heart valves receive oral anticoagulant therapy. Use of the parenteral penicillin or penicillin-streptomycin regimens requires intramuscular injections, which are relatively contraindicated in such individuals. Experienced physicians, including hematologists and coagulation experts, differ considerably in their evaluation of the risk of serious hematoma formation under such circumstances. Options open to the attending physician include: utilizing intramuscular injections with appropriate precautions and careful observation; discontinuing anticogulation briefly prior to the procedure;[48] administering intravenous vancomycin; utilizing forms of penicillin and aminoglycosides which may be given by the intravenous route, or depending upon oral prophylaxis. The decision must be individualized.

In the penicillin-allergic patient who requires antibiotic prophylaxis prior to dental procedures, the currently recommended regimen consists of an initial dose of erythromycin, 1.0 gram orally, followed by 500 mg.

every 6 hours for 2 days. This represents a doubling of the previously recommended erythromycin dose. Occasionally, physicians have reported that their patients exhibit gastrointestinal intolerance to the large initial dosage. The alternative agent, vancomycin, is not practical in the usual case because of the cost of the drug: currently in excess of $20 per gram to pharmacists in the Memphis area. The cost to the consumer, including attendant costs of intravenous administration, will be significantly more than this. The drug should be administered under professional supervision and would certainly need to be given in a physician's office, outpatient clinic or hospital. This problem becomes virtually insoluble in the patient requiring multiple, frequently-spaced dental visits. While such expense and inconvenience may well be tolerable in the case of penicillin-allergic patients with prosthetic heart valves, it is unlikely to be acceptable in most other instances. Some consideration should be given to the use of oral cephalosporins in erythromycin-intolerant individuals whose prior penicillin reaction was not anaphylactic in type. Calculating the risk-benefit ratio of such prophylaxis is difficult because of the poor performance of oral cephalosporins in the rabbit model and because of uncertainty as to the safety of oral cephalosporins in penicillin-allergic patients.

Prophylaxis for "below the belt" procedures is directed primarily against enterococci. The necessity for synergistic combinations of cell-wall active antibiotics is well-documented. Current recommendations, therefore, (Table 9) call for combinations of ACPG or ampicillin plus either gentamicin or streptomycin. Vancomycin plus streptomycin is prescribed for penicillin allergic patients.

Krogstad et al[49] have demonstrated that high level resistance to streptomycin and kanamycin among some clinical isolates of enterococci is associated with a 45 megadalton plasmid, and that the same plasmid is also responsible for the resistance observed in these strains to penicillin aminoglycoside synergy. Such high-level resistant strains (minimum inhibitory concentration >2000 μgm/ml to streptomycin and kanamycin) have been reported to comprise 25 to 50 percent of clinical isolates from several cities in the U.S. (chapter 6). Almost all these strains are still susceptible *in vitro* to the synergistic bactericidal effect of penicillin and gentamicin. Moreover, Murillo et al[50] administered streptomycin, gentamicin or amikacin, each in combination with ampicillin, to six healthy adult volunteers in a crossover manner and determined the serum bactericidal activity against 16 strains of enterococci. The gentamicin–ampicillin combination produced higher serum bactericidal titers for a longer duration that the other two regimens. This effect was noted not only against the 3 strains which were highly streptomycin-resistant but also against 13 strains which were only moderately streptomycin-resistant, despite the lower serum levels attained with gentamicin in comparison to the other aminoglycosides tested. These observations raise the question of

Table 9. Antimicrobial Prophylaxis for Gastrointestinal and Genitourinary Tract Surgery and Instrumentation*

1. Adults who are not allergic to penicillin**

   Aqueous crystalline penicillin G, 2,000,000 units intramuscularly or intravenously

   or

   Ampicillin, 1.0 gram intramuscularly or intravenously

   plus

   Gentamicin, 1.5 mg/kg (not to exceed 80 mg) intramuscularly or intravenously

   or

   Streptomycin, 1.0 gram intramuscularly

   Give initial doses 30 minutes to 1 hour prior to procedure. If gentamicin is used, then give a similar dose of gentamicin and penicillin (or ampicillin) every 8 hours for 2 additional doses. If streptomycin is used then give a similar dose of streptomycin and penicillin (or ampicillin) every 12 hours for two additional doses.

2. Adults who are allergic to penicillin**

   Vancomycin, 1.0 gram intranveously given over 30 to 60 minutes

   plus

   Streptomycin, 1.0 gram intramuscularly.

   A single dose of these antibiotics begun 30 to 60 minutes prior to the procedure is probably sufficient, but the same dose may be repeated in 12 hours.

*Adapted from AHA (1).

**For children's dosages and important footnotes, see appendix I.

whether streptomycin should be omitted from the prophylactic regimen for genitourinary and gastrointestinal surgery or instrumentation.

The issue is more complex than it might seem at first blush, however. In chapter 7 of this volume, Kaye points out the paucity of data indicating penicillin-streptomycin treatment failures in endocarditis due to highly streptomycin-resistant enterococci, and, by the same token, the lack of clear-cut data supporting the efficacy of penicillin-gentamicin in treatment of infections due to such organisms. Durack et al[39] reported only modest success (50% cure rate) in treating experimental endocarditis due to a highly streptomycin-resistant strain of *S. faecalis* with repeated doses of ampicillin plus gentamicin. Finally, Moellering et al[51] have recently reported an enterococcal strain resistant to penicillin-gentamicin (but not penicillin-tobramycin or penicillin-kanamycin) synergism, and French workers[52] have reported isolation of enterococci with transmissible high-level gentamicin resistance. Obviously, the situation regarding enterococcal suspectibility to multiple aminoglycoside antibiotics is in flux, and any recommendation for prophylaxis will remain open to challenge. Because there is no compelling evidence to suggest prophylactic combinations containing gentamicin are *less* effective that those containing streptomycin, and because gentamicin is much more widely used today and can be administered either intravenously or intramuscularly, simplicity would suggest the virtue of using this agent exclusively until changing susceptibility patterns dictate otherwise.

Special Considerations

Patients receiving oral or high dose parenteral penicillin therapy harbor in their oral cavities alpha hemolytic streptococci which are modestly or even highly resistant to penicillin. This is also true of patients receiving continuous oral penicillin for rheumatic fever prophylaxis. On the other hand, the very low level of penicillinemia achieved by monthly intramuscular benzathine penicillin G prophylaxis is not ordinarily associated with major changes in the penicillin-susceptibility of oral streptococci, nor is continuous rheumatic fever prophylaxis with oral sulfadiazine.[53] There are examples in the medical literature of endocarditis due to penicillin-resistant viridans streptococci occurring in patients on penicillin therapy or oral penicillin prophylaxis.[33,54]

Patients requiring endocarditis prophylaxis who are receiving or have recently completed therapeutic courses of penicillin should probably delay elective dental procedures for two or more weeks to allow restoration of penicillin-sensitive oral microflora.[53] If dental prophylaxis is required in patients receiving penicillin (excepting those on intramuscular benzathine penicillin G) consideration should be given to alternative regimens such as vancomycin, parenteral penicillin-streptomycin, or oral erythromycin. (The efficacy of the latter regimen is, of course, on theoretical and experimental grounds, less secure.)

Patients undergoing cardiac surgery employing extracorporeal circulation – especially if such surgery involves placement of prosthetic intravascular devices – are at risk of developing endocarditis in the perioperative period. "Early-onset" prosthetic valve endocarditis (PVE) (chapter 12) is most frequently due to *Staphylococcus epidermidis* or *Staphylococcus aureus,* although a variety of other organisms may also be responsible. Controlled, prospective studies[55,56] have failed to confirm a beneficial effect of prophylactic antibiotics in preventing early-onset PVE, but interpretation of these data are hampered by early termination of the study in one case[55] and the absence of any cases of PVE in the placebo group in another.[56]

It is currently routine in cardiovascular surgery units with which this author is familiar to administer prophylactic antibiotics in the perioperative period to patients undergoing valve replacement. It is impossible to design a regimen which would "cover" all potential pathogens, and prolonged use of broad-spectrum antibiotics may predispose to suprainfection with highly-antibiotic resistant organisms, if not on the valve itself then at distant body sites (e.g., post-operative pneumonia, urinary tract infection, sternotomy infection). Prophylaxis at the time of open heart surgery should be directed primarily towards staphylococci, should be started immediately before the procedure, and should be brief.[57] Designing an appropriate regimen is complicated by the fact that many *Staphylococcus epidermidis* strains, particularly hospital strains, may be resistant to semi-synthetic penicillinase-resistant penicillins (methicillin, oxacillin, nafcillin); infections with such strains often do not respond well to cephalosporins, regardless of *in vitro* sensitivities. For adults, Durack[58] recommends cefazolin 2 grams intramuscularly or intravenously 30 minutes preoperatively and repeated every 8 hours for 5 additional doses; gentamicin, 1.5 mg /kg intramuscularly or intravenously may be given by the same dosage schedule. For children the dosage of cefazolin is 30 mg/kg and of gentamicin is 2.0 mg/kg, given in the same dosage schedule. In most instances, I believe a cephalosporin alone should suffice.

Despite all that has been written concerning rational prophylaxis of bacterial endocarditis, considerable confusion remains. For example, only 14.5% of 359 Michigan dentists recently surveyed[59] actually follow the 1977 AHA guidelines for oral penicillin V prophylaxis! Moreover, physicians and dentists alike tend to confuse prophylaxis for prevention of rheumatic fever with that for endocarditis. The former consists of continuous low doses of penicillin, sulfadiazine, or erythromycin designed to prevent upper respiratory infections with group A streptococci[60] and is inadequate to prevent endocarditis. Thus, patients with valvular heart disease receiving rheumatic prophylaxis require endocarditis prophylaxis as well when undergoing dental or surgical procedures. Indeed, if the rheumatic prophylaxis consists of daily oral penicillin, this may well affect the endocarditis prophylactic regimen prescribed (see above).

Although this review has focused upon prevention of bacterial endocarditis by antimicrobial agents, there are a number of other measures which may actually be more effective. These include maintenance of an optimal state of oral hygiene, prompt detection and eradication of peripheral foci of infection (skin, oral cavity, urinary tract, etc.) which might lead to bacteremia and endocarditis, and minimization of the use of indwelling intravascular catheters during periods of hospitalization in patients at increased risk of developing endocarditis.

REFERENCES

1. American Heart Association, Committee on Rheumatic Fever and Bacterial Endocarditis: Prevention of Bacterial Endocarditis. Circulation 56:139A, 1977.
2. Petersdorf, R.G.: Antimicrobial prophylaxis of bacterial endocarditis: prudent caution or bacterial overkill? Amer J Med 65:220, 1978.
3. Kaye, D.: Prophylaxis against bacterial endocarditis: a dilemma, in Kaplan, E.L., and Taranta, A.V., eds., Infective Endocarditis: AHA Monograph No. 52, Dallas, Tex., 1977. p. 67.
4. Hook, E.W., and Kaye, D.: Prophylaxis of endocarditis. J Chron Dis 15:635, 1962.
5. Hilson, G.R.F.: Is chemoprophylaxis necessary? Proc. Royal Soc. Med. 63:267, 1970.
6. Okell, C.C., and Elliot, S.D.: Bacteremia and oral sepsis with special reference to the aetiology of subacute endocarditis: Lancet 2:869, 1935.
7. Everett, E.D., and Hirschmann, J.V.: Transient bacteremia and endocarditis prophylaxis. A review. Medicine 56:61, 1977.
8. Crawford, J.J., Scorryers, J.R., Moriarity, J.D., King, R.C., West, J.F.: Bacteremia after tooth extraction studied with the aid of prereduced anaerobically sterilized culture media. Appl. Micro. 27:927, 1974.
9. Elliott, S.D.: Bacteraemia following tonsillectomy. Lancet, 2:589, 1939.
10. Burman, S.O.: Bronchoscopy and bacteremia. J. Thorac. Cardiovasc. Surg. 40:635, 1960.
11. Pereira, W., Kovnat, D.M., Kahn, M.A., Iacovino, J.R., Spivack, M.L. and Snider, G.L.: Fever and pneumonia after flexible fiberoptic bronchoscopy. Amer. Rev. Respir. Dis., 112:59, 1975.
12. Baltch, A.L., Buhac, I., Agrawal, A., O'Connor, P., Bram, M. and Malatino, E.: Bacteremia following endoscopy. Presented at the 15th Interscience Conference on Antimicrobial Agents and Chemotherapy, Sept. 1975, Washington, D.C. (Abstract 165).

13. Dickman, M.D., Farrell, R., Higgs, R.H., Wright, L.E., Humphries, T.J., Wojcik, J.D and Chappelka, R.: Colonoscopy associated bacteremia. Surg. Gynecol. Obstet., 142:173, 1976.
14. LeFrock, J., Ellis, C.A., Klainer, A.S. and Weinstein, L.: Transient bacteremia associated with barium enema. Arch. Intern. Med., 135:835, 1975.
15. Marshall, A.: Bacteraemia following retropubic prostatectomy. Br. J. Urol. 33:25, 1961.
16. Sullivan, N.M., Sutter, V.L., Mims, M.M., Marsh, V.H. and Finegold, S.M.: Clinical aspects of bacteremia after manipulation of the genitourinary tract. J. Infect. Dis. 127:49, 1973.
17. McCormack, W.M., Rosner, B., Lee, Y.H., Rankin, J.S. and Lin, J.S.: Isolation of genital mycoplasmas from blood obtained shortly after vaginal delivery. Lancet, 1:596, 1975.
18. Starkebaum, M., Durack, D., and Beeson, P.: The "incubation period" of subacute bacterial endocarditis. Yale J. Biol. Med. 50:49, 1977.
19. Devereaux, R.B., Perloff, J.K., Reichek, N., Josephson, M.E.: Mitral valve prolapse. Circulation 54:3, 1976.
20. Markiewicz, W., Stomer, J., London, E., Hunt, S.A., Topp, R.L.: Mitral valve prolapse in one hundred presumably healthy young females. Circulation 53:464, 1976.
21. Procacci, P.M., Savran, S.V., Schreiter, S.L. et al: Prevalence of clinical mitral valve prolapse in 1169 young women. New Eng. J. Med. 294:1086, 1976.
22. Allen, E.,Harris, A.,and Leatham, A.: Significance and prognosis of an isolated late sytolic murmur: a 9 to 22 year follow-up. Brit. Heart J. 36:525, 1974.
23. Mills, P., Rose, J., Hollingsworth, J., Amara, I., and Craige, E.: Long-term prognosis of mitral valve prolapse. New Eng. J. Med 297:3, 1977.
24. Corrigall, D., Bolen, J., Hancock, E.W., and Popp, R.L.: Mitral valve prolapse and infective endocarditis, Amer. J. Med. 63:215, 1977.
25. Garvey, G.J., and Neu, H.C.: Infective endocarditis - an evolving disease. Medicine 57:105, 1978.
26. Sipes, J.N., Thompson, R.L., and Hook, E.W.: Prophylaxis of infective endocarditis: a reevaluation. Ann. Rev. Med. 28:371, 1977.
27. McGowan, D.A.: Failure of prophylaxis of infective endocarditis following dental treatment. J. Antimicrobial Chemother. 4:486, 1978.
28. McCarthy, V.P., Cho, C.T., Diehl, A.M., and Ramsey, B.W.: Bacterial endocarditis due to penicillin-resistant *Streptococcus viridans.* Clin. Pediat. 18:263, 1979.
29. Dormer, A.E.: Bacterial endocarditis. Survey of patients between 1945 and 1956. Brit. Med. J. 2:846, 1974.
30. Barnes, C.G., and Hurley, R. Antibiotic cover for dental extractions. Brit. Med. J. 2:1205, 1963.

31. Neutze, J.M., and Arter, W.J.: Bacterial endocarditis and the dentist. New Zealand Dent. J. 67:79, 1981.
32. Durack, D.T., and Littler, W.A.: Case of a failure of penicillin prophylaxis. Brit. Med. J. 2:846, 1974.
33. Garrod, L.P., and Waterworth, P.M.: The risks of dental extraction during penicillin treatment. Brit. Heart J. 24:39, 1962.
34. Geraci, J.E., Hermans, P.E., and Washington, J.A., II: *Eikenella corrodens* endocarditis: report of a cure in two cases. Mayo Clin. Proc. 49:950, 1974.
35. Durack, D.T., Kaplan, E.L., and Bisno, A.L.: Twenty five cases of apparent endocarditis prophylaxis failure: results of a national survey. Clin. Res. 29:384A, 1981.
36. Garrison, P.K., and Freedman, L.R.: Experimental endocarditis: I. Staphylococcal endocarditis in rabbits resulting from placement of a polyethylene catheter in the right side of the heart. Yale J. Biol. Med. 42:394, 1970.
37. Durack, D.T., and Petersdorf, R.G.: Chemotherapy of experimental streptococcal endocarditis: I. Comparison of commonly recommended prophylactic regimens. J. Clin. Invest. 52:592, 1973.
38. Pelletier, L.L., Durack, D.T., and Petersdorf, R.G.: Chemotherapy of experimental streptococcal endocarditis. IV. Further observations on prophylaxis. J. Clin. Invest. 56:319, 1975.
39. Durack, D.T., Starkebaum, M.K., and Petersdorf, R.G.: Chemotherapy of experimental streptococcal endocarditis. VI. Prevention of enterococcal endocarditis. J. Lab. Clin. Med. 90:171, 1971.
40. Durack, D.T.: Experience with prevention of experimental endocarditis, in Kaplan, E.L., and Taranta, A.V., ed., Infective Endocarditis, American Heart Association Monograph No. 52, Dallas, 1977, p. 28.
41. Oakley, C.M., Darrell, J.H.: Antibiotic prophylaxis for bacterial endocarditis. Amer. J. Cardiol. 46:1073, 1980.
42. Oakley, C.M.: Prevention of infective endocarditis. Thorax 34:711, 1979.
43. Oakley, C., and Somerville, W.: Prevention of infective endocarditis. Brit. Heart J. 45:233, 1981.
44. Kaye, D.: Prophylaxis of endocarditis, in Kaye, D., ed., Infective Endocarditis, University Park Press, Baltimore, 1976, p. 245.
45. Kaplan, E.L., Rich, H., Gersony, W., and Manning, J.: A collaborative study of infective endocarditis in the 1970's: emphasis on infections in patients who have undergone cardiovascular surgery. Circulation 59:327, 1979.
46. Sugrue, D., Blake, S., Troy, P., and McDonald, D.: Antibiotic prophylaxis against infective endocarditis after normal delivery - is it necessary? Brit. Heart J. 44:499, 1980.
47. Medical Letter on Drugs and Therapeutics: Antimicrobial prophylaxis for surgery 21:73, 1979.

48. Tinker, J.H., and Tarhan, S.: Discontinuing anticoagulant therapy in surgical patients with cardiac valve prostheses. JAMA 239:738, 1978.
49. Krogstad, D.J., Dorfhagen, R.R., Moellering R.C., Jr., Wennersten, C., and Swartz, M.N.: Plasmid-mediated-resistance to antibiotic synergism in enterococci. J. Clin. Invest. 61:1645, 1978.
50. Murillo, J., Standiford, H.C., Holley, H.P., Tatem, B.A., and Caplan, E.S.: Prophylaxis against enterococcal endocarditis: comparison of the aminoglycoside component of parenteral antimicrobial regimens. Antimicrob. Agents Chemother. 18:448, 1980.
51. Moellering, R.C., Jr., Murray, B.E., Schoenbaum, S.C., Adler, J., and Wennersten, C.B.: A novel mechanism of resistance to penicillin-gentamicin synergism in *S. faecalis*. J. Inf. Dis. 141:81, 1980.
52. Horodniceanu, T., Bouqueleret, L., El-Salh, N., Bieth, G., and Delbos, F.: High-level, plasmid-borne resistance to gentamicin in *Streptococcus faecalis* subsp. *zymogenes*. Antimicrob. Agents Chemother. 16:686, 1979.
53. Sprunt, K.: Role of antibiotic resistance in bacterial endocarditis, in Kaplan, E.L., and Taranta, A.V., eds., Infective Endocarditis, AHA Monograph No. 52, Dallas, Tex., 1977, p. 17.
54. Doyle, E.F., Spagnuolo, M., Taranta, A., Kuttner, A.G., and Markowitz, M.: The risk of bacterial endocarditis during rheumatic fever prophylaxis. JAMA 201:129, 1967.
55. Goodman, J.S., Schaffner, W., Collins, H.A., Battersby, E.J. and Koenig, M.G.: Infection after cardiovascular surgery: clinical study including examination of antimicrobial prophylaxis. New Engl. J. Med. 278:117, 1968.
56. Fekety, F.R., Cluff, L.E., Sabiston, D.E., Seidl, L.G., Smith, J.W., Thoburn, R.: A study of antibiotic prophylaxis in cardiac surgery. J. Thorac. Cardiovasc. Surg. 57:757, 1969.
57. Conte, J.E., Cohen, S.N., Roe, B.B., and Elashoff, R.M.: Antibiotic prophylaxis and cardiac surgery: a prospective double-blind comparison of single dose versus multiple-dose regimens. Ann. Intern. Med. 76:943, 1972.
58. Durack, D.T.:Prophylaxis of infective endocarditis, in Mandell, G.L., Douglas, R.G., Jr., and Bennett, J.E., eds., Principles and Practice of Infectious Diseases. J. Wiley and Sons, New York, 1979, p. 701.
59. Brooks, S.L.: Survey of compliance with American Heart Association guidelines for prevention of bacterial endocarditis, J. Am. Dent. Assoc. 101:41, 1980.
60. Committee on Rheumatic Fever and Bacterial Endocarditis, American Heart Association: Prevention of rheumatic fever, Circulation 55:1A, 1977.

APPENDIX I.

PREVENTION OF BACTERIAL ENDOCARDITIS

Bacterial endocarditis remains one of the most serious complications of cardiac disease. The morbidity and mortality remain significant despite advances in antimicrobial therapy and cardiovascular surgery. This infection occurs most often in patients with structural abnormalities of the heart or great vessels. Effective measures for prevention of this infection by physicians and dentists are highly desirable.

Prevention of Bacterial Endocarditis

Dental treatment, or surgical procedures or instrumentation involving the upper respiratory tract, genitourinary tract, or lower gastrointestinal tract, may be associated with transitory bacteremia. Bacteria in the blood stream may lodge on damaged or abnormal valves such as are found in rheumatic or congenital heart disease or on endocardium near congenital anatomic defects, causing bacterial endocarditis or endarteritis. However, it is not possible to predict specific patients with structural heart disease in whom this infection will occur, nor the specific causal event.

Prophylaxis is recommended in those situations most likely to be associated with bacteremia since bacterial endocarditis cannot occur without a preceding bacteremia. Certain patients (e.g., those with prosthetic heart valves) appear to be at higher risk to develop endocarditis than are others (e.g., those with mitral valve prolapse syndrome). Likewise, certain dental (e.g., extractions) and surgical (e.g., genitourinary tract surgery) procedures appear to be much more likely to initiate significant bacteremia than are others. These factors, although difficult to quantitate, have been considered in developing these recommendations.

Since there have been no controlled clinical trials, adequate data for comparing various methods for prevention of endocarditis in man are not available. However, an experimental animal model permitting consistent induction of bacterial endocarditis with microorganisms which often cause the infection in man has allowed experimental evaluation of both prophylaxis and treatment. Data from these studies, although derived from animal rather than clinical investigations, represent the only direct information on the efficacy of prophylaxis that is presently available. This information has influenced formulation of the current recommendations. The significant morbidity and mortality associated with infective endocarditis and the paucity of conclusive clinical studies emphasize the need for continuing research into the epidemiology, pathogenesis, prevention, and therapy of infective endocarditis.

When selecting antibiotics for bacterial endocarditis prophylaxis one should consider both the variety of bacteria that is likely to enter the blood stream from any given site and those organisms most likely to cause this infection. Certain species of microorganisms cause the majority of cases of infective endocarditis, and their antimicrobial sensitivity patterns have been defined. The present recommendations are based on a review of available information about the organisms responsible for endocarditis including their *in vivo* and *in vitro* sensitivity to specific antibiotics and the pharmacokinetics of these drugs.

In general, *parenteral administration* of antibiotics provides more predictable blood levels and is preferred when practical, especially for patients thought to be at high risk. Optimal prophylaxis requires close cooperation between physicians, and between physicians and dentists.

DENTAL PROCEDURES AND UPPER RESPIRATORY TRACT SURGICAL PROCEDURES

Patients at risk to develop infective endocarditis should maintain the highest level of oral health to reduce potential sources of bacterial seeding. Even in the absence of dental procedures, poor dental hygiene or other dental disease such as periodontal or periapical infections may induce bacteremia. Patients without natural teeth are not free from the risk of bacterial endocarditis. Ulcers caused by ill-fitting dentures should be promptly cared for since they may be a source of bacteremia.

Antibiotic prophylaxis is recommended with **all** dental procedures (including routine professional cleaning) that are likely to cause gingival bleeding. Chemoprophylaxis for dental procedures in children should be managed in a similar manner to the way in which it is handled in adults. Although not a procedure, one exception to this is the spontaneous shedding of deciduous teeth; there are no data to suggest a significant risk of bacteremia accompanying this common event.

Devices which utilize water under pressure to clean between teeth, and dental flossing may improve dental hygiene, but they also have been shown to cause bacteremia. However, bacterial endocarditis associated with the use of these devices has not been reported. Present data are insufficient to make firm recommendations with regard to their use in patients susceptible to endocarditis. However, caution is advised in their use by patients with cardiac defects, especially when oral hygiene is poor.

Several studies suggest that *local gingival degerming* immediately preceding a dental procedure provides some degree of protection against bacteremia. However, use of this technique is controversial, since gingival sulcus irrigation itself could theoretically induce bacteremia. If local degerming is employed, it should be used only as an adjunct to antibiotic prophylaxis.

Since alpha hemolytic streptococci (e.g., viridans streptococci) are the organisms most commonly implicated in bacterial endocarditis following dental procedures, antibiotic prophylaxis should be specifically directed toward them. Certain procedures on the upper respiratory tract (e.g., tonsillectomy or adenoidectomy, bronchoscopy—especially with a rigid bronchoscope—and surgical procedures involving respiratory mucosa) also may cause bacteremia. Since bacteria entering the blood stream after these procedures usually have similar antibiotic sensitivities to those recovered following dental procedures, the same regimens are recommended.

The following table contains suggested regimens for chemoprophylaxis for dental procedures, or surgical procedures and instrumentation of the upper respiratory tract. The order of listing does not imply superiority of one regimen over another although parenteral administration is favored when practical. The committee also favors the combined use of penicillin and streptomycin or the use of vancomycin in the penicillin allergic patient (regimen B) in those patients felt to be at high risk (e.g., prosthetic valves).

FOR DENTAL PROCEDURES AND SURGERY OF THE UPPER RESPIRATORY TRACT

Prophylaxis for Dental Procedures and Surgical Procedures of the Upper Respiratory tract

	Most congenital heart disease;[3] rheumatic or other acquired valvular heart disease; idiopathic hypertrophic subaortic stenosis; mitral valve[4] prolapse syndrome with mitral insufficiency.	Prosthetic heart valves[5]
All dental procedures that are likely to result in gingival bleeding.[1,2]	Regimen A or B	Regimen B
Surgery or instrumentation of the respiratory tract.[6]	Regimen A or B	Regimen B

[1] *Does not include shedding of deciduous teeth.*

[2] *Does not include simple adjustment of orthodontic appliances.*

[3] *E.g., ventricular septal defect, tetralogy of Fallot, aortic stenosis, pulmonic stenosis, complex cyanotic heart disease, patent ductus arteriosus or systemic to pulmonary artery shunts. Does not include uncomplicated secundum atrial septal defect.*

[4] *Although cases of infective endocarditis in patients with mitral valve prolapse syndrome have been documented, the incidence appears to be relatively low and the necessity for prophylaxis in all of these patients has not yet been established.*

[5] *Some patients with a prosthetic heart valve in whom a high level of oral health is being maintained may be offered oral antibiotic prophylaxis for routine dental procedures except the following: parenteral antibiotics are recommended for patients with prosthetic valves who require extensive dental procedures, especially extractions, or oral or gingival surgical procedures.*

[6] *E.g., tonsillectomy, adenoidectomy, bronchoscopy, and other surgical procedures of the upper respiratory tract involving disruption of the respiratory mucosa. (See text).*

Regimen A - Penicillin

1. *Parenteral-oral combined:*

Adults: Aqueous crystalline penicillin G (1,000,000 units intramuscularly) **mixed with** *Procaine Penicillin G* (600,000 units intramuscularly). Give 30 minutes to 1 hour prior to procedure and then give penicillin V (formerly called phenoxymethyl penicillin) 500 mg orally every 6 hours for 8 doses.†

Children: Aqueous crystalline penicillin G* (30,000 units/kg intramuscularly) **mixed with** *Procaine Penicillin G* (600,000 units intramuscularly). Timing of doses for children is the same as for adults. For children less than 60 lbs. the dose of penicillin V is 250 mg orally every 6 hours for 8 doses.†

2. *Oral:‡*

Adults: Penicillin V (2.0 gm orally 30 minutes to 1 hour prior to the procedure and then 500 mg orally every 6 hours for 8 doses.)†

Children: Penicillin V* (2.0 gm orally 30 minutes to 1 hour prior to procedure and then 500 mg orally every 6 hours for 8 doses.† For children less than 60 lbs. use 1.0 gm orally 30 minutes to one hour prior to the procedure and then 250 mg orally every 6 hours for 8 doses.)†

For Patients Allergic to Penicillin:

Use *either Vancomycin* (see Regimen B)

or use

Adults: Erythromycin (1.0 gm orally 1½-2 hours prior to the procedure and then 500 mg orally every 6 hours for 8 doses.)†

Children: Erythromycin (20 mg/kg orally 1½-2 hours prior to the procedure and then 10 mg/kg every 6 hours for 8 doses.)†

Regimen B - Penicillin plus Streptomycin

Adults: *Aqueous crystalline penicillin G* (1,000,000 units intramuscularly)

mixed with

Procaine penicillin G (600,000 units intramuscularly)

PLUS

Streptomycin (1 gm intramuscularly)

Give 30 minutes to 1 hour prior to the procedure; then penicillin V 500 mg orally every 6 hours for 8 doses.†

*Children:** *Aqueous crystalline penicillin G* (30,000 units/kg intramuscularly)

mixed with

Procaine penicillin G (600,000 units intramuscularly)

PLUS

Streptomycin (20 mg/kg intramuscularly).
Timing of doses for children is the same as for adults. For children less than 60 lbs. the recommended oral dose of penicillin V is 250 mg every 6 hours for 8 doses. †

For Patients Allergic to Penicillin:

Adults: Vancomycin (1 gm intravenously over 30 minutes to 1 hour). Start initial vancomycin infusion ½ to 1 hour prior to procedure; then *erythromycin* 500 mg orally every 6 hours for 8 doses.†
*Children:** *Vancomycin* (20 mg/kg intravenously over 30 minutes to 1 hour).** Timing of doses for children is the same as for adults. *Erythromycin* dose is 10 mg/kg every 6 hours for 8 doses.†

Footnotes to Regimens:

† *In unusual circumstances or in the case of delayed healing, it may be prudent to provide additional doses of antibiotics even though available data suggest that bacteremia rarely persists longer than 15 minutes after the procedure. The physician or dentist may also choose to use the parenteral route of administration for all of the doses in selected situations.*

* *Doses for children should not exceed recommendations for adults for a single dose or for a 24-hour period.*

** *For vancomycin the total dose for children should not exceed 44 mg/kg/24 hours.*

‡ *For those* patients receiving continuous oral penicillin for secondary prevention of rheumatic fever, *alpha hemolytic streptococci which are relatively resistant to penicillin are occasionally found in the oral cavity. While it is likely that the doses of penicillin recommended in Regimen A are sufficient to control these organisms, the physician or dentist may choose one of the suggestions in Regimen B or may choose oral erythromycin.*

GENITOURINARY TRACT AND GASTROINTESTINAL TRACT SURGERY OR INSTRUMENTATION

Bacteremia may be caused by surgery or instrumentation of the genitourinary tract (especially urethral or prostatic manipulations, including urethral catheterization whether the urine is infected or not). It may also accompany surgery and instrumention of the lower gastrointestinal tract and of the gall bladder, and may be associated with obstetrical infections such as septic abortion or peri-partum infection. Documented cases of bacterial endocarditis have been recorded following these procedures and antibiotic prophylaxis to prevent this infection should be employed.

Endocarditis following uncomplicated vaginal delivery is extremely rare; the necessity for antibiotic prophylaxis has not been firmly established. Likewise, upper gastrointestinal endoscopy (without biopsy), percutaneous liver biopsy, proctoscopy, sigmoidoscopy, barium enema, pelvic examination, dilatation and curettage of the uterus, and uncomplicated insertion or removal of intrauterine devices (IUDs) - although occasionally associated with bacteremia - have only very rarely, if ever, been associated with development of infective endocarditis. Based upon currently available evidence, they do not require antibiotic prophylaxis in most patients with underlying heart disease. However, since the patient with a prosthetic valve appears to be at especially high risk, it may be wise to administer antibiotic prophylaxis with these procedures. This empiric recommendation is based more upon concern than definitive data.

Enterococci (e.g., *Streptococcus fecalis*) are frequently responsible for endocarditis following genitourinary tract and gastrointestinal tract surgery or instrumentation. Although bacteremia and even sepsis with gram-negative bacteria may follow instrumentation of the genitourinary tract or gastrointestinal tract, these organisms only rarely cause bacterial endocarditis. Thus, antibiotic prophylaxis to prevent endocarditis following these procedures should be directed primarily against enterococci. Because these procedures are usually performed in a hospital or clinic, parenteral antibiotics are recommended.

Suggested antibiotic regimens for gastrointestinal and genitourinary tract surgery and instrumentation are shown below:

FOR GASTROINTESTINAL AND GENITOURINARY TRACT SURGERY AND INSTRUMENTATION‡

Adults: *Aqueous crystalline penicillin G* (2,000,000 units intramuscularly or intravenously) or

Ampicillin (1.0 gm intramuscularly or intravenously)

PLUS

Gentamicin [1.5 mg/kg, (not to exceed 80 mg) intramuscularly or intravenously]

or

Streptomycin (1.0 gm, intramuscularly).

Give initial doses 30 minutes to 1 hour prior to procedure. If gentamicin is used then give a similar dose of gentamicin and penicillin (or ampicillin) every 8 hours for two additional doses.† If streptomycin is used then give a similar dose of streptomycin and penicillin (or ampicillin) every 12 hours for two additional doses.†

*Children:** *Aqueous crystalline penicillin G* (30,000 units/kg intramuscularly or intravenously)

or

Ampicillin (50 mg/kg intramuscularly or intravenously)

plus

Gentamicin (2.0 mg/kg intramuscularly or intravenously)

or

Streptomycin (20 mg/kg intramuscularly). Timing of doses for children is the same as for adults.†

For Those Patients who are Allergic to Penicillin†

Adults: Vancomycin (1.0 gm intravenously given over 30 minutes to 1 hour) **plus** *Streptomycin* (1.0 gm intramuscularly). A single dose of these antibiotics begun 30 minutes to one hour prior to the procedure is probably sufficient, but the same dose may be repeated in 12 hours.†

Children: Vancomycin*** (20 mg/kg given intravenously over 30 minutes to 1 hour) **plus** *Streptomycin* (20 mg/kg intramuscularly). Timing of doses for children is the same as for adults.†

Footnotes:

† *During prolonged procedures, or in the case of delayed healing, it may be necessary to provide additional doses of antibiotics. For brief outpatient procedures such as uncomplicated catheterization of the bladder one dose may be sufficient.*

* *Doses for children should not exceed recommendations for adults for a single dose or for a 24-hour period.*

** *For vancomycin the total dose for children should not exceed 44 mg/kg/24 hours.*

‡ *In patients with significantly compromised renal function, it may be necessary to modify the dose of antibiotics used. Some of these doses may exceed manufacturer's recommendations for a 24-hour period. However, since they are only recommended for a 24-hour period in most cases, it is unlikely that toxicity will occur.*

CARDIAC SURGERY

Patients undergoing cardiac surgery utilizing extracorporeal circulation—especially those requiring placement of prosthetic heart valves or needing prosthetic intravascular or intracardiac materials - are at risk to develop infective endocarditis in the perioperative and postoperative periods. Because the morbidity and mortality of infective endocarditis in such patients are high, maximal preventive efforts are indicated, including the use of prophylactic antibiotics.

Early postoperative infective endocarditis following these surgical procedures is most often due to *Staphylococcus aureus* (coagulase positive) or *Staphylococcus epidermidis* (coagulase negative). Streptococci, gram negative bacteria, and fungi are less frequently responsible. No single antibiotic regimen is effective against all these organisms. Futhermore, the prolonged use of broad spectrum antibiotics may itself predispose to superinfection with unusual or highly resistant microorganisms. Therefore, antibiotic prophylaxis at the time of open heart surgery should be directed primarily against staphylococci and should be of short duration. The choice of antibiotic should be influenced by each individual hospital's antibiotic sensitivity data, but *penicillinase resistant penicillins* or *cephalosporin antibiotics* are most often selected. Antibiotic prophylaxis should be started shortly before the operative procedure and usually is continued for no more than three to five days postoperatively to reduce the likelihood of emergence of resistant microorgansims. The physician or surgeon should consider the effects of cardiopulmonary bypass on serum antibiotic levels and time the doses accordingly.

Careful pre-operative dental evaluation is recommended so that any required dental treatment can be carried out *several weeks prior* to cardiac surgery whenever possible. Such measures may decrease the incidence of late post-operative endocarditis (occuring later than 6-8 weeks following surgery) which is often due to the same organisms which are responsible for causing infective endocarditis in the unoperated patient.

STATUS FOLLOWING CARDIAC SURGERY

Following cardiovascular surgery the same precautions should be observed that have been outlined for the unoperated patient undergoing dental, gastrointestinal, genitourinary, and other procedures. As far as is known, the risk of endocarditis probably continues indefinitely; it appears particularly significant in patients with prosthetic heart valves. Exceptions are patients with an uncomplicated secundum atrial septal defect repaired by direct suture without a prosthetic patch, and patients who have had ligation and division of a patent ductus arteriosus; these patients do not appear to be at increased risk of developing endocarditis. For these two defects, prophylaxis for prevention of infective endocarditis is not necessary following a healing period of six months after surgery. Although prophylactic antibiotics are often given intraoperatively, there is no evidence to suggest that patients who have undergone coronary artery operations are at risk to develop endocarditis in the months and years following surgery unless there is another cardiac defect present; prophylactic antibiotics to protect against endocarditis are not needed in these postoperative patients.

OTHER INDICATIONS FOR ANTIBIOTIC PROPHYLAXIS TO PREVENT ENDOCARDITIS

In susceptible patients chemoprophylaxis to prevent endocarditis is also indicated for surgical procedures on *any infected or contaminated tissues,* including incision and drainage of abscesses. Antibiotic prophylaxis for the indicated dental and surgical procedures should also be given to those patients who have had a documented previous episode of infective endocarditis, even in the absence of clinically detectable heart disease.

Indwelling vascular catheters, especially those which reside in one of the cardiac chambers, present a continual danger. Particular care should be given to maintaining the sterility of these catheters and to avoiding unnecessarily prolonged use.

Indwelling transvenous cardiac pacemakers appear to present a low risk of endocarditis; however dentists and physicians may choose to employ prophylactic antibiotics to cover dental and surgical procedures in these patients. The same recommendations apply to renal dialysis patients with implanted arteriovenous shunt appliances. Although no firm recommendation can be made on the basis of current information, antibiotic prophylaxis for preventing bacteremia provoked by dental and surgical procedures also deserves consideration in patients with ventriculoatrial shunts placed to relieve hydrocephalus since there are documented cases of infective endocarditis in these patients.

Prophylactic antibiotics are *not* required in diagnostic cardiac catheterization and angiography since, with standard techniques, the occurrence of endocarditis following these procedures has proven to be extremely uncommon.

It is important to recognize that antibiotic doses used to prevent recurrences of acute rheumatic fever ("secondary" rheumatic fever prophylaxis) are *inadequate* for the prevention of bacterial endocarditis (see reference). Special attention should be paid to these patients and appropriate antibiotics should be prescribed *in addition* to the antibiotic they are receiving for prevention of group A beta hemolytic streptococcal infections (the addition of an aminoglycoside to appropriate doses of penicillin, or the use of erythromycin or vancomycin).

WARNING

The committee recognizes that it is not possible to make recommendations for all possible clinical situations. Practitioners should exercise their clinical judgment in determining the duration and choice of antibiotic(s) when special circumstances apply. Furthermore, since endocarditis may occur despite antibiotic prophylaxis, physicians and dentists should maintain a high index of suspicion in the interpretation of any unusual clinical events following the above procedures. Early diagnosis is important to reduce complications, sequelae, and mortality.

Selected References

1. American Heart Association Committee on Prevention of Rheumatic Fever: Prevention of Rheumatic Fever. Circulation 55: 1,1977
2. Durack DT, Petersdorf RG: Chemotherapy of experimental streptococcal endocarditis. I. Comparison of commonly recommended prophylactic regimens. J Clin Invest 52: 592,1973
3. Durack DT, Starkebaum MS, Petersdorf RG: Chemotherapy of experimental streptococcal endocarditis. VI. Prevention of enterococcal endocarditis. J Lab Clin Med 90: 171,1977
4. Editorial: Prophylaxis of bacterial endocarditis. Faith, Hope, and Charitable Interpretations. Lancet 1: 519,1976
5. Everett ED, Hirschman JV: Transient Bacteremia and Endocarditis Prophylaxis. A review. Medicine 56: 61,1977
6. Finland M: Current problems in infective endocarditis. Mod Con Cardiovasc Dis 41: 53,1972
7. Parker MT, Ball LC: Streptococci and aerococci associated with systemic infection in man. J Med Microbiol 9: 275,1976
8. Pelletier LL Jr, Durack DT, Petersdorf RG: Chemotherapy of experimental streptococcal endocarditis IV. Further observations on prophylaxis. J Clin Invest 56: 319,1975
9. Sande MA, Levison ME, Lukas DS, Kaye D: Bacteremia associated with cardiac catheterization. N Eng J Med 281: 1104,1969
10. Sande MA, Johnson WS, Hook EW, Kaye D: Sustained bacteremia in patients with prosthetic cardiac valves. N Eng J Med 286: 1067,1972
11. Scopp IW, Orvieto LD: Gingival degerming by povidone-iodine irrigation. Bacteremia reduction in extraction procedures. J Am Dent Assoc 83: 1294,1971

12. Sipes JN, Thompson RL, Hook EW: Prophylaxis of infective endocarditis: A reevaluation. Ann Rev Med 28: 371,1977
13. Sullivan NM, Sutter VL, Mims MM, Marsh VH, Finegold SM: Clinical aspects of bacteremia after manipulation of the genitourinary tract. J Infect Dis 127: 49,1973

BOOKS

1. Infective Endocarditis - An American Heart Association Symposium, edited by E.L. Kaplan and A.V. Taranta, American Heart Association Monograph Series, No. 52, American Heart Association, Dallas, Texas, 1977
2. Infective Endocarditis, edited by Donald Kaye, University Park Press, Baltimore, Maryland. 1976
3. Subacute Bacterial Endocarditis, by Andrew Kerr, Jr., Charles C. Thomas, publisher, Springfield, Illinois. 1955

This statement was prepared by the Committee on Rheumatic Fever and Bacterial Endocarditis of the Council on Cardiovascular Disease in the Young of the American Heart Association. Membership of the Committee at the time of this statement was prepared.

Edward L. Kaplan, M.D., *Chairman*
Bascom F. Anthony, M.D.
Alan Bisno, M.D.
David Durack, M.B., D. Phil.
Harold Houser, M.D.
H. Dean Millard, D.D.S.
Jay Sanford, M.D.
Stanford T. Shulman, M.D.
Max Stillerman, M.D.
Angelo Taranta, M.D.
Nanette Wenger, M.D.

Reprinted from Circulation 56:139A, 1977, with permission.

APPENDIX II.

TREATMENT OF INFECTIVE ENDOCARDITIS DUE TO VIRIDANS STREPTOCOCCI

This statement was prepared by the ad hoc Subcommittee on Treatment of Bacterial Endocarditis of the American Heart Association Council on Cardiovascular Disease in the Young

INFECTIVE ENDOCARDITIS is caused by microbial infection of the endocardial surface of the heart and occurs in patients of all ages. It most frequently involves the heart valves, but may occur on the mural endocardium. A similar clinical illness, termed endarteritis, develops when there is infection of arteriovenous shunts, patent ductus arteriosus, the great vessels, or aneurysms. Depending primarily upon the virulence of the infecting microorganism, the clinical course of infective endocarditis may be prolonged and indolent, or it may be abrupt and fulminant. Infective endocarditis is characterized by fever, cardiac murmurs, splenomegaly, anemia, hematuria, petechiae, and systemic emboli. The disease is fatal unless cured by antimicrobial and/or surgical means.

Viridans streptococci are the most common etiologic agents in bacterial endocarditis superimposed upon congenital or acquired heart lesions, and such infections ordinarily pursue a subacute clinical course. A wide variety of different antibiotic regimens have been advocated for treatment, and, consequently, considerable confusion has arisen concerning the most appropriate forms of therapy. This report, based upon analysis of published clinical and experimental data, sets forth recommendations for treatment of bacterial endocarditis due to viridans streptococci; the recommendations also apply to infection with *Streptococcus bovis,* a closely related organism.

Diagnosis

Specific etiologic diagnosis requires isolation of the infecting agent from the blood stream or, on occasion, from peripheral emboli. Although the bacteremia associated with endocarditis is usually low-grade (less than 100 colony-forming units per ml of blood), it is continuous. Ordinarily, all or nearly all of the blood cultures obtained will be positive. Previous antibiotic therapy may decrease the frequency of positive cultures. Some viridans streptococci have special nutritional requirements that may hinder their growth in routine laboratory culture media. Such thiol-requiring organisms may require broth supplemented with pyridoxal hydrochloride and/or cysteine.

Once the infecting organism is isolated by the laboratory, the clinician should be aware that errors in classification are possible. In particular, *S. bovis* belongs to Lancefield's serogroup D, but it can be distinguished from enterococci by appropriate biochemical tests. *S.bovis* endocarditis is frequently associated with pathologic conditions of the gastrointestinal tract, including carcinoma of the colon. *Streptococcus mutans,* a common inhabitant of the oral cavity, may also at times be confused with enterococci on the basis of certain biochemical characteristics, although it does not belong to the family of group D organisms and is readily distinguished by appropriate laboratory tests. Distinguishing these organisms from enterococci is important, because both *S. bovis* and *S. mutans* are readily killed by penicillin, whereas adequate killing of enterococci in cardiac vegetations requires the use of an aminoglycoside antibiotic (e.g., streptomycin, gentamicin) in combination with penicillin for prolonged periods of time.

It is important that the organism isolated from the patient's blood be saved by the laboratory for antibiotic sensitivity testing. Disc diffusion susceptibility studies, such as are performed in many clinical laboratories, may not be adequate in this instance. Where possible, both the minimal inhibitory and minimal bactericidal concentrations (MIC and MBC) of the antibiotic for the infecting organism should be determined using broth dilution techniques. The penicillin sensitivity of an organism may be helpful in suggesting errors in identification. All enterococci are resistant to 0.2 μgm/ml of penicillin G, while 90 percent or more of viridans streptococci are inhibited by 0.2 μgm/ml or less.

Treatment

To achieve optimal cure rates in treatment of bacterial endocarditis, it is necessary that the antibiotics selected exert a bactericidal effect on the infecting organism. It is important to achieve antibiotic levels in the patient's serum which exceed the MBC for the particular etiologic agent. Fortunately, the majority of strains of viridans streptococci causing endocarditis are readily killed by low concentrations of penicillin G. Although cases of endocarditis have been cured with oral penicillin therapy, the generally higher and more predictable serum levels obtainable with intramuscular or intravenous injection make parenteral therapy preferable for this life-threatening diease.

High cure rates can be anticipated with a variety of different regimens in treatment of cases of endocarditis caused by penicillin-sensitive viridans streptococci. Penicillin alone, in doses of 10,000,000 to

20,000,000 units a day for four weeks, can be anticipated to cure 95 to 99 per cent of adult patients. Penicillin plus streptomycin exert a synergistic killing effect upon viridans streptococci *in vitro*. Moreover, in an experimental model of endocarditis in rabbits, addition of streptomycin to penicillin results in more rapid sterilization of cardiac vegetations. Excellent cure rates, approaching 99 per cent, have been achieved in man with the use of such combination therapy, in which streptomycin is added during the first two weeks of the usual four week course of penicillin. Because the incidence of relapse may possibly be greater in individuals who have been ill for three months or longer prior to the institution of therapy, the synergism offered by penicillin-streptomycin therapy may theoretically be advantageous in this group of patients. On the other hand, it should be emphasized that combination therapy has not been established to be superior to penicillin alone in treating endocarditis due to viridans streptococci in man.

Considerable experience has now been accumulated with the use of short-course (two-week) combination therapy with penicillin and streptomycin. Although older reports indicated higher failure rates (6 to 11 per cent) with this two-week regimen, others have reported excellent results with cure rates as high as 99 per cent. While the total experience with short-course regimens is less extensive than that with the four-week forms of treatment, it does seem clear that the two-week regimen is efficacious, and its use could greatly decrease the duration of hospitalization and the medical costs associated with endocarditis due to viridans streptococci. The two-week regimen appears to be acceptable for uncomplicated cases of endocarditis due to viridans streptococci occurring in patients at low risk of streptomycin toxicity. At present, the two-week regimen is not recommended for patients with complications, e.g., shock, extra-cardiac foci of infection, prosthetic valve infections, or for those infected with nutritionally-deficient variants of viridans streptococci.

Specific recommendations for treatment of endocarditis due to penicillin-sensitive viridans streptococci in patients who are not allergic to penicillin are presented in table 1. While all three regimens in table 1 are acceptable, each has advantages and disadvantages. The advantages are: the two-week regiman is the most cost effective and appreciably shortens the period of hospitilization; the penicillin alone regimen avoids use of streptomycin, which is ototoxic; and the four-week regimen with streptomycin added is, theoretically, the most effective. The disadvantages are: the regimens including streptomycin introduce the risk of ototoxicity, especially in older individuals or those with impaired renal function; the penicillin alone and the two-week regimen have been associated with more reported relapses; and the four-week regimens require a longer hospitalization.

In the penicillin-allergic patient, vancomycin is an effective alternative (table 2). Prolonged intravenous use of this drug may be complicated by the occurrence of thrombophlebitis, ototoxicity, or,

Table 1. *Suggested Regimens for Therapy of Endocarditis Due to Penicillin-Sensitive Viridans Streptococci and Streptococcus bovis (MIC less than 0.2 μgm/ml)*[1,2]

	Antibiotic	Dosage	Route	Duration	Comment
1.	Aqueous crystalline penicillin G	10 million to 20 million units/day either continuously or in equally divided doses every 4 hours.	Intravenous	4 weeks	Preferred in most patients more than 65 years of age or with impairment of VIIIth nerve function. Regimens employing four weeks of penicillin alone are preferred in patients with impaired renal function; however, the penicillin dose may have to be reduced, based upon the level of renal function.
2.	Aqueous crystalline penicillin G	10 million to 20 million units/day either continuously or in equally divided doses every 4 hours.	Intravenous	4 weeks	
	or Procaine penicillin G	1.2 million units every 6 hours.	Intramuscular	4 weeks	Age more than 65 years or renal or VIIIth nerve impairment serve as relative contraindications to the use of streptomycin.
	plus Streptomycin[3]	10 mg/kg body weight (not to exceed 500 mg) every 12 hours.	Intramuscular	2 weeks	

3.	Aqueous crystalline penicillin G	10 million to 20 million units/day either continuously or in equally divided doses every 4 hours.	Intravenous	2 weeks	Age more than 65 years or renal or VIIIth nerve impairment serve as relative contraindications to the use of streptomycin. Not recommended for patients with shock, extracardiac foci of infection, prosthetic valve endocarditis or for patients infected with nutritionally-deficient variants of viridans streptococci.
	or				
	Procaine penicillin G	1.2 million units every 6 hours.	Intramuscular	2 weeks	
	plus				
	Streptomycin[3]	10 mg/kg body weight (not to exceed 500 mg) every 12 hours.	Intramuscular	2 weeks	

[1]FOR CHILDREN, THE RECOMMENDED DOSAGES ARE AQUEOUS CRYSTALLINE PENICILLIN G, 150,000 UNITS/KG/DAY INTRAVENOUSLY EITHER CONTINUOUSLY OR IN EQUALLY DIVIDED DOSES EVERY 4 HOURS; STREPTOMYCIN, 15 MG/KG INTRAMUSCULARLY (NOT TO EXCEED 500 MG) EVERY 12 HOURS. PROCAINE PENICILLIN G IS NOT RECOMMENDED FOR TREATMENT OF ENDOCARDITIS DUE TO VIRIDANS STREPTOCOCCI IN CHILDREN.

[2]For penicillin-allergic patients, see table 2. For patients with impaired renal function, appropriate modification should be made in the doses of penicillin and streptomycin.

[3]Streptomycin should be given concurrently with penicillin for the first two weeks of treatment.

Table 2. *Therapy of Endocarditis Due to Penicillin-Sensitive Viridans Streptococci and S. bovis in Patients Allergic to Penicillin*

Antibiotic	Dosage	Route	Duration	Comment
Vancomycin	10 mg/kg body weight (not to exceed 500 mg) every 6 hours.	Intravenous	4 weeks	Thrombophlebitis, VIIIth nerve toxicity, and, occasionally, nephrotoxicity may occur.
Cephalothin[1,2]	2.0 gm every 4 hours.	Intravenous	4 weeks	Potential cross-allergenicity between penicillins and cephalosporins. (See text).

[1]FOR CHILDREN, THE RECOMMENDED DOSE OF CEPHALOTHIN IS 100—150 MG/KG/DAY IN EQUALLY DIVIDED DOSES EVERY 4 HOURS.

[2]Other cephalosporin antibiotics in equivalent doses may also be effective; *in vitro* susceptibility of the infecting organism should be confirmed. Adequate comparative data regarding clinical efficacy of the various cephalosporin derivatives in endocarditis are lacking.

occasionally, nephrotoxicity. Cephalothin is also effective. Other cephalosporin antibiotics in equivalent doses may be effective, but *in vitro* susceptibility of the infecting organism should be confirmed. The safety of cephalosporin antibiotics in patients with a history of penicillin allergy remains a matter of debate, but the risk of cross-reaction is low. Cephalosporins should not be used for treatment of streptococcal endocarditis in patients with a history of immediate-type hypersensitivity reactions to penicillin drugs. If cephalosporins are used in penicillin-allergic patients, they should be initiated cautiously in a setting in which serious allergic reactions may be dealt with expeditiously.

When endocarditis is due to viridans streptococci requiring more than 0.2 μgm/ml of penicillin for inhibition, combination therapy with penicillin and streptomycin is indicated (table 3). When penicillin cannot be used because of hypersensitivity (especially immediate reactions), vancomycin for four weeks is the substitute of choice (table 2). Cephalothin or other cephalosporins may also be considered (see caution in preceding paragraph). Although addition of streptomycin to these drugs causes more rapid bactericidal activity *in vitro*, there is insufficient clinical information available to determine whether or not streptomycin should be added to vancomycin or a cephalosporin antibiotic in these patients.

Monitoring Adequacy of Antibiotic Therapy

Careful daily observation is a most important aspect of monitoring adequacy of therapy. Persistent or recurrent fever may be a manifestation of therapeutic failure but may also be due to a variety of other causes, including thrombophlebitis, sterile embolization, or hypersensitivity reactions to drugs.

The serum bactericidal titer is also useful for monitoring adequacy of therapy. This is the dilution of the patient's serum, obtained while he is receiving antibiotic therapy, which kills a standard inoculum of the patient's organism *in vitro*. Although the test has not been fully validated under clinical circumstances and varies from laboratory to laboratory in the way in which it is performed, most authorities agree that serum bactericidal titers of 1:8 or greater are highly desirable in treatment of bacterial endocarditis. Whether such titers are necessary only at the peak of antibiotic activity or should be maintained throughout the day remains controversial. This test may find its greatest utility in the evaluation of therapy of endocarditis caused by streptococci which are moderately resistant to penicillin, when less well established antibiotic regimens are being used, and when the response to therapy has been suboptimal.

All patients with infective endocarditis should have assiduous follow-up, including additional blood cultures once or twice during the eight weeks following completion of antibiotic treatment. Relapses, should they occur, can be promptly detected by clinical and bacteriologic means and do respond to retreatment.

Table 3. *Therapy of Endocarditis Due to Strains of Viridans Streptococci and S. bovis Relatively Resistant to Penicillin G (MIC Greater Than 0.2 μgm/ml)*[1,2]

Antibiotic	Dosage	Route	Duration
Aqueous crystalline penicillin G	20 millions units/day given continuously or in equally divided doses every 4 hours.	Intravenous	4 weeks
plus Streptomycin	10 mg/kg body weight (not to exceed 500 mg) every 12 hours.	Intramuscular	4 weeks[3,4]

[1]FOR CHILDREN, THE RECOMMENDED DOSAGES ARE AQUEOUS CRYSTALLINE PENICILLIN G, 150,000 UNITS/KG/DAY INTRAVENOUSLY EITHER CONTINUOUSLY OR IN EQUALLY DIVIDED DOSES EVERY 4 HOURS; STREPTOMYCIN, 15 MG/KG INTRAMUSCULARLY (NOT TO EXCEED 500 MG) EVERY 12 HOURS.

[2]For penicillin-allergic patients, see text.

[3]Although the published data are limited, some authorities feel that for viridans streptococci whose minimal inhibitory concentration of penicillin is greater than 0.2 μgm/ml, but less than or equal to 0.5 μgm/ml, it may be unnecessary to give streptomycin for more than two weeks.

[4]Streptomycin should be given concurrently with penicillin. For patients with impaired renal function, appropriate modification should be made in the doses of penicillin and streptomycin.

Indications for Surgery

Surgical intervention may at times be life-saving in patients with infective endocarditis. The major indications for surgery in endocarditis due to viridans streptococci are valvular dysfunction, causing heart failure which is not readily controlled by medical therapy, and repeated major emboli. Once indications for surgery are clear-cut, intervention should be prompt, without regard to duration of prior antimicrobial therapy.

Treatment of Patients with Intracardiac Prostheses

The same principles of therapy outlined above apply to patients who have prosthetic valve endocarditis caused by viridans streptococci and *S. bovis*. However, eradication of the intracardiac infection is more difficult in these patients, and, therefore, treatment should be continued for a minimum of four weeks. More prolonged therapy may be necessary. In addition to the indications for surgical intervention listed above, failure to respond to appropriate antimicrobial therapy or evidence of myocardial abscess formation should lead to consideration of surgical replacement of the prosthetic valve.

References

Books

1. Bisno AL (ed), Treatment of Infective Endocarditis. New York, Grune & Stratton, 1981.
2. Kaye D (ed),Infective Endocarditis. Baltimore, University Park Press, 1976
3. Kaplan EL, Taranta AV (eds),Infective Endocarditis. An American Heart Association Symposium, Monograph 52. Dallas, American Heart Association, 1977
4. Rahimtoola SH (ed), Infective Endocarditis. New York, Grune & Stratton, 1978

Articles

1. Karchmer AW, Moellering RC Jr, Maki DG, Swartz MN: Single-antibiotic therapy for streptococcal endocarditis. JAMA 241: 1801-1806, 1979

2. Malacoff RF, Frank E, Andriole VT: Streptococcal endocarditis (non-enterococcal, non-group A): single vs combination therapy. JAMA 24:1807-1810, 1979
3. Phair JP, Tan JS: Therapy of streptococcus viridans endocarditis. *In* Kaplan EL, Taranta AV (eds) Infective Endocarditis. An American Heart Association Symposium, Monograph 52. Dallas, American Heart Association, pp 55-57, 1977
4. Moellering RC Jr, Watson BK, Kunz LJ: Endocarditis due to group D streptococci. Comparison of disease caused by *Streptococcus bovis* with that produced by the enterococci. Am J Med 57: 239-250, 1974
5. Tan JS, Terhune CA Jr, Kaplan S et al: Successful two-week treatment schedule for penicillin-sensitive *Streptococcus viridans* endocarditis. Lancet 2: 340-1343, 1971
6. Wilson WR, Geraci JE, Wilkowske CJ, Washington JA: Short-term intramuscular therapy with procaine penicillin plus streptomycin for infective endocarditis due to viridans streptococci. Circulation 57: 1158-1161, 1979
7. Wilson WR, Thompson RL, Wilkowske CJ, Washington JA, Giuliani ER, Geraci JE: Short term therapy of streptococcal infective endocarditis. JAMA 245: 360-363, 1981
8. Wolfe JD, Johnson WD: Penicillin-sensitive streptococcal endocarditis: *In vitro* and clinical observations on penicillin-streptomycin therapy. Ann Intern Med 81: 178-181, 1974

This statement was prepared by the ad hoc Subcommittee on Treatment of Bacterial Endocarditis of the American Heart Association Council on Cardiovascular Disease in the Young:

Alan L. Bisno, M.D., *Chairman*
William E. Dismukes, M.D.
David T. Durack, M.B., D. Phil.
Edward L. Kaplan, M.D.
Adolf W. Karchmer, M.D.
Donald Kaye, M.D.
Merle A. Sande, M.D.
Jay P. Sanford, M.D.
Walter R. Wilson, M.D.

Reprinted from Circulation 63:730A, 1981, with permission.

INDEX

a b c d e f g h 1 i 8 2 j